**This book is to be returned on or before
the last date stamped below.**

LIBREX

D0540415

BONE

Volume 4: Bone Metabolism and Mineralization

Brian K. Hall
Department of Biology
Dalhousie University
Halifax, Nova Scotia
Canada

CRC Press
Boca Raton Ann Arbor London

Library of Congress Cataloging-in-Publication Data
(Revised for volume 4)

Bone.
    Includes biobliographical references and index.
    Contents: v. 1. The osteoblast and osteocyte — v. 2. The osteoclast — v. 3. Bone
matrix and bone specific products — v. 4. Bone metabolism and mineralization.
    1. Bones. I. Hall, Brian Keith, 1941–
[DNLM: 1. Bone and Bones.   WE 200/B7113]
QP88.2.B58 1991 599'.01852   89-20391
ISBN 0-93692-324-5 (v. 1)
ISBN 0-8493-9922-8 (v. 2)
ISBN 0-8493-8823-6 (v. 3)
ISBN 0-8493-8824-4 (v. 4)

Developed by Telford Press

This book represents information obtained from authentic and highly regarded sources. Reprinted material is quoted with permission, and sources are indicated. A wide variety of references are listed. Every reasonable effort has been made to give reliable data and information, but the authors and the publisher cannot assume responsibility for the validity of all materials or for the consequences of their use.

Direct all inquiries to CRC Press, Inc., 2000 Corporate Blvd., N.W., Boca Raton, Florida, 33431.

International Standard Book Number 0-8493-8824-4

Library of Congress Card Number 89-20391

Printed in the United States of America   1 2 3 4 5 6 7 8 9 0

Preface

This is the fourth of seven volumes devoted to bone. The impetus for initiating this series was to fill the need for an up-to-date, comprehensive, and authoritative treatment of all aspects of bone. Cartilage has been covered in the three volume series, *Cartilage* (Hall, 1983), and in *Cartilage: Molecular Aspects* (Hall and Newman, 1991), published by CRC Press.

The seven volumes in this series are organized thematically, each volume integrating structure, function, biochemistry, metabolism, and the molecular and clinical aspects of a particular aspect of the biology of bone. The chapters are written by authors actively engaged in basic, applied, and/or clinical research upon bone, ensuring that each chapter is both authoritative and up-to-date.

Bone-forming cells were covered in *Volume 1: The Osteoblast and Osteocyte.* The second volume, *The Osteoclast,* dealt with bone-resorbing cells, both multicellular osteoclasts that resorb the mineral and organic phases of bone and mononuclear cells that resorb only the latter. The third volume, *Bone Matrix and Bone Specific Products,* extended coverage from bone-forming and -resorbing cells to the synthesis of bone specific products and their deposition into the extracellular matrix. This volume, *Bone Metabolism and Mineralization,* summarizes the current status of knowledge on bone metabolism and mineralization of the bone matrix.

Volume 4 begins with an analysis of the cells that line "inactive" bone surfaces. These bone lining cells, derived from osteoblasts, may spend anywhere from six months to the lifespan of the individual in an inactive state. They represent a resident population of determined osteogenic precursor cells (see Volume 1, Chapter 2) that form a cellular membrane between endosteum and hematopoietic marrow. They are the "gate-keepers" of bone resorption and the functional bone membrane.

The second chapter surveys the Haversian systems, the structural units of lamellar (Haversian) bone. They represent the structural legacy of the balance between resorption and deposition and the physical record of stress- and strain-generated bone turnover.

Chapter 3 takes us beneath the structure of bone and its lining cells to the role played by growth factors and cytokines in the local regulation of bone metabolism, growth, and repair. Calcium-regulating hormones act, in part, through their effects on growth factors. The local production of such factors begins to provide an explanation for control of bone metabolism and mineralization at the microenvironmental level, a theme that is continued in Chapter 4 with a discussion of calcium metabolism. It is such microscopic remodeling in bone turnover that enables the skeleton to act both as reservoir and as source of calcium. Chapter 4 discusses the mechanisms that maintain the Ca^{2+} equilibrium between blood and bone fluids and the degree of bone mineralization in normality and how that balance is perturbed in conditions requiring excess calcium mobilization from the skeleton.

Bone metabolism can be approached from the viewpoint of energy metabolism of bone cells as discussed in Chapter 5. The metabolic importance of the juxtaposition of metabolically active cells and the vascular system is emphasized. This juxtaposition facilitates access to ions, nutrients, oxygen, blood-borne hormones, and local growth factors, all of which are required for mineral formation.

Vitamins play an important role in bone metabolism and mineralization as discussed in Chapter 6. Vitamins A, C, D, and K are emphasized, with discussions of mechanisms of vitamin action, hyper- and hypovitaminosis, and the relationship between vitamin levels and regulation of such bone matrix proteins as osteocalcin and matrix Gla proteins.

Chapter 7 provides a comparative survey of mineralization of the integumental skeleton in fishes, amphibians, and reptiles, with a concentration on extant forms. The integumental skeleton consists of several skeletal tissues along with dental tissues such as dentine and enamel. This chapter raises such questions as "what is bone?", "what cells can produce bone?", and "is such mineralization regulated as is endoskeletal mineralization?".

The final chapter provides an evaluation of *in vitro* approaches to the study of mineralization of extracellular matrices and the metabolic processes involved in that mineralization. Differences between mineralization of bone and of cartilage are emphasized, especially the role of nucleators for hydroxyapatite aggregation.

In summary, Volume 4 provides an up-to-date authoritative overview of our current knowledge of bone metabolism and mineralization in respect to bone structure, bone cells, factors that activate bone cells, energy requirements, and the importance for mineralization of cellular and matricial context. Along with Volume 3, it provides an analysis of bone matrix products, structure, metabolism, and mineralization. Volumes 1 through 4 provide an encyclopedic overview of bone cells, matrix, metabolism, and mineralization and a background for the subsequent volumes that explore bone repair, regeneration, and growth.

Brian K. Hall
Halifax, 1991

The Editor

Brian K. Hall, Ph.D., D.Sc, is Izaak Walton Killam Research Professor in the Department of Biology, Faculty of Science, Dalhousie University, Halifax, N. S., Canada. He also holds an appointment as Professor of Physiotherapy, Faculty of Health Professions, Dalhousie University.

Professor Hall received his B.Sc. (Hons.) degree in 1965, his Ph.D. in Zoology in 1969, and a D.Sc. in Biological Sciences in 1978 from the University of New England, Armidale, N.S.W., Australia. He was appointed a Teaching Fellow in the Department of Zoology, UNE in 1965, Assistant Professor in the Department of Biology, Dalhousie University in 1968, Associate Professor in 1972, Professor in 1975, and Killam Research Professor in 1990. He served as Chair of the Biology Department, Dalhousie University from 1978 to 1985.

Professor Hall is a Fellow of the Royal Society of Canada and a member of the American Society of Zoologists, International Society for Differentiation, British Society for Developmental Biology, International Society for Developmental Biology, Society of Vertebrate Palaeontology, The Bone and Tooth Society, and the British Connective Tissue Society. He is an editor of *Anatomy and Embryology,* editorial board member of the *Journal of Craniofacial Genetics and Developmental Biology,* international advisory board member of the *Croatian Medical Journal,* past associate editor of the *Canadian Journal of Zoology,* and a past member of the advisory editorial board of *Bone.*

Professor Hall has worked on the development and differentiation of cartilage and bone for 25 years. He has presented invited lectures at international meetings and symposia and guest lectures at universities and institutes. He is the author or coauthor of 5 books, 130 papers in referenced scientific journals, and many chapters in edited works or conference proceedings. He edited a 3-volume series on cartilage (1983) and is coeditor of *Cartilage: Molecular Aspects* published by CRC Press in 1991. The current focus of his research is on the development and evolution of neural crest-derived craniofacial cartilage and bone.

Contents

1

Bone Lining Cells*

SCOTT C. MILLER and WEBSTER S. S. JEE

Division of Radiobiology
School of Medicine
University of Utah
Salt Lake City, Utah

Introduction

A relatively small fraction of the bone surface in the adult skeleton is undergoing bone remodeling at any one time. For example, active bone apposition usually occurs on less than about 15% of the trabecular bone surfaces of the iliac crest in the human (Merz and Schenk, 1970; Parfitt, 1983) and dog (Marotti, 1976), although this will vary according to bone sampling site and age (Schulz and Delling, 1976; Kimmel and Jee, 1982). The cells associated with bone remodeling (osteoblasts and osteoclasts) are phenotypes that are easily recognized and that have been extensively studied (Marks and Popoff, 1988; see Volumes 1 and 2). The remainder of the bone surfaces are considered as "inactive" or "resting" in terms of bone remodeling, but may be physiologically functional in terms of calcium exchange and mineral homeostasis.

The cells lining these "inactive" bone surfaces are best characterized on endosteal surfaces and are most commonly called "bone lining cells", al-

*Portions of work cited here were supported by Public Health Service Grant DE-06007 from
  the National Institutes of Health and U.S. Department of Energy Contract
  DEAC0276EV00119.

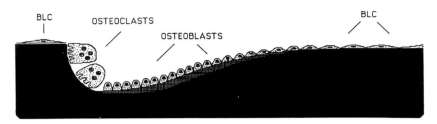

Fig. 1 Diagram of a bone remodeling unit, also known as a basic multicellular unit (BMU), illustrating the transition of osteoblasts to bone lining cells (BLC) that can be observed in histological sections.

though they have also been described by other names including "inactive osteoblasts", "resting osteoblasts", "surface osteocytes", and "flattened mesenchymal cells" (Miller *et al.*, 1980). While the name "bone lining cell" is generally accepted by most authors (Miller and Jee, 1987), it is occasionally used to generically describe all of the bone cells found on a bone surface (Deldar *et al.*, 1985). While the bone lining cell can be recognized as a distinct phenotype, on some bone surfaces it may be part of a cellular layer that separates bone from other tissue compartments, such as marrow. Although bone lining cells cover most of the bone surface in the adult skeleton and are the most common bone surface cells in the mature skeleton (Miller *et al.*, 1980), remarkably little is known about them.

Morphology and Ultrastructure of the Bone Lining Cell

The bone lining cell has some distinct morphological characteristics that allow it to be recognized as a distinct phenotype (Miller and Jee, 1987); however, it is a member of a functional continuum of the differentiation pathway of the osteoblast (Fig. 1). It is also an integral part of the surface barrier separating bone from other tissue compartments. On endosteal surfaces, for example, the bone lining cell is part of the endosteal tissues that may also include marrow sac cells, reticular cells, stromal cells, and osteoprogenitor cells. The bone lining cell has been best described on endosteal surfaces, particularly those from longer-lived species, although they have also been described lining the surfaces of Haversian canals (Cooper *et al.*, 1966). The lineal surface density of bone lining cells is reported to be about 19 cells/mm bone surface perimeter in fatty marrow sites in the young adult beagle and may decrease with age (Miller *et al.*, 1980). The surface density of bone lining cells in hematopoietic (red marrow) sites of the skeleton is likely to be greater than the value reported for fatty marrow, low bone turnover skeletal sites. The lineal surface density of bone lining cells on endosteal surfaces of adult male Japanese quail is reported to be about 21 cells/mm bone surface perimeter (Bowman and Miller, 1986).

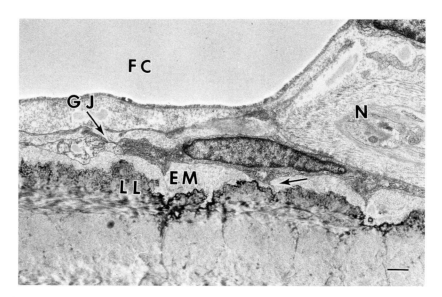

Fig. 2 Transmission electron micrograph of a bone lining cell on the endosteal surface from a fatty bone marrow site in an adult beagle. The cytoplasm contains few organelles but some profiles of rough endoplasmic reticulum can be seen. Bone lining cells often contact adjacent cells via gap junctions (GJ). Between the lamina limitans (LL) and the bone lining cell is a layer of connective tissue termed the "endosteal membrane" (EM). Cell processes can be seen extending into the bone (arrow). FC, fat cell; N, nerve. Decalcified section, bar = 1 μm. [From Miller, S. C. *et al.* (1980). *Anat. Rec.*, **198:** 163.]

Bone lining cells are very flat and elongated and are directly apposed to bone surfaces (Fig. 2). They may, however, be part of several layers of cells adjacent to the surface. Bone lining cell nuclei can be resolved in good light microscope preparations, but they can be confused with nuclei from fat cells, adventitial cells, reticular cells, stromal cells, marrow sac cells, osteoprogenitor cells, and endothelial cells (Miller *et al.*, 1980). Bone lining cell nuclear profiles are oval or flat and elongated, although younger bone lining cells may have thicker nuclei (Fig. 3). The nuclear profiles observed by electron microscopy generally range from 0.5 to 1.0 μm in thickness and up to about 12 μm in length in longer-lived species. In younger, more rapidly growing animals (e.g., rats and mice) where the bone has been recently formed, nuclear profiles may appear thicker than those observed in animals with longer lifespans and lower bone turnover rates. In rodents, for example, the age of the bone lining cells seen on mature bone surfaces may be measured in terms of weeks and months, whereas in longer-lived animals, the age of these cells at some sites may be measured in years.

The cytoplasm of the bone lining cell is generally so attenuated over the surface that detail is only resolved by electron microscopy (Vander Wiel *et al.*, 1978; Miller *et al.*, 1980; Doty and Nunez, 1985) (Figs. 4–6). The cytoplasm is often less than 0.1 μm in thickness, particularly in longer-lived

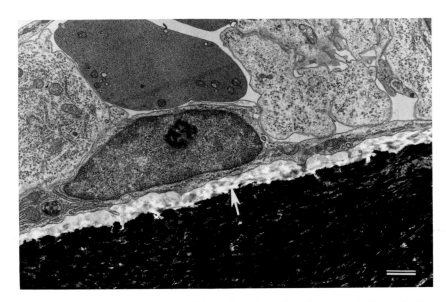

Fig. 3 Electron micrograph of a bone lining cell on the endosteal surface of a 2-month-old rat. The nuclear profiles of bone lining cells from younger animals may appear thicker than those from older animals and those with a longer lifespan (see Fig. 1). The endosteal membrane (arrow) is evident between the mineralized bone, which appears electron dense, and the bone lining cell. Undecalcified section, bar = 1 μm.

species. The cells contain few organelles, but profiles of endoplasmic reticulum, free ribosomes, and mitochondria can be seen usually located near the nucleus. In fatty bone marrow of the dog, bone lining cell nuclei are usually located near blood vessels (Miller *et al.,* 1980), while the cytoplasm extends for a considerable distance over the surface. Often several layers of bone lining cell cytoplasmic processes are observed. Cell processes from bone lining cells can be seen extending into canalicular channels of the bone matrix forming contacts with osteocytes (Doty and Nunez, 1985). Cell processes from adjacent bone lining cells are frequently joined by gap junctions (Miller *et al.,* 1980; Doty, 1981).

On resting bone surfaces, as observed by electron microscopy of decalcified sections, there is an osmiophilic dense region (see Fig. 2) that is commonly known as the "lamina limitans" (Scherft, 1972), although it is known by other names including "line of demarcation", "resting line", "dense line", "osmiophilic lamina", and "peripheral zone" (Vander Wiel *et al.,* 1978). The lamina limitans is not evident on all bone surfaces, however, particularly those that are mineralizing. During bone resorption, it is one of the first organic structures to disappear. These observations have led Scherft (1972) to suggest that the lamina limitans forms from the adsorption of organic material onto the surface of the mineralized matrix and thus is presumed to represent the mineralization front.

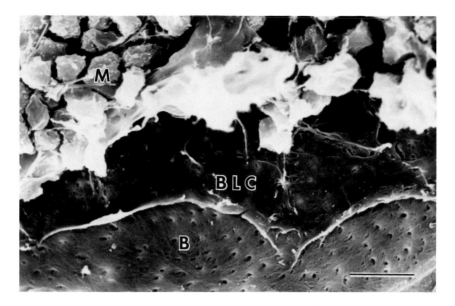

Fig. 4 Scanning electron micrograph of bone lining cells in the endocortical surface of a mouse femur. In this specimen, the interfaces between the bone surface (B), bone lining cells (BLC), and the bone marrow cells (M) are evident. The bone lining cells appear as a thin, sheet-like layer of cells over the bone surface. Perfusion fixation with formalin, critical point dried and coated with gold. Bar = 10 μm. (Courtesy of Dr. Louis de Saint-Georges.)

Between the lamina limitans and the bone lining cells is a layer of un-mineralized connective tissue, usually 100 to 500 nm in thickness. This layer may be present to some extent on all resting bone surfaces and has a different ultrastructural appearance than the osteoid which will normally mineralize. Termed the "endosteal membrane" (Parfitt, 1984), this layer contains amorphous material and some collagenous and reticular fibers that are morphologically different from the collagenous fiber bundles seen in bone (Miller *et al.*, 1980). The collagenous fibers in the endosteal membrane also lack the orientation that is typical of bone matrix collagenous fibers. While it has been a common practice to refer to this layer of unmineralized connective tissue as "osteoid", osteoid is a term that should be reserved specifically for unmineralized bone. The origin of this unmineralized tissue layer on the bone is not known, but it may be the final secretion product of osteoblasts as they cease their matrix synthesis function and become bone lining cells. The possible physiological significance of the endosteal membrane is discussed below. Similar appearing connective tissues, although in lesser amounts, have also been described on the other side of the bone lining cell, separating it from fat cells, reticular cells, and marrow cells (Miller *et al.*, 1980).

Ultrastructural studies have shown that in some species and at some endosteal sites there are several layers of flat cells separating osseous and hematopoietic tissues (Fig. 5). Menton *et al.* (1982) found that when marrow

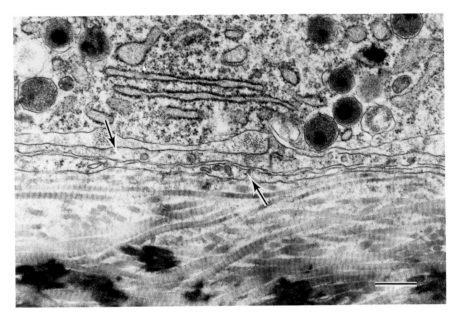

Fig. 5 Several layers of bone lining cell cytoplasm (arrows) separating a hematopoietic cell from the bone surface of an adult beagle. The bone lining cell cytoplasm is very thin and would be very difficult to resolve by light microscopy. The bone lining cell profiles contain a few free ribosomes and some vesicular structures. Decalcified section, bar = 0.5 μm.

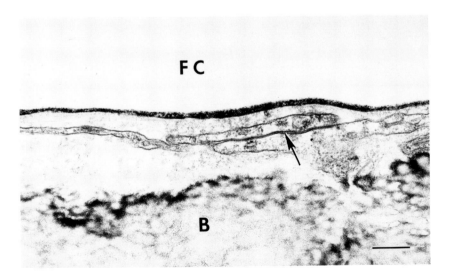

Fig. 6 Higher power electron micrograph illustrating the details of a gap injunction (arrow) between bone lining cell processes. This specimen was taken from an adult beagle. FC, fat cell; B, bone. Decalcified section, bar = 0.5 μm.

plugs were removed from diaphyseal shafts, there remained on the plug a pavement of squamous cells that invested the plug. These cells were called "marrow sac cells" and appeared to be separate from the bone lining cells that were directly apposed to the bone surface. The marrow sac cells were, however, considered an integral part of the endosteal cell layer. Marrow sac cells can be seen in samples obtained from rodents and rabbits (Menton *et al.*, 1982, 1984) as well as in some skeletal sites in dogs. Because the marrow sac cells are situated between the cells lining the bone surface and hematopoietic cells, it has been speculated that these cells could have important roles in the physiology of both the bone and the marrow, although this remains to be determined.

It is not clear if bone lining cells represent a continuous or discontinuous layer on resting bone surfaces. Some early light microscope studies suggested that inactive bone surfaces are incompletely covered by bone lining cells (Bleaney and Vaughan, 1971; Vaughan, 1972). Discontinuous bone lining cells or the absence of any surface cells have also been noted in the osteons of older persons (Cooper *et al.*, 1966), following starvation (Johnson, 1963) and after severe illness (Park, 1954). More recent electron microscope studies have not fully resolved this issue. Separations between bone lining cells have been noted in fatty bone marrow of the dog (Miller *et al.*, 1980; Miller and Jee, 1980) as well as in fatty bone marrow from hibernating bats (Doty and Nunez, 1985). On the other hand, Vander Weil *et al.* (1978) found no evidence of separations between bone lining cells or discontinuity of the bone lining cell covering of samples of iliac and femoral human bone. If "bare spots" were observed, they were attributed to poor fixation or artifact of preparation.

Origin and Fate of the Bone Lining Cell

It is generally accepted that bone lining cells are derived from osteoblasts that have become inactive, lost most of their cellular protein synthetic organelles, and spread over the bone surface. The transition from osteoblast to bone lining cell is apparent in histological sections, particularly those that use fluorochrome markers to distinguish states of bone formation activities. As bone formation at a given site decreases and the formation of a bone structural unit is nearly completed, the osteoblasts become less plump and flatten out (see Fig. 1). While there is some data on the kinetics of osteogenesis in modeling and remodeling systems, the kinetics of the transition of osteoblasts to bone lining cells as well as the maturation of recently formed bone surfaces is not understood. This view of the origin of the bone lining cells is based on morphological observations and does not preclude the possibility that some bone lining cells may be derived from other endosteal cells or stromal cell components.

The residence time or lifespan of bone lining cells is not known from direct experimental observations, but may be probabilistically estimated from local bone remodeling rates. The residence time of the bone lining cell on the bone surface would be equal to the predicted amount of time between remodeling cycles at a given site. In cancellous bone sites where annual turnover rates might equal 200%, for example, the average residence time of the bone lining cells would be about 180 days. On the other hand, if the annual turnover rate is 50%, then the average residence time would exceed 2 years. In cortical bone, where turnover rates might be very low, the potential longevity of the bone lining cells might approach the lifespan of the organism. The differences in residence time and estimated lifespan of these cells may account for some of the anatomical differences that have been described in bone lining cells among different species. For example, in young rodents the bone lining cells cannot exceed the age of the animal (which may be measured in months), whereas in studies of longer-lived species the lining cells may be measured in years, perhaps even over a decade at some sites.

Because the transition from osteoblast to bone lining cell can be observed in histological sections, bone lining cells have some similarities with osteocytes in that both cell types are derived from the osteoblast. Bone lining cells and osteocytes appear to represent further differentiated phenotypes (or perhaps dedifferentiated phenotypes) of osteoblasts. Because these cells share a common origin as well as some functional characteristics, the term "surface osteocyte" has been used by some investigators to describe the bone lining cell (Miller *et al.*, 1980). While there may be some differences in the proliferation and differentiation potential of bone lining cells and osteocytes, they do appear to form a functional syncytium that is important in the maintenance of bone, as described below.

The proliferative capacity or differentiation potential, if any, of the bone lining cell under normal physiological conditions is poorly understood. Mature osteoblasts and other bone surface cells and osteocytes rarely incorporate a ^{3}H-thymidine label, indicating that they are not actively dividing, as observed in rodents (Tonna and Cronkite, 1961; Young, 1962; Simmons, 1962) and young rabbits (Owen and MacPherson, 1963). Using electron microscopic autoradiography, ^{3}H-thymidine labels were not observed in bone lining cells in adult birds (Bowman and Miller, 1986). However, endosteal bone lining cells in adult male birds can be induced to proliferate by estrogen administration (Kusuhara and Schraer, 1982; Bowman and Miller, 1986) (Fig. 7). In this model, the bone lining cells may also appear to contribute to the pool of osteogenic cells that rapidly appear on bone surfaces, forming medullary bone deposits (Miller and Bowman, 1981) in response to the estrogenic stimulus. The bone lining cells were considered to first become preosteoblasts and then to differentiate into osteoblasts (Ohashi *et al.*, 1987). From these studies it was concluded that the bone lining cell is an inducible osteogenic precursor cell because it differentiates into the osteoblast phen-

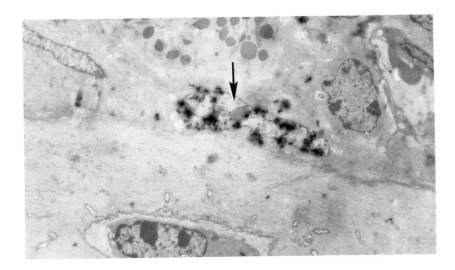

Fig. 7 Electron microscopic autoradiograph illustrating the incorporation of a ³H-thymidine label in an endosteal bone lining cell nucleus (arrow) at 20 hours after estrogen administration to an adult male Japanese quail. This demonstrates that bone lining cells have proliferative capacity following an inductive stimuli. [From Bowman, B. M. and Miller, S. C. (1986). *Bone*, **7:** 351. With permission.]

otype in response to an inductive signal. If these observations made in birds could be extrapolated to other species, then bone lining cells could represent a pool of osteogenic precursors that may be involved in induced states of osteogenesis such as fracture repair, osteogenesis following marrow extirpation and radiation exposure, and the direct stimulation of osteogenesis by fluoride or prostaglandins. Because of the evidence suggesting that bone lining cells retain osteogenic potential, bone lining cells are considered as "target cells" for the induction of skeletal cancers from bone-seeking radionuclides (Polig and Jee, 1986). As discussed in the next section, some investigators have even suggested that bone lining cells may represent a pool of totipotent hematopoietic stem cells.

While there is experimental evidence showing that bone lining cells can be induced to differentiate into osteoblasts, bone lining cells might also represent a population of "determined" osteogenic precursor cells. Determined osteogenic precursor cells are those cells that are capable of spontaneous bone formation (Owen, 1978). If the bone lining cell is a determined osteogenic precursor cell, then it may be considered as a preosteoblast or osteoprogenitor cell. During normal bone remodeling where resorption commences on inactive bone surfaces, and presuming that these surfaces were previously covered with bone lining cells, the fate of the bone lining cells as well as the source of the osteoblasts that appear later in the remodeling cycle are not understood. It is possible that as resorption commences on a bone surface, the bone lining cells may migrate or be forced away from the bone surface and become part of the stromal, reticular, mesenchymal, or osteoprogenitor cell compartment and be a source of preosteoblasts that will proliferate and differentiate at the completion of resorption and the beginning of the formation phase of the remodeling cycle. While there is no experimental evidence to support or contradict this scenario, this would be consistent with the possible role of the bone lining cell as a determined osteogenic precursor cell.

Bone Lining Cells, the Marrow Stromal System, and the Regulation of Hematopoiesis

Depending on one's vantage point, bone lining cells can be viewed as the outer investment layer of the bone tissue and thus implicated in the regulation of bone metabolism (Miller and Jee, 1987), or they can be considered as the outermost layer of cells investing the hematopoietic tissues, perhaps even involved in the regulation of hematopoietic functions (Deldar et al., 1985). Noting that endosteal cells interfaced the osseous and hematopoietic tissues, McLean and Urist (1968) suggested that they were the peripheral layer of the marrow stromal system with both osteogenic and hematopoietic capacities. Based on morphological findings, bone lining cells and other cells of the endosteal layer are thought to be continuous with the stromal system of the bone marrow (Weiss and Sakai, 1984). This view is supported by the observation that cells isolated from the marrow stroma can express osteogenic potential (Owen, 1985). Experimental data also suggest that bone lining cells retain osteogenic potential in the adult skeleton of birds (Bowman and Miller, 1986). These results collectively demonstrate some functional capabilities between these bone lining cell and stromal cell populations.

Bone marrow stromal cells are considered to be a heterogeneous population of cells that include cells classified under a number of different names including marrow fibroblasts, reticular cells, dendritic cells, preosteoblasts, vascular pericytes, and in some cases endothelial cells. One model of the marrow stromal system is that stromal stem cells provide progenitors that are committed to give rise to different cell lines (Owen, 1985), including reticular cells, marrow fibroblasts, and other differentiated cells of the marrow stroma. The precise origin and lineage of hematopoietic stromal cells is, however, controversial and may include some species variability (Perkins and Fleischman, 1988). While endothelial cells are sometimes included as a component of the marrow stromal system, there is little evidence that they arise from stromal stem cells.

Friedenstein et al. (1968) were the first to demonstrate that cells derived from colonies of marrow stromal cells had osteogenic potential. In their studies, fibroblastic colonies from stromal components were first grown in culture and then transplanted in diffusion chambers in vivo where the formation of bone then occurred. The formation of bone was also noted when suspensions of total bone marrow were implanted in the diffusion chamber. This led Friedenstein to suggest that bone marrow stromal cell populations contain osteogenic precursor cells. These osteogenic precursor cells were considered to be "determined osteogenic precursor cells" if they formed osteogenic tissues without a heterogenic inductive stimuli (Friedenstein, 1973). They were considered to be inducible osteogenic progenitors if a heterogenic inductive stimulus was necessary. Inducible osteogenic and chondrogenic precursor cells have been found in other tissues including spleen (Friedenstein, 1973) and embryonic muscle (Nogami and Urist, 1970). More recent studies have demonstrated that marrow stromal cells retain both chondrogenic and osteogenic potential (Ashton et al., 1980) and may conceivably be involved in fracture repair, regeneration of bone and marrow tissue, and in certain disease states (Owen, 1985). Components of the marrow stromal system may also be "determined osteogenic progenitors" and be involved in normal bone remodeling, as discussed above.

There are distinct developmental and perhaps functional relationships between osseous and hematopoietic tissues, and these relationships may be mediated by components of the stromal system and cells of the endosteal surface, perhaps including bone lining cells. The interrelations of the histogenesis of hematopoietic tissues in the marrow cavities of developing bone are well known. Under normal circumstances, the development of hematopoietic tissues follows an ordered sequence involving endochondral and intramembranous ossification to develop a suitable site (the marrow cavity) for seeding and development of the hematopoietic tissues. This relationship has also been defined in several experimental settings. For example, the regeneration of bone marrow following marrow extirpation or ablation occurs after the formation of new cancellous bone (Steinberg and Hufford, 1947; Patt and Maloney, 1975). The formation of a new cancellous network of bone appears to be a necessary prerequisite for the reconstruction of hematopoietic tissues. The cells responsible for the regeneration of the marrow stroma following marrow ablation appeared to arise from the endosteal surface of the bone (Patt and Maloney, 1970, 1975). Cells on the endosteal surfaces of this newly formed bone, perhaps including bone lining cells, may also interact with and perhaps regulate the vascular ingrowth that occurs prior to reconstitution of the hematopoietic cells (Branemark et al., 1964; Amsel et al., 1969). The formation of bone trabeculae has also been reported prior to marrow reconstitution of ectopic implants of whole bone marrow (Patt and Maloney, 1972a). In this case, the reticular cells of the marrow transplants appear to give rise to the osteogenic cells that form bone trabeculae in the implant (Tavossoli and Crosby 1968, 1970). From these studies, it appears that the formation of bone, and perhaps resorption of bone (Patt and Maloney, 1972b), is a necessary prerequisite for both normal marrow development and reconstitution of bone marrow in experimental situations. The formation of osseous tissue may be necessary to establish a suitable stromal system to support hematopoiesis.

In recent years it has become apparent that stromal domains exist within the bone marrow, each of which commits the resident pluripotent hematopoietic cells to a particular differentiation pathway (Lambertsen and Weiss, 1984). The proliferation and differentiation of the hematopoietic cells within these microenvironmental compartments appears to be regulated by the marrow stromal system (Gidali and Lajtha, 1972). It is also recognized that pluripotent stem cells in the bone marrow, particularly CFU-C, are most concentrated along the bone surface (Lord et al., 1975). The stem cells near endosteal surfaces also proliferate more rapidly than those away from bone (Shackney et al., 1975). The association of stem cells with endosteal surfaces has led to the suggestion that endosteal bone surface cells, perhaps including the bone lining cell, are totipotent stem cells capable of giving rise to proliferating progenitors of hematopoietic cells, stromal cells, as well as osteogenic cells (Islam, 1985).

Detailed morphological descriptions of the relationships of bone lining cells with hematopoietic cells (Weiss and Sakai, 1984) have led Deldar et al. (1985) to suggest that bone lining cells contribute to or perhaps even regulate the hematopoietic inductive microenvironment. This could involve direct cell to cell interactions or the elaboration of paracrine factors that control hematopoiesis. There is some evidence that hematopoiesis is regulated through direct cell contact with cells of the stromal system via growth factors bound to their cell surface (Roberts et al., 1988).

Bone Lining Cells and the Activation of Bone Remodeling

Bone remodeling consists of an ordered and predictable sequence of bone resorption followed by bone formation. The initiation of the remodeling sequence and birth of new basic multicellular units (BMUs) occur on inactive bone surfaces. This initiation process is termed "activation" and occurs on surfaces presumed to be covered by bone lining cells. The first histologic indication of BMU activation is the appearance of osteoclasts on the bone surface followed by the appearance of a resorption space. Prior to this, however, osteoclast progenitors would have to be recruited to the bone remodeling site, and the progenitors would have to fuse and then differentiate into the mature phenotype.

Very little is known about how activation of new bone remodeling units occurs, but there is increasing evidence that cells of the osteoblastic lineage play a role in the regulation and modulation of osteoclast activities, including bone resorption and osteoclast recruitment and differentiation. These interactions between osteogenic and osteoclastic cells may provide, at least in part, the physiological and anatomical basis for the "coupling" of bone formation and resorption. The coupling of bone formation and resorption allows the skeleton to normally maintain an appropriate balance between the amount of bone resorption and formation. There is some evidence that bone remodeling units may be activated to repair or prevent fatigue damage (Martin and Burr, 1982; Parfitt, 1984) and to allow the skeleton to adapt to mechanical usage (Frost, 1986 and 1987). However, the response of bone to microdamage is largely unknown at this time (Parfitt, 1988). Regardless if microdamage or local fatigue is responsible for the initial signal for bone activation, a signal must be transmitted to the bone surface where osteoclast progenitors can be recruited. Because of the location of the bone lining cell, it may be involved in the propagation or transduction of the activation signal that initiates bone remodeling (Miller and Jee, 1987).

Cells of the osteoblastic lineage, which would include bone lining cells, could possibly be involved in the activation and initiation of new remodeling units in a variety of ways (as reviewed by Rodan and Martin, 1981; Parfitt, 1984; Burger et al., 1984; Jilka, 1986; Vaes, 1988). Bone lining cells could release factors that are chemotactic for osteoclasts or their progenitors and perhaps control their differentiation. Osteoclasts have been shown to be derived from hematopoietic stem cells (Schneider et al., 1986) and the mechanisms of osteoclast regulation may be similar to those that may be involved in the regulation of hematopoietic cell proliferation and differentiation, as discussed in the previous section.

Cells of osteogenic lineage may also be involved in the regulation of osteoclastic functions and expression of the osteoclast phenotype. For example, bone resorption by isolated osteoclasts on devitalized bone slices was not affected by interleukin-1 (Thompson et al., 1986), tumor necrosis factor-α and 1-β (Thompson et al., 1987), parathyroid hormone (McSheehy and Chambers, 1986), or 1,25-dihydroxyvitamin D_3 (McSheehy and Chambers, 1987) unless the osteoclasts were co-cultured with osteoblasts. In these studies there was a significant increase in the number of resorption cavities, suggesting increased cellular efficiency and/or increased osteoclast activation in the presence of osteoblastic cells. In addition, the prostaglandins PGE_1, PGE_2, and PGI_2 were found to be inhibitors of isolated osteoclasts, but when co-cultured with osteoclasts these substances caused a considerable increase in cell spreading (Chambers et al., 1984 and see Chapter 6 in Volume 2). These observations have been interpreted as implicating a role for osteogenic cells in the regulation of osteoclastic activities.

Bone lining cells may serve as "gate-keepers" on the bone surface by restricting or permitting the osteoclasts or their progenitors from coming in contact with the bone surface. It is possible that the bone lining cells may retract and expose the "bare" bone surface and thus initiate the signal for the chemoattraction of osteoclasts and/or their progenitors. There is evidence that osteoclasts are activated upon exposure to the "bare" mineralized bone surface, but not the intact endosteal surface (Chambers et al., 1984). As noted earlier, the mineralized bone surface is covered by the endosteal membrane and this may function as a protective barrier over the mineralized tissue. When this membrane is removed, the mineralized matrix may facilitate the recruitment and attachment of osteoclast progenitors (Chambers and Fuller, 1985). Bone lining cells, or other cells that come in contact with the bone surface, may secrete enzymes to remove the unmineralized endosteal membrane on the bone surface. In this regard, osteogenic cells have been demonstrated to synthesize collagenase (Heath et al., 1984; Sakamoto and Sakamoto, 1984) as well as plasminogen activator (Hamilton et al., 1985). Plasminogen activator is considered to be a potentially potent activator of procollagenase (Vaes, 1988). It should be noted, however, that most of the evidence that demonstrates interactions between osteogenic and osteoclastic cell populations has been gathered in culture systems that use fetal or neonatal tissues or transformed cell lines. It is not clear if the "signals" that might regulate these rapidly developing and transformed systems would be the same as those encountered in the mature skeleton.

As noted earlier, the formation of bone appears to be a necessary prerequisite for the formation of bone marrow, providing evidence that the formation of the osseous tissue establishes a suitable microenvironment for hematopoiesis. There is also evidence that the opposite is also true — that is, a normal hematopoietic stromal system is necessary for normal bone remodeling. In studies using the op/op osteopetrotic murine mutant, Wiktor-Jedrzejczak et al. (1981 and 1982) have found that the resorption defect appears to be caused by an abnormal bone marrow microenvironment that results in impaired differentiation of osteoclasts from the hematopoietic stem cells. The defect appears to be caused by a reduced production of colony stimulating factors (CSFs) by components of the marrow stromal system. In vitro, CSFs will promote the differentiation of the hematopoietic stem cells and restore bone resorption by the osteoclasts. These data provide evidence that the stromal system, of which the bone lining may be an integral part, plays an important role in the activation of bone remodeling by producing a paracrine factor that promotes the differentiation of the osteoclast.

The Bone Lining Cell and the "Functional Bone Membrane"

Early studies by Neuman and his co-workers established that the electrolyte composition of the bone fluid compartment was different from that of the interstitial fluids (Neuman and Neuman, 1958). These findings supported the notion that there was a functional "membrane" on the bone surfaces that separated and likely regulated the exchange of electrolytes and molecules between compartments (Neuman and Ramp, 1971). The barriers that are considered to be important in bone are the endothelial cells that separate the blood fluids from the interstitial fluids and the bone lining cells that

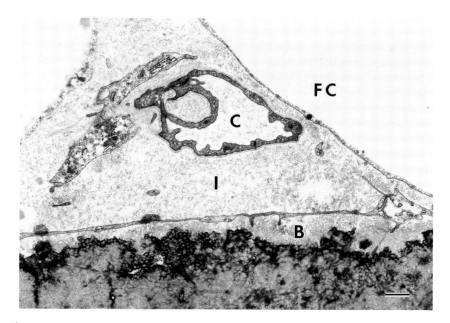

Fig. 8 The cytoplasm of a bone lining cell extends over a trabecular bone surface from a fatty marrow site in a beagle. This micrograph illustrates the morphological representation of the barriers between the different fluid compartments. Near the bone is a capillary, which in fatty marrow is a true capillary (C) representing the blood fluid compartment. Between the capillary and the bone lining cell are the interstitial tissues, representing the interstitial fluid compartment (I). The bone fluid compartment (B) is bordered by the bone lining cell. FC, fat cell cytoplasm. Decalcified section, bar = 1 μm. [From Miller, S. C. *et al.* (1980). *Metab. Bone Dis. Rel. Res.*, **2**: 239. With permission.]

separate the interstitial fluids from the bone fluids. The anatomical representations of the fluid compartment barriers in bone are illustrated in Fig. 8. All bone surface cells, however, can be considered as components of the "functional bone membrane" (Matthews *et al.*, 1978).

Bone lining cell processes extend into canaliculi and contact osteocytes via gap junctions. Bone lining cells also make contact with each other by gap junctions (Miller *et al.*, 1980). Gap junctions are also observed between osteoblasts, but have not been observed on osteoclasts (Doty, 1988). Gap junctions function in intercellular communication by allowing the movement of ions and small molecules between cells (Bennett and Goodenough, 1978). The coupling of bone lining cells with osteocytes and perhaps osteogenic cells via gap junctions suggests that regions of bone volume might act as a functional syncytium (Doty, 1981). This metabolic and electrical coupling of cells within bone might facilitate a number of physiological functions including the conversion of mechanical signals into remodeling activity and/ or the movement of mineral in and out of bone.

Experimental evidence suggests that osteoblasts, osteocytes, and bone lining cells play an important role in the regulation of mineral homeostasis, independent of any role in bone remodeling (Canas *et al.*, 1969; Talmage, 1970; Matthews and Talmage, 1981). Because bone lining cells cover most of the bone surfaces in the adult skeleton, they might be the most important cell in the minute-to-minute regulation of mineral homeostasis (Miller and Jee, 1987). Bone surface cells do not, however, appear to present an actual physical barrier for certain tracer molecules. For example, lanthanum easily penetrates intercellular spaces between bone surface cells, leading to the suggestion that mineral exchange might occur via intercellular channels and involve membrane pumps (Matthews and Talmage, 1981). This is further documented by observations that bone-seeking radionuclides are incorporated on all bone surfaces, although to a greater extent on mineralizing surfaces as well as resting surfaces in more highly vascularized areas (Smith *et al.*, 1984). It should be noted that most of the studies that have examined the functional capacity of bone surface cells have been conducted in young rodents where many of the bone surfaces are covered by osteoblasts or very young bone lining cells. The actual role of the bone lining cell in mineral homeostasis in longer-lived animals remains to be determined.

References

Amsel, S., Maniatis, A., Tavassoli, M., and Crosby, W. H. (1969). The significance of intra-medullary cancellous bone formation in the repair of bone marrow tissue. *Anat. Rec.*, **164**: 101.

Ashton, B. A., Allen, T. D., Howlett, C. R., Eagleson, C. C., Hattori, A., and Owen, M. (1980). Formation of bone and cartilage by marrow stromal cells in diffusion chambers in vivo. *Clin. Orthop.*, **151**: 294.

Bennett, M. V. L. and Goodenough, D. A. (1978). Gap junctions, electric coupling and inter-cellular communications. *Neurosci. Res. Program Bull.*, **16**: 373.

Bleaney, D. and Vaughan, J. (1971). Distribution of ^{239}Pu in the bone marrow and on the endosteal surface of the femur of adult rabbits following injection of ^{239}Pu(NO$_3$)$_4$. *Br. J. Radiol.*, **44**: 67.

Bowman, B. M. and Miller, S. C. (1986). The proliferation and differentiation of the bone-lining cell in estrogen-induced osteogenesis. *Bone*, **7**: 351.

Branemark, P. I., Breine, U., Johnansson, B., Roylance, P. J., Rockert, H., and Yoffey, J. M. (1964). Regeneration of bone marrow: a clinical and experimental study following removal of bone marrow by currettage. *Acta Anat.*, **59**: 1.

Burger, E. H., Van der Meer, J. W. M., and Nijweide, P. J. (1984). Osteoclast formation from mononuclear phagocytes: role of bone-forming cells. *J. Cell Biol.*, **99**: 1901.

Canas, F., Terepka, A. R., and Neuman, W. F. (1969). Potassium and milieu interieur of bone. *Am. J. Physiol.*, **217**: 117.

Chambers, T. J., Fuller, K., and Athanasou, N. A. (1984). The effect of prostaglandins I$_2$, E$_1$, E$_2$ and dibutyryl cyclic AMP on the cytoplasmic spreading of rat osteoclasts. *Br. J. Exp. Pathol.*, **65**: 557.

Chambers, T. J., Thompson, B. M., and Fuller, K. (1984). Effect of substrate composition on bone resorption by rabbit osteoclasts. *J. Cell Sci.*, **70**: 61.

Chambers, T. J. and Fuller, K. (1985). Bone cells predispose bone surfaces to resorption by exposure of mineral to osteoclastic contact. *J. Cell Sci.*, **76**: 155.

Cooper, R. R., Milgram, J. W., and Robinson, R. A. (1966). Morphology of the osteon. An electron microscopic study. *J. Bone Joint Surg. (Am.)*, **48**: 1239.

Deldar, A., Lewis, H., and Weiss, L. (1985). Bone lining cells and hematopoiesis: an electron microscopic study of canine bone marrow. *Anat. Rec.*, **213**: 187.

Doty, S. B. (1981). Morphological evidence of gap junctions between bone cells. *Calcif. Tissue Int.*, **33**: 509.

Doty, S. B. and Nunez, E. A. (1985). Activation of osteoclasts and the repopulation of bone surfaces following hiberation in the bat, *Myotis lucifugus*. *Anat. Rec.*, **213**: 481.

Doty, S. B. (1988). *Biological Mechanisms of Tooth Eruption and Root Resorption*, Ohio State University, Columbus, 61–69.

Friedenstein, A. J., Petrakova, K. V., Kurolesova, A. I., and Frolova, G. P. (1968). Heterotopic transplants of bone marrow. Analysis of precursor cells for osteogenic and hematopoietic tissues. *Transplantation*, **6**: 230.

Friedenstein, A. J. (1973). Hard tissue growth, repair, and remineralization. In: *Ciba Foundation Symposium*, Elsevier-Excepta Medica, Amsterdam, 169–182.

Frost, H. M. (1987). Bone mass and the mechanostat: a proposal. *Anat. Rec.*, **219**: 1.

Frost, H. M. (1986). *Intermediary Organization of the Skeleton*, CRC Press, Boca Raton, Florida.

Gidali, J. and Lajtha, L. G. (1972). Regulation of hematopoietic stem cell turnover in partially irradiated mice. *Cell Tissue Kinet.*, **5**: 147.

Hamilton, J. A., Lingelbach, S., Partridge, N. C., and Martin, T. J. (1985). Regulation of plasminogen activator production by bone-resorbing hormones in normal and malignant osteoblasts. *Endocrinology*, **116**: 2186.

Heath, J. K., Atkinson, S. J., Meikle, M. C., and Reynolds, J. J. (1984). Mouse osteoblasts synthesize collagenase in response to bone resorbing agents. *Biochim. Biophys. Acta*, **802**: 151.

Islam, A. (1985). Haemopoietic stem cell: a new concept. *Leukemia Res.*, **9**: 1415.

Jilka, R. L. (1986). Are osteoblastic cells required for the control of osteoclast activity by parathyroid hormone? *Bone Miner.*, **1**: 261.

Johnson, L. C. (1963). *Bone Dynamics*, Little and Brown, Boston, 543–654.

Kimmel, D. B. and Jee, W. S. S. (1982). A quantitative histological study of bone turnover in young adult beagles. *Anat. Rec.*, **203**: 21.

Kusuhara, S. and Schraer, H. (1982). Cytology and autoradiography of estrogen-induced differentiation of avian endosteal cells. *Calcif. Tissue Int.*, **34**: 352.

Lambertsen, R. H. and Weiss, L. (1984). A model of intramedullary hematopoietic microenvironments based on stereologic study of the distribution of endocloned marrow colonies. *Blood*, **63**: 287.

Lord, B. E., Testa, N. G., and Hendry, J. H. (1975). The relative spatial distributions of CFU-S and CFU-C in the normal mouse femur. *Blood*, **46**: 65.

Marks, S. C. Jr. and Popoff, S. N. (1988). Bone cell biology: the regulation of development, structure and function in the skeleton. *Am. J. Anat.*, **183**: 1.

Marotti, G. (1976). *Bone Morphometry*, University of Ottawa Press, Ottawa, 202–207.

Martin, R. B. and Burr, D. B. (1982). A hypothetical mechanism for the stimulation of osteonal remodeling by fatigue damage. *J. Biomech.*, **15**: 137.

Matthews, J. L., Vander Wiel, C., and Talmage, R. V. (1978). Bone lining cells and the bone fluid compartment, an ultrastructural study. *Adv. Exp. Med. Biol.*, **103**: 451.

Matthews, J. L. and Talmage, R. V. (1981). Influence of parathyroid hormone on bone cell ultrastructure. *Clin. Orthop.*, **156**: 27.

McLean, F. C. and Urist, M. R. (1968). *Bone: Fundamentals of the Physiology of Skeletal Tissue*, 3rd ed., University of Chicago Press, Chicago, 3–17.

McSheehy, P. M. J. and Chambers, T. J. (1986). Osteoblastic cells mediate osteoclastic responsiveness to parathyroid hormone. *Endocrinology*, **118**: 824.

McSheehy, P. M. J. and Chambers, T. J. (1987). 1,25-Dihydroxyvitamin D$_3$ stiulates rat osteoblastic cells to release a soluble factor that increases osteoclastic bone resorption. *J. Clin. Invest.*, **80**: 425.

Menton, D. N., Simmons, D. J., Orr, B. Y., and Plurad, S. B. (1982). A cellular investment of bone marrow. *Anat. Rec.*, **203**: 157.

Menton, D. N., Simmons, D. J., Chang, S. L., and Orr, B. Y. (1984). From bone lining cell to osteocyte. *Anat. Rec.*, **209**: 29.

Merz, W. and Schenk, R. (1970). A quantitative histological study on bone formation in human cancellous bone. *Acta Anat.*, **76**: 1.

Miller, S. C., Bowman, B. M., Smith, J. M., and Jee, W. S. S. (1980). Characterization of endosteal bone-lining cells from fatty marrow bone sites in adult beagles. *Anat. Rec.*, **198**: 163.

Miller, S. C. and Jee, W. S. S. (1980). The microvascular bed of fatty bone marrow in the adult beagle. *Metab. Bone Dis. Rel. Res.*, **2**: 239.

Miller, S. C. and Bowman, B. M. (1981). Medullary bone osteogenesis following estrogen administration to mature male japanese quail. *Dev. Biol.*, **87**: 52.

Miller, S. C. and Jee. W. S. S. (1987). The bone lining cell: a distinct phenotype? *Calcif. Tissue Int.*, **41**: 1.

Neuman, W. F. and Neuman, M. W. (1958). *Chemical Dynamics of Bone Mineral*, Chicago University Press, Chicago, 1–38.

Neuman, W. F. and Ramp, W. K. (1971). *Cellular Mechanisms for Calcium Transfer and Homeostasis*, Academic Press, New York, 197–206.

Nogami, H. and Urist, M. R. (1970). A substratum of bone matrix for differentiation of mesenchymal cells into chondro-osseous tissues in vitro. *Exp. Cell Res.*, **63**: 404.

Ohashi, T., Kusuhara, S., and Ishida K. (1987). Effects of oestrogen and anti-oestrogen on the cells of the endosteal surface of male japanese quail. *Br. Poul. Sci.*, **28**: 727.

Owen, M. and MacPherson, S. (1963). Cell population kinetics of an osteogenic tissue. II. *J. Cell Biol.*, **19**: 33.

Owen, M. (1978). Histogenesis of bone cells. *Calcif. Tissue Int.*, **25**: 205.

Owen, M. (1985). *Bone and Mineral Research*, Vol. 3, Elsevier Science Publishers, Amsterdam, 1–25.

Parfitt, A. M. (1983). *Bone Histomorphometry: Techniques and Interpretation*, CRC Press, Boca Raton, Florida, 143–223.

Parfitt, A. M. (1984). The cellular basis of bone remodeling: the quantum concept reexamined in light of recent advances in the cell biology of bone. *Calcif. Tissue Int.*, **36(suppl.)**: S37.

Parfitt, A. M. (1988). *Osteoporosis: Etiology, Diagnosis and Management*, Raven Press, New York, 45–93.

Park, E. A. (1954). Bone growth in health and disease. *Arch. Dis. Child.*, **29**: 269.

Patt, H. M. and Maloney, M. A. (1970). *Hemopoietic Cellular Proliferation*, Grune and Stratton, New York, 56–66.

Patt, H. M. and Maloney, M. A. (1972a). Evolution of marrow regeneration as revealed by transplantation studies. *Exp. Cell Res.*, **71**: 307.

Patt, H. M. and Maloney, M. A. (1972b). Bone formation and resorption as a requirement for marrow development. *Proc. Soc. Exp. Biol.*, **140**: 205.

Patt, H. M. and Maloney, M. A. (1975). Bone marrow regeneration after local injury: a review. *Exp. Hematol.*, **3**: 135.

Perkins, S. and Fleischman, R. A. (1988). Hematopoietic microenvironment. Origin, lineage, and transplantability of the stromal cells in long-term bone marrow cultures from chimeric mice. *J. Clin. Invest.*, **81**: 1072.

Polig, E. and Jee, W. S. S. (1986). Cell-specific radiation dosimetry in the skeleton. *Calcif. Tissue Int.*, **39**: 119.

Roberts, R., Gallagher, J., Spooncer, E., Allen, T. D., Bloomfield, F., and Dexter, T. M. (1988). Heparan sulphate bound growth factors: a mechanism for stromal cell mediated haemopoiesis. *Nature (London)*, **332**: 376.

Rodan, G. A. and Martin, T. J. (1981). Role of osteoblasts in hormonal control of bone resorption — a hypothesis. *Calcif. Tissue Int.*, **33**: 349.

Sakamoto, M. and Sakamoto, S. (1984). Immunocytochemical localization of collagenase in isolated mouse bone cells. *Biomed. Res.*, **5**: 29.

Shackney, S. E., Ford, S. S., and Wittig, A. B. (1975). Kinetic-microarchitectural correlations in the bone marrow of the mouse. *Cell Tissue Kinet.*, **8**: 505.

Scherft, J. P. (1972). The lamina limitans of the organic matrix of calcified cartilage and bone. *J. Ultrastruct. Res.*, **38**: 318.

Schneider, G. B., Relfson, M., and Nicolas, J. (1986). Pluripotent hemopoietic stem cells give rise to osteoclasts. *Am. J. Anat.*, **177**: 505.

Schulz, A. and Delling, G. (1976). *Bone Morphometry*, University of Ottawa Press, Ottawa, 189–196.

Simmons, D. J. (1962). Cellular changes in the bones of mice as studied with tritiated thymidine and the effects of estrogen. *Clin. Orthop. Rel. Res.*, **26**: 176.

Smith, J. M., Miller, S. C., and Jee, W. S. S. (1984). The relationship of bone marrow type and microvasculature to the microdistribution and local dosimetry of plutonium in the adult skeleton. *Radiat. Res.*, **99**: 324.

Steinberg, B. and Hufford, V. (1947). Development of bone marrow in adult rabbits. *Arch. Pathol.*, **43**: 117.

Talmage, R. V. (1970). Morphological and physiological consideration in a new concept of calcium transport in bone. *Am. J. Anat.*, **129**: 467.

Tavossoli, M. and Crosby, W. H. (1968). Transplantation of marrow to extramedullary sites, *Science*, **161**: 54.

Tavossoli, M. and Crosby, W. H. (1970). Bone marrow histogenesis: a comparison of fatty and red marrow. *Science*, **169**: 291.

Thompson, B. M., Mundy, G. R., and Chambers, T. J. (1987). Tumor necrosis factors α and β induce osteoblastic cells to stimulate osteoclastic bone resorption. *J. Immunol.*, **138**: 775.

Thompson, B. M., Saklatvala, J., and Chambers, T. J. (1986). Osteoblasts mediate interleukin 1 stimulation of bone resorption by rat osteoclasts. *J. Exp. Med.*, **164**: 104.

Tonna, E. A. and Cronkite, E. P. (1961). Autoradiographic studies of cell proliferation in the periosteium of intact and fractured femora of mice utilizing DNA labeling with H^3-thymidine. *Soc. Exp. Biol. Med. Proc.*, **107**: 719.

Vaes, G. (1988). Cell biology and biochemical mechanism of bone resorption. A review of recent developments on the formation, activation, and mode of action of osteoclasts. *Clin. Orthop.*, **231**: 239.

Vander Wiel, C. J., Grubb, S. A., and Talmage, R. V. (1978). The presence of lining cells on surfaces of human trabecular bone. *Clin. Orthop.*, **134**: 350.

Vaughan, E. (1972). *Radiobiology of Plutonium*, J.W. Press, Salt Lake City, 323–332.

Weiss, L. and Sakai, H. (1984). The hematopoietic stroma. *Am. J. Anat.*, **170**: 447.

Wiktor-Jedrzejczak, W., Ahmed, A., Szczylik, C., and Skelly, R. R. (1982). Hematological characterization of congenital osteopetrosis in op/op mouse. *J. Exp. Med.*, **156**: 1516.

Wiktor-Jedrzejczak, W., Skelly, R.R., and Ahmed, A. (1981). *Immunologic Defects in Laboratory Animals*, Plenum Press, New York, 51–77.

Young, R. W. (1962). Cell proliferation and specialization during endochondral osteogenesis in young rats. *J. Cell Biol.*, **14**: 357.

2

Haversian Systems and Haversian Bone

Z. F. G. JAWORSKI
Department of Medicine, Faculty of Health Sciences
University of Ottawa and Ottawa General Hospital
Ottawa, Ontario, Canada

Introduction

On the semi-microscopic scale, bones of the mature human skeleton consist of discrete packets or basic structural units of lamellar bone (BSUs*). Within the diaphyses of long bones of larger long-lived animals they are represented by the Haversian systems (secondary osteons) forming Haversian bone (Currey, 1960). In adult mammals, regardless of size, similar units of lamellar bone are seen on the periosteal and endosteal cortical and trabecular surfaces; in the diaphyses they are referred to as the external and internal circumferential lamellae (Fig. 1).

The formation of Haversian bone begins in man early during postnatal growth. It is a product of discrete spatially (circumscribed) and temporally (transient) coupled activity of osteoclast and osteoblast populations, forming the basic multicellular unit or Haversian BMU. This process, the formation of Haversian bone or internal modeling, appears to be distinct from subsequent turnover which the Haversian bone undergoes by means of similar Haversian BMUs, a part of what is referred to as internal remodeling, and which continues throughout life. Since periosteal and endosteal cortical and trabecular surfaces eventually also undergo a similar piecemeal lamellar bone turnover, one refers to this process globally as the lamellar bone turnover system or LBTS (Frost, 1963).

Such packets of lamellar bone or skeletal second order structures (Table 2) derive from a process quite distinct from that which first establishes and then maintains, as the bones grow, their respective sizes, shapes and architectures, that is, their first order structure (see Table 2). This is referred to as external modeling (Lacroix, 1971); it subsides with growth.

Haversian bone as a structure as well as the processes of which it is a product continue to be a subject of numerous studies and speculations as to their respective functions and controls. One of the reasons for this may be that the evolving Haversian system constitutes a relatively simple *in vivo* model allowing us to study several fundamental problems of bone physiology. In this chapter I propose first to review the current notions concerning Haversian systems and Haversian bone and, second, to review the contributions resulting from such studies to present knowledge of bone physiology in general.

Haversian Systems and Haversian Bone

Haversian bone consists of a network of osteons aligned parallel to the diaphysis long axis and running a slightly spiral course (Cohen and Harris, 1958; Tappen, 1977).

---

* See Table 1 for list of abbreviations used in this chapter.

Table 1.

Abbreviations

BMU	Basic multicellular unit of lamellar bone turnover
BSU	Basic structural unit of lamellar bone
EO LBTS	Effector organ of lamellar bone turnover system
LBT	Lamellar bone turnover
LMS	Locomotor system
MCSk	Mechanical competence of the skeleton
MDE	Mean depth of erosion within BMU
MES	Minimum effective strain
MU	Mechanical usage (mechanical loading)
MWT	Mean wall thickness of BSU

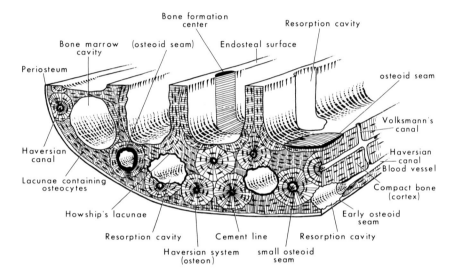

Fig. 1 A cross and longitudinal section of tubular bone (rib) shows the structural units of bone tissue (BSU) and the active remodeling sites (BMU) in cortical bone and on the endosteal envelope. [From Duncan, H. and Jaworski, Z. F. G. (1970). In: *Practice of Medicine*, Vol. 5. With permission.]

Individual osteons are identifiable over the course of several millimeters. Individual osteons measure only a fraction of the total length of the diaphysis (Cohen and Harris, 1958). Consequently the diaphyses are made of Haversian type of bone tissue (Currey, 1960, 1984). Osteons measure from 200 to 300 μm in diameter; the diameter of their central canal varies from 20 to 50 μm and their wall thickness measures up to 80 μm (Johnson, 1964, 1966). Individual osteons are separated from the adjacent tissue by a thin protein-aceous membrane which in cross section (see Fig. 1) is referred to as the

Table 2.
Elements of Skeleton's Mechanical Competence (MCSk)

I. Structural
   1. 1st order
      a. The respective shapes and sizes of bones
      b. Architecture (distribution of the bone tissue within the bone space)
      c. Mass (volume of bone tissue within the bone space)
   2. 2nd order
      BSUs and LB wall thickness
   3. 3rd order
      a. Lamellae
      b. Collagen fibrils bundles

II. Material
   1. Basic material
      a. Bone matrix
      b. Mineral
   2. Mean bone age (mineral content)

---

cement or reversal line. Their canals are joined every few millimeters by transversally running Volksmann's canals; together they form a network containing the innervated blood vessels, which communicate both with the blood circuit on the periosteal surface and with one within the bone marrow (Hert and Liskova, 1966; Brooks, 1971).

The walls of the osteons consist of several lamellae between 2 and $2^{1}/_{2}$ μm thick. Lamellae with high and low density collagen fibers alternate, giving them respectively bifringent (dense fibers) and dark (loose fibers) appearance under the polarized microscope (Marotti and Muglia, 1988). Until recently the bifringent lamellae were thought to be composed of fibril bundles aligned transversely while the dark ones run longitudinally or parallel to the osteon's long axis (Portigliatti Barbos et al., 1984). Furthermore, the transverse orientation of the collagen fibers was thought to predominate in osteons located in the areas subjected to mechanical compressive forces and the longitudinal one where the tensile mechanical forces would prevail.

Thus, while the osteons constitute the skeleton's second order structures, the collagen fibers within the lamellae form the third order structure (see Table 2); both the osteons and the lamellae within are aligned parallel to the long axis of the diaphysis.

The surface of the Haversian canals is covered by the lining cells connected by gap junctions between themselves and with the osteocytes located in the canalicular-lacunar space (Whitson, 1972; Matthews et al., 1977; see Chapter 1).

Evolutionary Aspects

Haversian bone is best developed in larger long-lived mammals, including man (Currey, 1970). Such a bone (that is, a system of osteons interconnected by the Haversian canals) should be distinguished from the isolated osteons or a few evolving Haversian-like systems in smaller animals such as a rat or a rabbit (Ruth, 1953). In such instances, the appearance of the Haversian-like resorption cavities or osteons, usually in paramedullary diaphyseal cortex, is conditioned by the demands of calcium ion homeostasis in the body fluids and consequently by the overall organism's mineral economy, which is under hormonal control (Parfitt, 1981). This points to a variety of factors which can prompt osteoclasts to form Haversian-like cavities and via coupling with the osteoblasts ensure their subsequent transformation into the residual osteon-like units.

Ontogeny

Formation of the Haversian Bone (Osteonalization)

The process which installs Haversian bone within the diaphyseal compacta, that is, internal modeling, appears to be operationally distinct from the piecemeal turnover which Haversian bone subsequently undergoes, although both are accomplished by the Haversian BMUs.

The creation of Haversian bone or the "osteonalization" of the diaphyseal compacta begins in man early during the first year of postnatal growth, as a process whereby the primary woven or plexiform bone tissue becomes replaced by lamellar bone. The first osteons appear in the regions located close to the muscle and tendon insertions on the periosteal surface (Enlow, 1962a), although eventually the whole width of the diaphysis becomes "osteonalized".

The osteonalization continues during growth as new tissue forms in the subperiosteal and endosteal locations, a result of both transverse growth and formation drifts (Enlow, 1963). On the other hand, some already osteonalized bone tissue may be removed by resorption drifts, which along with the formation drifts maintain the shape and architecture of growing bones.

The resorption cavities and hence the resulting osteons formed in the osteonalization process assume configurations not seen in the adult Haversian remodeling. They may form a double-ended column composed of two cutting cones moving in opposite direction or divide and move separately in parallel, forming forked osteons, etc. (Johnson, 1966).

Haversian Bone Turnover

In certain areas as soon as the Haversian bone is formed it begins to undergo a turnover by means of the same type of Haversian BMUs which formed it. The turnover, from the beginning in the dog (Amprino and Marotti, 1964) and very likely in man (Podenphant and Engel, 1987), assumes a characteristic pattern or topography, which maintains itself throughout life, although the rate of new BMUs activation within this pattern is faster during growth. It is this pattern that Marotti (1976a) referred to as the (internal) remodeling map.

As mentioned, with the onset of maturity, similar packets of lamellar bone or BSUs appear on the periosteal and endosteal surfaces in the diaphyses and in the spongy parts of the skeleton; in the latter they appear once the microresorption and formation drifts, which during growth establish and maintain the trabecular pattern, subside. Here too the BMU-based lamellar bone turnover exhibits a specific distribution or topography (Kimmel and Jee, 1982). Since the diaphyses of all long bones become osteonalized and all the periosteal and endosteal surfaces are covered by BSUs, but the BMU-based LBT shows local variations in intensity, the activation of BMUs for the purpose of osteonalization and turnover appears to be under different controls.

Formation of the Osteon

Haversian BMU

Activation and Formation of the Cutting Cone

Formation of the secondary osteon, requiring by definition first the removal of the pre-existing bone tissue, begins with the appearance of osteoclasts somewhere on the surface of a Volksmann's canal (or later within the Haversian bone on the surface of the existing Haversian canal) (Fig. 2). This event, referred to as the BMU activation (Frost, 1969), implies assembly of multinuclear osteoclasts from the dividing, differentiating and fusing mononuclear precursors (Jaworski et al., 1981). The standard appearance of the Haversian BMUs, both in the osteonalization and the subsequent internal remodeling process, suggests that local factors not operating in vitro mold the Haversian BMUs.

Some nine osteoclasts, each containing eight to nine nuclei, align to form the resorption front or a cutting cone (Johnson, 1964), some 250 to 300 μm long and 200 to 250 μm in diameter at the base (Fig. 3). The osteoclasts are supported by the capillary loop, an outgrowth of the vessels within the Volksmann's (or the Haversian) canal, the loop following the cutting cone as it advances parallel to the long axis of the diaphysis.

Cutting Cone

As the cutting cone moves, at a speed of some 40 to 50 μm/day (Jaworski

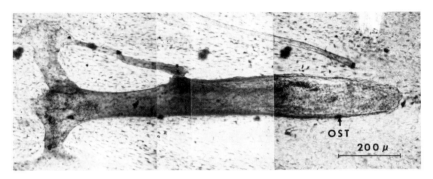

Fig. 2 A microphotograph of an early evolving Haversian system with the cutting cone containing osteoclasts in front and the closing cone behind with the layers of freshly deposited osteoid and bone tissue. The cutting cone is still close to the Volksmann's canal on the surface of which it originated. [From Jaworski, Z. F. G. and Lok, E. (1976). In: *Bone Morphometry*, Jaworski, Z. F. G., Ed., University of Ottawa Press. With permission.]

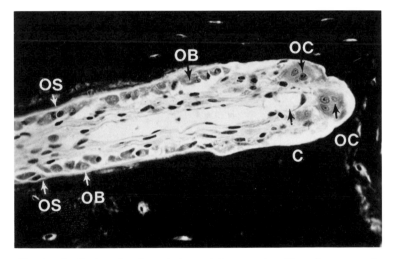

Fig. 3 This longitudinal section through the evolving secondary Haversian system shows the osteoclast front (OC) and the monolayer of osteoblasts (OB) on the surface of the eroded cavity. Behind the osteoclasts, capillaries (C) and supporting tissue can be identified. The whole unit moves across the bone (to the right) at 40 to 50 μm/day. [From Jaworski, Z. F. G. *et al.* (1981). *J. Anat.*, **133**: 397–405. With permission.] (Photomicrograph courtesy of Dr. R. K. Schenk, Bern University, Switzerland.)

and Lok, 1972), the osteoclast population within the front undergoes a turnover; new mononuclear cells join the osteoclasts at random replacing those nuclei which die or leave the population (Jaworski *et al.*, 1981). In other words, the osteoclast population is maintained during its lifespan by a continuous recruitment of new mononuclear cells.

The configuration, and dimensions, as well as the distance of the cutting

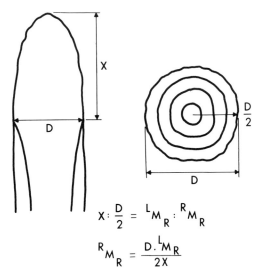

$$X : \frac{D}{2} = {}^LM_R : {}^RM_R$$

$${}^RM_R = \frac{D \cdot {}^LM_R}{2X}$$

Fig. 4 A schematic representation of the longitudinal (left) and cross section (right) of a cutting cone, illustrating the rationale for calculating the radial bone resorption rate. X = length of the cutting cone. D = cone's largest diameter; D/2 = cone's largest radius. [From Jaworski, Z. F. G. and Lok, E. (1972). *Calcif. Tissue Res.*, **10**: 103–112. With permission.]

cone's advance, could be determined (and limited) by the supply of oxygen and nutrients which the capillary loop provides. The advance of the cutting cone parallel to the long axis of the diaphysis appears to be determined by biomechanical requirements since their alignment (bone grain) follows the strain distribution (Currey, 1984).

The rate of the cutting cone longitudinal advance (some 40 to 50 μm/day) and the radial resorption rate are obviously related (Fig. 4). Thus, the time it takes to resorb the Haversian cavity in the cross-sectional sense equals the time it takes the cutting cone to move its own length from the tip to its largest diameter at the base, hence some 6 to 7 days (Jaworski and Lok, 1972). This time is referred to as Sigma R (Frost, 1969). The latter represents only a fraction of the actual lifespan of the cutting cone which equals the time it takes to resorb the whole length of the Haversian tunnel (see Chapter 9, Volume 1).

Transitional Zone

The surface of the resorbed tunnel located immediately behind the cutting cone (that is, the transitional zone) (Baron *et al.*, 1980) is a site of osteoblast precursor intense division and differentiation. They seem to originate from the connective tissue surrounding the capillary loop which supports the osteoclasts (see Fig. 3). Thus, contrary to the osteoclasts, the activation of osteoblasts, that is the onset of division and differentiation of their precursors, is clearly seen in the longitudinal section of the Haversian BMU (Fig. 5A).

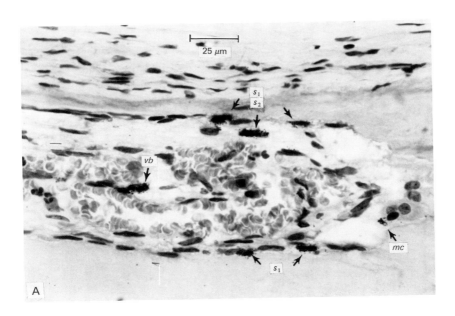

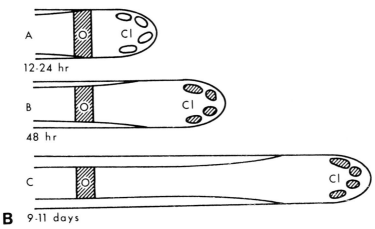

Fig. 5 **(A)** Labeled cells found in the longitudinal section through the system one hour after ³HtdR administration. Labeled spindle cells (S₁) at the base of the cutting cone (transitional zone) correspond to dividing pre-osteoblasts. **(B)** Schematic representation of migration of labeled cells within the evolving secondary Haversian system: (A) at 12 to 24 hours, (B) at 48 hours and (C) at 9 to 11 days after the tritiated thymidine injection. At 12 to 24 hours (A) the zone with labeled osteoblasts (○) is located in the most proximal part of the closing clone (shaded area). The first labeled nuclei are found in the osteoclasts (Cl) at 48 hours (B), when the cutting cone (shaded area) has moved some 50 to 100 μm since the time of ³HtdR administration. The zone of labeled osteoblasts is now seen left behind the advancing cutting cone. At 9 to 11 days (C), further separation occurred between the cutting cone with the labeled osteoclasts' nuclei (which has now advanced some 450 to 500 μm since the time of ³HtdR injection) and the zone with the originally labeled osteoblasts. [From Jaworski, Z. F. G. and Hooper, C. (1980). *J. Anat.*, **131**: 91–102. With permission.]

A coupling factor, a cytokine released presumably from the bone matrix during its resorption (Mohan *et al.*, 1984), would account for the onset, the rate and the duration of precursor division and differentiation and hence for the recruitment of the functional osteoblasts forming and maintaining the closing cone.

Closing Cone

The newly differentiated cuboid osteoblasts connected by gap junctions (Whitson, 1972) form a monolayer, lining the surface of the just-resorbed tunnel with an initial surface density of some 4000 cells/mm² (Jaworski and Wieczorek, 1985). As soon as it is formed the monolayer begins to deposit lamellae, 2–2½ μm thick, aligning parallel to the tunnel surface and into which some osteoblasts become incorporated as osteocytes. Since the density of the osteocytes in the lamellar bone remains constant (Frost, 1960a), the rate of their incorporation is proportional to the rate of osteoid formation. The rate of osteoid apposition is initially 2 to 3 μm/day, decreasing as the osteon closes (Frost, 1969).

The osteoid becomes mineralizable only after a few days of "maturation", after which the mineralization front follows in parallel the osteoid apposition, at a distance of some 8 to 10 μm. This accounts for the presence of the osteoid seams (see Fig. 3) in sites of lamellar bone formation.

Since the osteoblasts do not move, while their monolayer continues to deposit lamellae, they become more and more separated from the advancing cutting cone in front by the newly recruited osteoblasts in the transitional zone and from the original tunnel surface by the lamellae deposited underneath (see Fig. 3). This segment of the evolving Haversian system is, therefore, referred to as a closing cone (Johnson, 1964). Thus, in contradistinction to the motile osteoclasts in the cutting cone, osteoblasts in the closing cone remain stationary. The closing cone only appears to move *en bloc* behind the cutting cone (and in doing so maintains the same configuration and length, some 1200 to 1500 μm, as well as the rate of bone formation) because the newly recruited osteoblasts in the transitional zone replace the cells that either are lost as osteocytes from the monolayer in the closing cone or that finally become the lining cells (Jaworski *et al.*, 1981). Thus, the cutting and closing cone longitudinal advance is due to a different mechanism: in the first instance to the motility of osteoclasts and in the second to continuous ostseoblast recruitment, that is, to cell kinetics (Fig. 5B).

Haversian BMU Turnover Time (Sigma) and Volume of Lamellar Bone Turned Over

The Haversian BMU turnover time or Sigma of Frost (1969) should be distinguished from the time it takes to form the whole new osteon. The former equals, as mentioned, the time it takes for the BMU to move longitudinally its whole length (some 1500 μm), which in the cross section equals the time it takes to resorb centrifugally the Haversian cavity (Sigma R) (some 6 to 7 days) and to refill it (Sigma F) (some 30 to 60 days). The ratio of Sigma R to Sigma F is the same as the ratio of the cutting cone to closing cone lengths (see Fig. 4). Both reflect indirectly the respective efficiency of osteoclasts and osteoblasts. In fact, it is the difference in osteoclast and osteoblast efficiency (volume of bone resorbed or formed respectively per cell nucleus in a unit time) which also accounts, under normal circumstances, for exactly the same time it takes the shorter cutting cone to resorb the whole length of the tunnel and the much longer closing cone to refill it; the efficiency of some 9 osteoclasts in the cutting cone (or a population of some 80 mononuclear cells forming the 9 multinuclear osteoclasts) equals the efficiency of some 4000 osteoblasts in the closing cone, and the respective lengths of the cutting and closing cones reflect that difference (Jaworski, 1986). The time required to form the whole osteon, several millimeters long, is also longer than the Haversian BMU turnover time or Sigma, and similarly the volume of the osteon formed is several times greater than the volume of the bone turned over (some 0.05 mm^3) by the Haversian BMU during its Sigma. Similarly, the lifespan of the Haversian BMU (that is, of the osteoclast and osteoblast populations forming it) is several times longer than the BMUs Sigma as defined; it depends on the duration of recruitment of new functional cells necessary to maintain the Haversian BMU during the formation of the whole osteon (Jaworski, 1981).

During its lifespan, the Haversian BMU constitutes a unit of remodeling space (RMSp), that is, of a temporary bone deficit, some 0.05 mm^3, as shown in Fig. 6A (Jaworski, 1981).

Thickness of the Lamellar Bone Depots (MWT)

The mode of osteoblast recruitment and lamellar bone apposition, associated with the progressive loss of osteoblasts from the monolayer as osteocytes, may explain the constancy of the Haversian system wall thickness (and in fact of lamellar bone packets elsewhere) as well as of its limitation to some 80 μm (Ham, 1952).

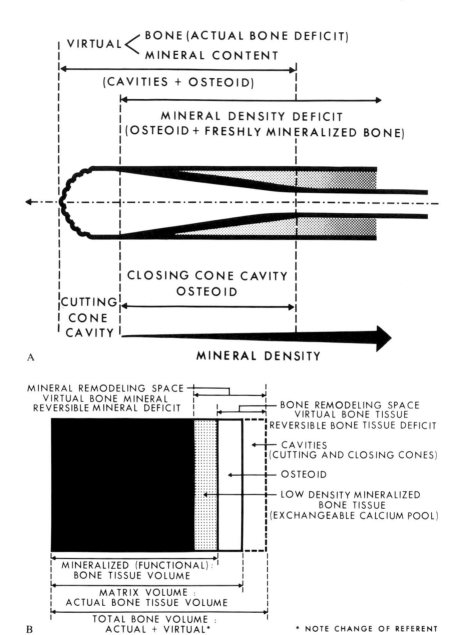

Fig. 6 (A) This schematic representation of an evolving Haversian system shows its various components that contribute to the bone remodeling space and bone tissue. (B) This global representation of bone tissue and mineral compartments is based on the contribution of individual remodeling sites to it as shown in Figure 6A. [From Jaworski, Z. F. G. (1981). *Rheumatology*, **33**: 233–246. With permission.]

Because of the progressive depletion of osteoblasts from the original monolayer and because the cells are connected by gap junctions, the remaining
surface osteoblasts elongate and flatten as they continue to deposit layers of
osteoid. Simultaneously, as the rate of osteoid apposition, and the separation
of the successive rows of osteocytes, decrease, the osteocytes and their lacunae
elongate (Marotti, 1977). Finally, the apposition of osteoid terminates and
the residual osteoid becomes mineralized while the remaining osteoblasts on
the surface, now of a Haversian canal, become lining cells. Their final density
is some $2000/mm^2$. Thus, the osteocytes incorporated in the osteon wall
appear to account for the difference between the surface density of osteoblasts
in the original monolayer, some $4000/mm^2$ and the density of the lining cells
(Jaworski and Wieczorek, 1985). Since their original density may be less but
cannot normally exceed some 4000 cells/mm^2, assuming their customary
efficiency, this may set the limit to the thickness of the osteon wall which
can be achieved.

Osteon Bone Balance

Since the osteon wall thickness (MWT) is limited by a potential maximum,
the diameter of the cutting cone at the base or its radius (mean depth of
erosion or MDE) determines the bone balance within the completed osteon;
the lumen of the Haversian canal reflects the difference between the MDE
and MWT (Fig. 7). The number of osteoclasts in the cutting cone in turn
determines the radius of the cavity or its MDE; that number may be limited
by the supply of oxygen and nutrients provided by the capillary loop supporting the advancing resorption front. For instance, the lumen of the Haversian canals in the paramedullary systems which communicate with the
bone marrow cavity are larger than the canals in the remaining two thirds
of the diaphyseal cortex. This implies an excess of MDE over MWT. The
negative bone balance in individual paramedullary osteons thus may account
for the progressive trabeculation of the inner cortex and, along with the
negative bone balance in the BSUs on the endosteal cortical and trabecular
surfaces, for the continuous expansion of bone marrow cavity throughout life
(Arnold, 1970).

Osteon: Its Microstructure and Evolution

Lamellar Bone Grain

Lamellar bone constitutes a composite and anisotropic material; composite
because it consists of collagenous matrix impregnated by the apatite crystals
and anisotropic because of the alignment of the lamellae (grain). The grain
of the lamellar bone is consequently one of the factors (the other being the
bone mineral content or BMC) which determine the mechanical properties

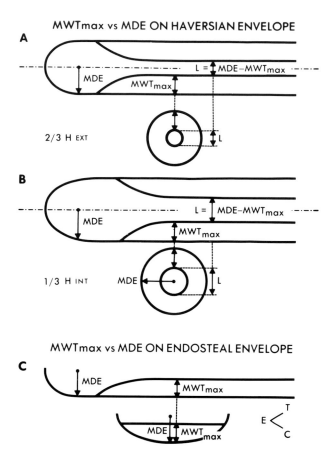

Fig. 7 Schematic representation of longitudinal and cross section of the evolving Haversian system (A and B) and similar turnover site on the endosteal bone surface (C) demonstrating the effect of mean bone depth of bone erosion (MDE) and mean wall thickness (MWT) on the osteon's bone balance. The MWT being limited by a maximum, the osteons balance (in the Haversian system reflected by the lumen of Haversian canal) is mainly determined by MDE.

of lamellar bone as a material (Currey, 1984). These properties vary, therefore, according to the osteon's mineral content and how the osteons and lamellae align with respect to the strain pattern within the bone tissue. Thus, alignment of the osteons and their lamellae, parallel to the long axis of bones, may contribute to the strength of the material under mechanical loading (Currey, 1984).

Lining Cells — Osteocytic System

The lining cells on the surface of the Haversian canal connected with the osteocytes within the osteon's wall by the protoplasmic processes form a syncytium. On the microscopic level there is therefore a space between the bone surface and the lining cells communicating with the canalicular and lacunar system which is filled with the bone fluid. This fluid, on the one hand in contact with the apatite crystals, is separated on the other from the extracellular fluid by the loose membrane consisting of lining cells (Matthews *et al.*, 1977). The composition of the bone fluid, while tending to equilibrate with the crystalline phase, is affected also by exchange with the extracellular fluid across the lining cell's membrane. The activity of the lining cells-osteocytic syncytium regulated by hormones allows for the influx of mineral for mineralization of the osteoid and crystal growth (accretion) during the lamellar bone formation as well as for the efflux of calcium for support of the calcium ion concentration (homeostasis) in the body fluids.

In addition to the function just mentioned, it was postulated that the lining cells-osteocytic system may operate as a sensor of the strain range within the bone tissue, resulting from the application of mechanical loads (Currey, 1984). Recent demonstration of biochemical changes taking place within the osteocytes and in the organic matrix following the application of a single mechanical load supports this hypothesis (Binderman *et al.*, 1984; Pead *et al.*, 1988). Such biochemical imprints related to strain could constitute a part of the afferent loop of the feedback mechanism, which adjusts bone structure and its materials properties to mechanical demands (Bassett, 1971; Frost, 1987).

Evolution and Aging of the Osteon

The BMC of new osteons due first to primary mineralization (that is, the advance of the mineralization front through the osteoid) continues to increase as the apatite crystals grow, a process referred to as accretion or secondary mineralization (Marotti *et al.*, 1972; Marotti, 1976b) and clearly seen on microradiographs (Amprino and Engstrom, 1952; Vincent, 1957; Rowland *et al.*, 1959; Lee *et al.*, 1965).

The BMC determines several osteonal materials properties. As the BMC increases, bone tissue compliance tends to decrease, while the increasing stiffness contributes to the bone strength. If the BMC exceeds the optimal value, bone strength decreases and bone becomes brittle (Smith and Walmsley, 1960; Currey, 1969; Lipson and Katz, 1984; Katz *et al.*, 1984). The proper balance between strength and compliance depends, therefore, on the BMC. When it is right, bone tissue at an ultrastructural level under mechanical loading would undergo only elastic reversible deformation and sustain a minimum of mechanical fatigue. The upper range of elastic reversible deformation appears also to generate signals and stimuli prompting bone cells to affect the appropriate structural and materials adjustments (Frost, 1983). If that happens, strains return to the safe range. On the other hand, bones (osteons) with excessive BMC when overstrained, because of the loss of compliance, first tend to undergo the plastic irreversible deformation resulting in the production and accumulation of mechanical fatigue (Evans, 1970; Reilly and Burnstein, 1974), and second lose the strain range necessary to generate stimuli and signals to activate the feedback mechanism. Thus, adjustments of the bone structure and its materials properties in response to the mechanical demands may fail to occur and a vicious circle becomes installed, whereby the production and accumulation of mechanical fatigue continues causing bone fragility.

BMC varies with the osteon's age, probably because the function or the number of viable osteocytes decreases with the osteon's age, preventing overmineralization. The important role of the lining cells-osteocytic system in maintaining the optimal mineral content of the osteon is demonstrated by the massive inflow of mineral into the canalicular-lacunar system following death of the osteocytes, referred to as micropetrosis (Frost, 1960b).

The changes in the BMC due to aging of the osteon have to be distinguished from changes within osteons resulting from the decline of the proliferative potential of the aging organism. Thus, Dhem and Robert (1986) noted that in the diaphyses of old dogs, the intracortical porosis is due to the decreased thickness of the osteon's wall, resulting in a large lumen of the Haversian canal. In some such osteons a layer of newly deposited lamellar bone can be seen, as if the radial closure took place in two stages, separated by a long time interval. This is shown clearly on a microradiograph because of the high optical density of the first layer and a low one of the second. In humans the decrease in the MWT with age (Lips *et al.*, 1978; Kragstrup *et al.*, 1983) may reflect such a decrease in cell proliferative potential and/or function.

The proportion of old osteons within bone tissue, while reflecting mean bone age, depends on, in addition to the intrinsic changes in the osteons with aging, the rate of Haversian BMU lamellar bone turnover (Jerome, 1989) and hence on BMUs activation frequency and in disease also on the BMU turnover time (Sigma) (Jaworski, 1986). Since the activation frequency decreases with age, the mean bone age and BMC tend to increase with age too. In general, therefore, the areas where the mechanical competence of the skeleton depends particularly on the materials properties become particularly vulnerable and prone to fractures (vertebrae, ribs, lower radius, upper femur), if the process of bone tissue renewal becomes impaired.

The changes in the structural and materials properties which the evolving Haversian systems undergo translate, however, into tissue level effects through the local Haversian BMU activation frequency, that is, the internal remodeling map.

Tissue Level Effects of the Haversian BMUs

Osteonalization

The final replacement of more primitive bone tissue by lamellar bone, which includes the osteonalization of the diaphyseal compacta by Haversian BMUs, may invest the skeleton with biomechanical advantages (Currey, 1984). While woven bone is grainless, lamellar bone is anisotropic, that is, it exhibits grain. Thus, the alignment of the osteons themselves (second order structures), the lamellae and the collagen fibers within (third order structures), according to the strain pattern may contribute to bone tissue strength while saving on weight and the amount of materials, as seen, for instance, in the trabecular pattern in the upper femur. Any device which reduces the skeleton's weight while not depriving it of strength may offer a distinct advantage since it saves on the organism's energy expenditure.

Haversian Turnover

In addition to their role in osteonalization, the BMUs in the Haversian turnover process appear to contribute to the maintenance of the quality of the lamellar bone tissue.

The number of BMUs (A) operating at any given time per unit of bone volume, considering their standard volume of bone turned over and its time or Sigma (σ), depends on the BMUs activation frequency (μ), as shown in the following equation (Frost, 1969).

$$A = \sigma \times \mu$$

Since the space which the BMU occupies within the bone tissue and volume of bone it turns over (some 0.05 mm^3) is also more or less standard, and since each BMU represents a unit of temporary deficit within the bone's space, collectively they constitute the bone remodeling space (RMSp), as shown in Fig. 6. They also collectively determine the volume of bone turned over, expressed as a fraction of a total bone volume during the convenient time unit (Frost, 1969). The standard intra-BMU events initiated by the BMU activation and the activation frequency, which varies in different parts of the skeleton, consequently may represent independent variables of LBT.

The BMUs activation frequency, apart from determining the volume of the RMSp, produces several other tissue level effects. First, it determines the mean bone age and hence its quality because of replacing the pre-existing "old" bone tissue (with high BMC and accumulated microdamage) by new fresh osteons with relatively low BMC; it in turn enhances the bone tissue compliance. As a consequence, this increases the strain range while producing within the bone tissue elastic reversible deformation and little mechanical fatigue, and, on the other hand, by enhancing the strain generated signals and stimuli, the optimal compliance may facilitate the operation of the feedback mechanism. Second, the high rate of activation frequency enables the osteons to realign (grain), and third, it allows bone mass to optimize because strains seem to mitigate resorption (MDE) and enhance bone formation

(MWT) within the osteons (Jaworski and Uhthoff, 1986). All these derivative effects of BMUs activation frequency thus tend to optimize the quality of bone tissue and the skeleton's mechanical competence.

Since the BMUs activation frequency in various bones and regions of bones may differ manyfold and exhibits a pattern referred to as the internal remodeling map (Amprino and Marotti, 1964; Marotti, 1976a; Kimmel and Jee, 1982), tissue level effects of Haversian LBT will vary accordingly.

Haversian Bone in a Larger Context

Haversian Bone and the Processes which Skeleton Undergoes

The installation of the Haversian bone and its subsequent turnover cannot be considered in isolation from the processes which establish, adjust and maintain the structure of the skeleton as an organ of physical support.

The development of the skeleton, a rigid articulated core of the locomotor system, proceeds through genetically determined stereotyped sequences (Enlow, 1962b; Gardner, 1956). First, the chondroblasts elaborate the skeleton's cartilagenous model whereby the gross shape and relative sizes of the bones are determined. Second, the growing cartilagenous skeleton's model becomes replaced by woven bone, which implies a prior removal of the mineralized matrix by osteoclasts in places such as the metaphyseal growth plates and the interior of short bones and epiphysis. This sequence, along with the installation of formation and resorption drifts, refines the bone's basic shape and determines its architecture, that is, the distribution of the bone tissues within the bone's space (diaphyseal compacta or spongiosa), and, with it, the anatomy of the bone marrow cavity housing the bone marrow. It appears logical, therefore, to call this process gross or external modeling.

The third and last sequence is also genetically determined, namely the replacement of the pre-existing woven or plexiform bone by lamellar bone. While not affecting significantly the shape or the architecture of bones, it subdivides them into units of lamellar bone by virtue of the limit to the thickness of lamellar bone which can be deposited. This is due, as previously discussed, to the manner by which lamellar bone is deposited on bone surfaces, whether primarily or secondarily, as on surfaces of cavities resorbed by the osteoclasts (Jaworski and Wieczorek, 1985). It is logical, therefore, to call the process replacing the woven or plexiform bone tissue and subdividing it into units of lamellar bone internal or micromodeling. The appearance of the Haversian systems forming the Haversian bone can be viewed as a part of internal modeling (osteonalization), its specific form being due to the local conditions in the diaphyseal compacta. As discussed earlier, lamellar bone, because of its anisotropy or grain, may invest bones with a biomechanical advantage (Currey, 1984).

Both external and internal modeling appear to follow the program stored in the genome during phylogeny, the program which unfolds by the forward feed principle, as it were, whereby each stage in the development prepares and enables the next one via emerging cell-tissue interactions (Hall, 1983). As sequences replacing one bone tissue by another, drifts and osteonalization proceed and bones continue to increase in size; consequently two superimposed processes go on simultaneously, referred to by Wolpert (1969) respectively as pattern development and pattern growth. Thus, external and internal modeling terminate with the completion of growth.

Although the basic bone structure unfolding as a result of external and internal modeling is genetically predetermined, the bone mass and architecture as well as its microstructure (grain) have the capacity to adjust to the actual mechanical demands which increase once the locomotor system begins to operate in the earth gravity environment shortly after birth. There is convincing evidence that these adjustments operate on the feedback principle (Bassett, 1971; Frost, 1987). Briefly, the excessive strains so produced appear to modulate the elaboration of the basic bone structure, that is, their mass, shape, architecture, and grain. The effector organ which allows for such mass and gross architectural adjustments during postnatal growth probably consists of cells already engaged in external modeling, tending globally to enhance bone formation and to mitigate its resorption (Jaworski and Uhthoff, 1986; Klein-Nulend et al., 1987). Thus, the individual enters maturity with a peak bone mass greater than what it would be if the skeleton were not subjected to mechanical loading. The potential to adjust decreases, however, with the completion of growth as the cellular mechanisms involved in external modeling subside. However, as the experiments of Lanyon (1984) and others have demonstrated, the external remodeling process can be reactivated in some form at any time afterward.

Insofar as the BMU-based remodeling, as distinct from the original osteonalization, is concerned, the excessive strains would activate the BMUs, that is, in the first place the local osteoclast populations, which via the coupling mechanism allow the osteoblasts to refill the resorbed cavity. A high activation frequency rate would be perpetuated, as discussed before, in areas where the bone mass does not reduce or neutralize the excessive strains (Jaworski, 1986). This in essence would explain the persistence throughout life of significant differences in the activation frequency and the BMU-based lamellar turnover rate in various bones and regions of bones referred to as the internal remodeling map (Marotti, 1976a). Thus, while the initial osteonalization would result from the process substituting the temporary bone tissue by lamellar bone, a part of the forward feed mechanism, the subsequent BMU-based lamellar bone turnover, would be determined mainly by the actual mechanical demands and operate on a feedback mechanism. There is some independent support for this view (Burr et al., 1988). The fact that a number of factors in addition may activate the BMUs (that is, in the first instance the osteoclast populations) does not detract from this point of view.

Cellular Mechanisms

Because the chondroblasts and osteoblasts which produce respectively cartilagenous and collagenous matrix or osteoid become incorporated as chondrocytes and osteocytes into their matrices, the formation of the latter requires a constant supply of new cells recruited from the dividing and differentiating committed precursors. The same applies to osteoclasts in sites where the replacement of one bone tissue by another is taking place or where resorption drifts operate.

The recruitment of new functional cells depends on the division and differentiation of committed precursors controlled by specific mitogens and cytokines (see Chapters 3 and 4 in Volume 1). They may constitute the final common path for all the processes in which the cells participate but their local release or activity would be triggered or modulated by a different combination of factors in each. For instance, pattern development (that is, the external and internal modeling) would be dependent upon their release as a result of unfolding cell-tissue interactions (Hall, 1983). Pattern growth during pre- but mainly postnatal growth, when the more or less formed bones increase in size, would depend in addition on systemic hormonal factors such as growth horomone, thyroxin, insulin, sex hormones, etc. (Reddi, 1983; Canalis, 1985; Vaes, 1988; Daughaday, 1989), while the external and internal remodeling (that is, the adaptation of the basic bone gross and microstructure to actual mechanical demands) would depend on the modulation of mitogens and cytokines already operating in the existing sites of cellular activity or insofar as the BMU-based lamellar bone turnover is concerned (that is, the activation of the BMUs) would depend on their local release. Ultimately such a reinforcement or release of the specific mitogens and cytokines would be related to effective strains (Frost, 1983). Thus, the actual load application on bones while producing strains which can be measured on the bone surface with the strain gauge would produce, according to their distribution within the bone tissue on the microscopic or ultrastructural levels, local alterations, such as the redistribution of the fluids (blood or bone fluid, the latter resulting in streaming potential), the deformation of intermolecular bonds (within crystals or collagen resulting possibly in piezoelectric potentials) and finally the distortion of the lining cell-osteocytic system (Basset, 1971). Biochemical changes in some of these elements as a result of loading have been demonstrated (Binderman et al., 1984; Pead et al., 1988). Which of these (if any) modulate or trigger the local release of specific mitogens and cytokines, prompting the effector organ (chondroblasts, osteoblasts and osteoclasts) via their recruitment and function to initiate the adequate structural adjustment in response to mechanical loads, remains to be established. The fact remains that we now know more about these cell kinetics and flow than about the factors which control them or about their mode of operation. Within the last few years, a number of such mitogens and cytokines have been isolated, identified and tested in *in vitro* systems both in terms of cells producing matrices as well as osteoclasts (Urist *et al.*, 1983; Reddi, 1983, Canalis, 1985; Chambers and Fuller, 1985; Vaes, 1988; Mundy, 1989), but how such factors affect the kinetics and function of the osteoclasts or osteoblasts under physiological conditions (that is, in the orderly and highly structured in space and time processes which elaborate the skeleton and maintain its mechanical competence) remains unknown (see Volume 7). There is still a large gap between the information which *in vitro* studies provide and what is observed *in vivo,* as shown by the formation of the Haversian systems and Haversian bone.

Summary

In this chapter, Haversian systems were viewed as the structural units of lamellar bone, constituting within the diaphyseal compacta the Haversian bone, that is, a system of interconnected Haversian systems oriented roughly parallel to the long axis of long bone diaphysis. Such an arrangement invests bones with structural advantages when bones are mechanically loaded.

Haversian systems are a product of discrete in space and time basic multicellular units or BMUs consisting basically of two types of self-renewing cell populations, the osteoclasts resorbing the Haversian cavity and the osteoblasts appearing next (coupling), refilling it with the lamellar bone. The Haversian systems and the Haversian BMUs would represent only a special variant of such units, encountered in all parts of the skeleton, which assume a special form in the diaphyseal compacta because of the local conditions.

The Haversian systems and BSUs on other bone surfaces appear first during the skeleton's development, as an outcome of the series of substitutions of temporary bone tissues, in this instance by the lamellar bone, which due to its mode of production, limiting the thickness of lamellar bone deposits to some 80 μm, subdivides bones into structural units (BSUs).

The BMU in general and Haversian BMU in particular appear to participate in two processes. The first is osteonalization, that is, installation of the Haversian bone in the diaphyseal compacta, which appears, as mentioned, to be a part of a genetically determined final substitution of temporary bone by lamellar bone. Lamellar bone may represent an evolutionary device which, because of its anisotropy or grain, by aligning according to strain distribution, may contribute to the mechanical competence on the skeleton as an organ of physical support.

The second process in which the Haversian BMUs, along with other BMUs, participate is lamellar bone turnover, again a part of a larger process, that is, the remodeling which allows the gross and microscopic structure of the skeleton to adapt to actual mechanical demands put on the locomotor system when it begins to operate, shortly after birth, in the earth gravity environment. It would operate by a feedback mechanism, whereby the signals generated by the excessive strains directing the cellular activities towards the structural adjustments in bone mass, shape, architecture, and grain, would bring the strains back to the safe level.

The excessive strains would also increase the activation of new BMUs and hence the lamellar bone turnover rate, but would persist only in regions of the skeleton where the bone mass becomes insufficient to reduce the strains. This is proposed as an explanation for the specific topography of the BMUs frequency activation and BMU-based lamellar bone turnover rate in the skeleton, referred to as the internal remodeling map.

The development of the skeleton, its growth and functional adaptations to actual mechanical demands depend on the constant supply of new cells recruited from the dividing and differentiating committed precursors, an activity controlled by specific local mitogens and cytokines. They would constitute a final common pathway through which other factors controlling skeleton development, growth and structural adaptations would operate. A number of such factors often encountered in pathological situations have been identified, isolated and tested *in vitro*. However, a large gap still exists between the information which the *in vitro* studies provide and the elucidation of their role in orderly operation of cellular mechanisms in the elaboration of the skeleton or its adaptation to mechanical demands observed *in vivo*.

References

Amprino, R. and Engstrom, A. (1952). Studies on X-ray absorption and diffraction of bone tissue. *Acta Anat.*, **15**: 1–22.

Amprino, R. and Marotti, G. (1964). A topographic quantitative study of bone formation and reconstruction. In: *Bone and Tooth Symposium,* Blackwood, E. J. J., Ed., Macmillan, New York, 21–23.

Arnold, J. S. (1970). Focal excessive endosteal resorption in aging and in senile osteoporosis. In: *Osteoporosis,* Barzel, U. S., Ed., Grune and Stratton, New York, 50.

Baron, R., Vignery, A., and Tran Van, P. (1980). The significance of lacunar erosion without osteoclasts: studies on the lacunar erosion of the remodeling sequence. *Metab. Bone Dis. Rel. Res.,* **25**: 35–40.

Bassett, C. A. L. (1971). Biophysical principles affecting bone structure. In: *The Biochemistry and Physiology of Bone. Vol. III* (2nd ed.), Bourne, G. H., Ed., Academic Press, New York, 1.

Binderman, I., Shimshoni, Z., and Somjen, D. (1984). Biochemical pathways involved in the translation of physical stimulus into biological message. *Calcif. Tissue Int.,* **36**: 82–85.

Brooks, M. (1971). *The Blood Supply of Bones,* Butterworths, London.

Burr, D. B., Martin, R. B., Lefever, S., Franklin, N., and Thompson, G. (1988). Repetitive loading to prevent osteoporosis in the vertebral column. In: *Current Concepts of Bone Fragility,* Uhthoff, H. K., Ed., Springer-Verlag, Berlin, 415.

Canalis, E. (1985). Effects of growth factors on bone cell replication and differentiation. *Clin. Orthop. Rel. Res.,* **193**: 246–263.

Chambers, T. J. and Fuller, K. (1985). Bone cells predispose bone surfaces to resorption by exposure of mineral to osteoclastic contact. *J. Cell. Sci.,* **76**: 155–165.

Cohen, J. and Harris, W. B. (1958). Three dimensional anatomy of Haversian systems. *J. Bone Jt. Surg.,* **40A**: 419–434.

Currey, J. D. (1960). Differences in the blood-supply of bone of different histologic types. *Quart. J. Microsc. Sci.*, **101**: 351–370.

Currey, J. D. (1969). The relationship between the stiffness and the mineral content of bone. *J. Biomech.*, **2**: 477–480.

Currey, J. D. (1970). The mechanical properties of bone. *Clin. Orthop. Rel. Res.*, **73**: 210–231.

Currey, J. (1984). *The Mechanical Adaptations of Bone*, Princeton University Press.

Daughaday, Wm. H. (1989). A personal history of the origin of the somatomedin hypothesis and recent challenges to its validity. *Persp. Biol. Med.*, **32**: 194–211.

Dhem, A. and Robert, V. (1986). Morphology of bone tissue aging. In: *Current Concepts of Bone Fragility*, Uhthoff, H. K., Ed., Springer-Verlag, Berlin, 364–370.

Duncan, H. and Jaworski, Z. F. G. (1970). Osteoporosis. In: *Practice of Medicine*, Vol. 5, 1.

Enlow, D.H. (1962a). Functions of the Haversian system. *Am. J. Anat.*, **110**: 269–306.

Enlow, D. H. (1962b). A study of the post-natal growth and remodeling of bone. *Am. J. Anat.*, **110**: 79–101.

Enlow, D. H. (1963). *Principles of Bone Remodeling*, Charles C Thomas, Springfield, IL.

Evans, F. G. (1970). *Mechanical Properties and Histologic Structure of Human Cortical Bone*. ASME 70-WA/BHF-7.

Frost, H. M. (1960a). Measurement of osteocytes per unit volume and volume components of osteocytes and canaliculae in man. *Henry Ford Hosp. Med. Bull.*, **8**: 208–211.

Frost, H. M. (1960b). Micropetrosis. *J. Bone Jt. Surg.*, **42A**: 144–150.

Frost, H. M. (1963). *Principles of Bone Remodeling*, Charles C Thomas, Springfield, IL.

Frost, H. M. (1969). Tetracycline-based histologic analysis of bone remodeling. *Calcif. Tissue Res.*, **3**: 211–237.

Frost, H. M. (1983). The minimum effective strain: a determinant of bone architecture. *Clin. Orthop. Rel. Res.*, **175**: 286–292.

Frost, H. M. (1987). The mechanostat: a proposed pathogenic mechanism of osteoporoses and the bone mass effects of mechanical and nonmechanical agents. *Bone and Mineral*, **2**: 73–85.

Gardner, E. (1956). Osteogenesis in the human embryo and fetus. In: *Biochemistry and Physiology of Bone*, Vol. III, Bourne, G. H., Ed., Academic Press, New York, 77–118.

Hall, B. K. (1983). Embryogenesis: cell-tissue interactions. In: *Skeletal Research — An Experimental Approach*, Vol. 2., Kunin, A. S. and Simmons, D. J., Eds., Academic Press, New York, 53.

Ham, A. W. (1952). Some histophysiological problems peculiar to calcified tissues. *J. Bone Jt. Surg.*, **34A**: 701–728.

Hert, J. and Liskova, M. (1966). Blood circulation in the compact Haversian bone of long bones. *Folia Morphologica*, **14**: 151–159.

Jaworski, Z. F. G. (1981). Osteoporosis revisited. *Rheumatologie*, **33**: 233–246.

Jaworski, Z. F. G. (1986). Cellular mechanisms underlying the skeleton's supportive function. In: *Current Concepts of Bone Fragility*, Uhthoff, H. K., Ed., Springer-Verlag, Berlin, 35–37.

Jaworski, Z. F. G., Duck, B., and Sekaly, G. (1981). Kinetics of osteoclasts and their nuclei in evolving secondary Haversian systems. *J. Anat.*, **133**: 397–405.

Jaworski, Z. F. G. and Hooper, C. (1980). Study of cell kinetics within evolving secondary Haversian systems. *J. Anat.*, **131**: 91–102.

Jaworski, Z. F. G. and Lok, E. (1972). The rate of osteoclastic bone erosion in Haversian remodeling sites in adult dog's rib. *Calcif. Tissue Res.*, **10**: 103–112.

Jaworski, Z. F. G. and Lok, E. (1976). The effect of moderate uremia and high phosphate-normal calcium diet on the linear erosion rate, measured in the Haversian turnover sites in the rib of the adult dog. In: *Bone Morphometry*, Jaworski, Z. F. G., Ed., University of Ottawa Press, Ottawa, 148.

Jaworski, Z. F. G. and Uhthoff, H. K. (1986). Disuse osteoporosis: current status and problems. In: *Current Concepts of Bone Fragility*, Uhthoff, H. K., Ed., Springer-Verlag, Berlin, 181.

Jaworski, Z. F. G. and Wieczorek, E. (1985). Constants in lamellar bone formation determined by osteoblasts kinetics. *Bone*, **6**: 361–363.

Jerome, C. P. (1989). Estimation of the bone mineral density variation associated with changes in turnover rate. *Calcif. Tissue Int.*, **44**: 406–410.

Johnson, L. C. (1964). Morphologic analysis: the kinetics of disease and general biology of bone. In: *Bone Biodynamics*, Frost, H. M., Ed., Little Brown, Boston.

Johnson, L. C. (1966). The kinetics of skeletal remodeling. In: *Structural Organization of the Skeleton*, Milch, R. A. and Robinson, R. M., Eds., National Foundation of the March of Dimes, New York, 66–142.

Katz, J. L., Yoon, H. S., Lipson, S., Maharidge, S., Meunier, A., and Christel, P. (1984). The effects of remodeling on the elastic properties of bone. *Calcif. Tissue Int.*, **36**: S31–S36.

Kimmel, D. B. and Jee, W. S. S. (1982). A quantitative histologic study of bone turnover in young adult beagles. *Anat. Rec.*, **203**: 31–45.

Klein-Nulend, J., Veldhuijen, J. P., Dejong, M., and Burger, E. H. (1987). Increased bone formation and decreased bone resorption in fetal mouse calvaria as a result of intermittent compressive force *in vitro*. *Bone and Mineral*, **2**: 441–448.

Kragstrup, J., Melsen, F., and Mosekide, L. (1983). Thickness of bone formed as remodeling sites in normal human iliac trabecular bone: variations with age and sex. *Metab. Bone Dis. Rel. Res.*, **5**: 17–21.

Lacroix, P. (1971). The internal remodeling of bones. In: *The Biochemistry and Physiology of Bone*, Vol. III, Bourne, G. H., Ed., Academic Press, New York, 119.

Lanyon, L. E. (1984). Functional strains as a determinant for bone remodeling. *Calcif. Tissue Int. Suppl.*, **36**: 56–61.

Lee, W. R., Marshall, J. H., and Sissons, H. A. (1965). Calcium accretion and bone formation in dogs. *J. Bone Jt. Surg.*, **47B**: 157–180.

Lips, P., Courpron, P., and Meunier, P. J. (1978). Mean wall thickness of trabecular bone packets in human iliac crest. Changes with age. *Calcif. Tissue Res.*, **26**: 13–17.

Lipson, S. F. and Katz, J. L. (1984). The relationship between elastic properties and micro-structure of bovine control bone. *J. Biomech.*, **17**: 231–240.

Marotti, G. (1976a). Map of bone formation range values recorded throughout the skeleton of the dog. In: *Bone Morphometry*, Jaworski, Z. F. G., Ed., University of Ottawa Press, Ottawa, 202.

Marotti, G. (1976b). What is the meaning of the terms primary and secondary mineralisation. In: *Bone Morphometry*, Jaworski, Z. F. G., Klosevych, S., and Cameron, E., Eds., University of Ottawa Press, Ottawa, 214.

Marotti, G. (1977). Decrement in volume of osteoblasts during osteon formation and its effect on the size of the corresponding osteocytes. In: *Bone Histomorphometry*, Meunier, P. J., Ed., Armour Montagu, Paris, 239.

Marotti, G., Favia, A., and Zallone, A. Z. (1972). Quantitative analysis on the rate of secondary mineralisation. *Calcif. Tissue Res.*, **10**: 67–81.

Marotti, G. and Muglia, M. A. (1988). A scanning electron microscopy of human bone lamellae. Proposal for a new model of collagen lamellar organisation. *Arch. Ital. Anat. Embriol.*, **93**: 163–175.

Matthews, J. L., Talmage, R. V., Martin, J. H., and Davis, W. L. (1977). Bone lining cells and the bone fluid compartment. In: *Bone Histomorphometry*, Meunier, P. J., Ed., Armour Montagu, Paris, 239.

Mohan, S., Linkhart, T., Farley, J., and Baylink, D. (1984). Bone derived factors active on bone cells. *Calcif. Tissue Int.*, **36**: S139–S145.

Mundy, G. R. (1989). Identifying mechanisms for increasing bone mass. *J. NIH Res.*, **1**: 65–68.

Parfitt, A. M. (1981). The integration of skeletal and mineral homeostasis. In: *Osteoporosis. Recent Advances in Pathogenesis and Treatment*, Deluca, H. F., Frost, H. M., Jee, W. S. S., Johnston, Jr., C. C., and Parfitt, A. M., Eds., University Park Press, Baltimore, 115–126.

Pead, M. J., Susvillo, R., Skerry, T. M., Vedis, S., and Lanyon, L. E. (1988). Increased ³H-uridine levels in osteocytes following a single short period of dynamic bone loading in vivo. *Calcif. Tissue Int.*, **43**: 92–96.

Podenphant, J. and Engel, U. (1987). Regional variations in histomorphometric bone dynamics from the skeleton of an osteoporotic woman. *Calcif. Tissue Int.*, **40**: 184–188.

Portigliatti Barbos, M., Bianco, P., Ascenzi, A., and Boyde, A. (1984). Collagen orientation in compact bone. II. Distribution of lamellae in the whole of the human femoral shaft with reference to its mechanical properties. *Metab. Bone Dis. Rel. Res.*, **5**: 309.

Reddi, A. H. (1983). Regulation of bone differentiation by local and systemic factors. In: *Bone and Mineral Research*, Vol. 3, Peck, Wm. A., Ed., Elsevier, 27–47.

Reilly, D. T. and Burnstein, A. H. (1974). The mechanical properties of cortical bone. *J. Bone Jt. Surg.*, **36A**: 1001–1002.

Rowland, R. E., Jowsey, J., and Marshall, J. H. (1959). Microscopic metabolism of calcium in bone. III. Microradiographic measurements of mineral density. *Radiat. Res.*, **10**: 234–242.

Ruth, E. B. (1953). Bone studies. II. An experimental study of the Haversian-type vascular channels. *Am. J. Anat.*, **93**: 429–456.

Smith, J. W. and Walmsley, R. (1960). Factor affecting the elasticity of bone. *J. Anat.*, **93**: 503–523.

Tappen, N. C. (1977). Three-dimensional studies of resorption spaces and developing osteons. *Am. J. Anat.*, **149**: 301–332.

Urist, M. R., DeLange, R. J., and Finerman, G. A. M. (1983). Bone cell differentiation and growth factors. *Science*, **220**: 680–686.

Vaes, G. (1988). Cellular biology and biochemical mechanism of bone resorption. *Clin. Orthop. Rel. Res.*, **231**: 239–271.

Vincent, J. (1957). Les remaniements de l'os compact marqué à l'aide de plomb. *Rev. Belge Path. Méd. Exp.*, **26**: 161–168.

Whitson, S. W. (1972). Tight junction formation in the osteon. *Clin. Orthop. Rel. Res.*, **86**: 206–213.

Wolpert, L. (1969). Positional information and the spatial pattern of cellular differentiation. *J. Theor. Biol.*, **25**: 1–47.

3

Growth Factors and Cytokines*

MICHAEL CENTRELLA, THOMAS L. McCARTHY, and ERNESTO CANALIS
Departments of Research and Medicine
Saint Francis Hospital and Medical Center
Hartford, Connecticut
  and
The University of Connecticut Health Center
Farmington, Connecticut

Introduction

Bone formation is a complex physiological event that is necessary for growth and fracture repair. During development and in the early years of

*This work was supported by National Institutes of Health Grants #AR-21707 and AR-39201 and Saint Francis Hospital and Medical Center.

47

life, bone mass increases as the organism grows. Throughout life, the bone matrix is actively metabolized or resorbed by osteoclasts and continuously replaced by the bone-forming osteoblasts. In addition, bone must regenerate following fracture; the process of fracture repair is likely to require biochemical events similar to those of *de novo* bone formation since bone healing occurs by the restoration of the original tissue, in contrast to scar formation in other connective tissues.

For most of the period of adult life, net bone mass within the body is continuously held in balance by systemic hormones, especially those that regulate blood calcium levels. However, results from numerous studies within the last several years have indicated that polypeptide growth factors also play an important, and likely a more direct, role in the activity of individual cells concerned with bone formation. More recent work further suggests an intricate interplay between the effects of systemic hormones and growth factors on bone cell function.

The purpose of this chapter is to discuss the role of growth factors and cytokines in bone formation and growth (see also Chapter 4 in Volume 1). A number of these agents are now known to be synthesized by bone cells and, accordingly, could have an autocrine or paracrine effect on bone growth. Other growth factors that have been shown to regulate bone cell activity *in vitro* are the products of blood cells. Considering both the production of many blood cell precursors in bone marrow and the infiltration of inflammatory cells into the site of trauma after fracture, blood cell-derived factors are also likely to function physiologically in bone formation or repair.

An even greater variety of growth factors have been isolated from the bone matrix; some of these matrix-derived factors are produced by bone cells and some are produced by peripheral or distant tissue and may localize to and become stored within the hydroxyapatite bone matrix. Growth factors stored within the bone matrix might be useful to signal new bone formation after their release during normal bone remodeling; furthermore, matrix-derived factors may help the process of bone repair after pathological resorption or fracture healing. The source of many of the growth factors thought to influence bone formation is summarized in Table 1.

Many growth factors have been examined for their effects on bone cell activity in organ and cell culture models. Indeed, most of the information available concerning the influence of growth factors on bone formation has been obtained from *in vitro* studies. We shall attempt to consider only those agents that appear to have well-defined and perhaps functional roles in bone formation. Where information is available, we shall address the receptors for these agents on the osteoblast and discuss the importance of each agent with regard to its effects on bone cell replication and on the production of bone cell-derived proteins. Since bone contains bone-forming cells at various stages of differentiation, we shall try to distinguish whether these factors

Table 1.

Growth Factors and Cytokines Shown to Influence Replication and/or Differentiated Cell Function in Bone and Bone Cell Cultures

Factors	Tissue Sources		
	Bone Cells	Blood Cells	Bone Matrix
TGF-β	+	+	+
IGFs	+	−	+
β₂m	+	+	+
PDGF	+	+	+
CFSs	+	+	−
TGF-α	−	+	−
ILs	−	+	−
TNFs	−	+	−
INF-γ	−	+	−
FGFs	+	−	+
BMP/OIF	−	−	+

The factors in each source are indicated by: (+), where the factor and/or mRNA has been demonstrated, or (−), where the factor has not been detected when examined for or has not yet been reported.

produce discrete effects within individual bone cell populations. Finally, very recent work has attempted to define a role for systemic hormones as modifiers of local growth factor activity; we shall try to place these studies into perspective with the observed influence of the local and systemic factor on bone cell function.

Growth Factors and Cytokines Produced by Bone Cells

Transforming Growth Factor Beta (TGF-β)

TGF-β was first detected in tumor and fetal tissue extracts and was thought initially to regulate neoplastic and embryonic tissue growth. Peripheral blood platelets were then shown to contain large amounts of TGF-β, suggesting that this agent might have a physiological function in wound healing (Sporn et al., 1987). TGF-β-like activity was subsequently detected in culture medium conditioned by fetal rat bone explants (Centrella and Canalis, 1985), and purification of this material revealed that it accounted for the bone-derived growth factor (BDGF) initially termed BDGF-I (Centrella and Canalis, 1987a). Bone cells have abundant levels of TGF-β mRNA (Gehron Robey et al., 1987; McCarthy et al., 1989a) and the amount of TGF-β in bone culture medium is about tenfold greater than that found in virus-transformed cell cultures (Centrella and Canalis, 1987a; Massague, 1984). Large amounts of TGF-β are also found in the extracellular bone matrix, constituting the largest reservoir of this growth factor in the intact organism (reviewed in Centrella *et al.*, 1988d). Consequently, TGF-β is likely to be important in regulating bone cell function.

To examine the role of TGF-β on tissue function, most studies have utilized platelet-derived TGF-β (human platelets contain a single form of TGF-β, composed of two identical polypeptides constituting a dimer of relative molecular mass (M_r) 25,000). Like a number of secreted proteins, TGF-β is synthesized in precursor form that requires proteolytic processing. It is released from the cell in an inactive high molecular weight complex composed of the processed dimer in combination with amino terminal fragments of each of the two TGF-β monomeric precursors and a third uncharacterized molecule. The physiological mechanism by which TGF-β is released from the inactive complex is uncertain, but may require specific enzyme activation (Sporn *et al.*, 1987; Miyazono *et al.*, 1988).

Platelet and bone-derived TGF-β have analogous stimulatory effects on DNA and collagen synthesis in cultured fetal rat calvariae (Centrella *et al.*, 1986), and histological evidence demonstrates that TGF-β increases nuclear ^{3}H-thymidine labeling in the osteoblast precursor cell zone (Hock *et al.*, 1988a). Studies with isolated bone cells show that TGF-β is a potent regulator of osteoblastic cell activity, and on a molar basis TGF-β is one of the most effective mitogens so far described for osteoblast-enriched cultures from fetal bone (Centrella *et al.*, 1987b, c). The mitotic response to TGF-β is biphasic: low concentrations (below 100 pM) are stimulatory, whereas higher levels produce less of a stimulatory effect. At higher, less mitogenic concentrations, TGF-β alters expression of various activities associated with the osteoblast phenotype in different ways; under these conditions TGF-β decreases alkaline phosphatase activity and, similar to its effects in a number of other connective tissue systems, enhances the synthesis of type I collagen, the major organic element in the bone matrix (Centrella *et al.*, 1987b; Rosen *et al.*, 1988). The metabolic effects of TGF-β may be somewhat more complex in adult bone and, unlike its effect in primary fetal bone cell cultures, TGF-β does not appear to enhance replication in certain osteoblast-like and osteosarcoma cell cultures, which presumably represent cells at later stages of differentiation. However, in osteosarcoma cultures, TGF-β enhances type I collagen synthesis, as well as the production of a variety of bone matrix-associated polypeptides such as osteonectin, osteopontin, and alkaline phosphatase (Noda and Rodan, 1986, 1987; Pfeilschifter *et al.*, 1987; Noda *et al.*, 1988), but decreases osteocalcin synthesis (Noda, 1989). These findings indicate that TGF-β enhances bone matrix accumulation and consequently the maintenance of bone mass. In general, the stimulatory influence of TGF-β on bone matrix protein synthesis may be attributed to effects at the transcriptional level (Centrella *et al.*, 1987b; Noda and Rodan, 1987; Rosen *et al.*, 1988; Rossi *et al.*, 1988). However, a direct relationship between the influence of TGF-β on type I collagen mRNA and polypeptide levels is not observed in isolated bone cells, suggesting that TGF-β has an additional supportive role in increasing bone matrix formation (Centrella *et al.*, 1987b).

Initial studies in neonatal mouse calvariae indicated that TGF-β enhanced bone resorption and that this effect was dependent on an increase in prostaglandin synthesis (Tashjian *et al.*, 1985). Subsequent studies in alternate *in vitro* models of bone resorption now suggest that this result is not universal. In fetal rat long bones, TGF-β decreases bone resorption (Pfeilschifter *et al.*, 1988), and this effect may be related to the ability of TGF-β to inhibit the formation of osteoclast-like cells *in vitro* (Chenu *et al.*, 1988). This difference may be a significant distinction in bone growth and development between the fetus and the newborn; within very early stages of bone formation, matrix formation may be more important to the organism than bone remodeling. These latter studies therefore suggest an additional, indirect role for TGF-β in increasing or maintaining net bone mass.

Similar to receptors on a variety of mammalian mesenchymal tissue-derived cells, TGF-β ligand/receptor complexes on fetal rat bone cells appear at M_r 65,000, 85,000, and >200,000 when analyzed by polyacrylamide gel electrophoresis. The affinity of each of these receptors for TGF-β varies between high and low affinity; consequently, binding to only one or a particular subset of these receptors may be responsible for each of the distinct biochemical effects induced by this growth factor (Centrella *et al.*, 1988a), but no studies are yet available to address this question.

Agents such as parathyroid hormone (PTH), interleukin-1 (IL-1), and 1,25-dihydroxyvitamin D_3 (1,25OH$_2$D$_3$) that induce bone resorption also increase TGF-β levels in bone explant culture medium (Pfeilschifter and Mundy, 1987). PTH does not appear to enhance TGF-β mRNA levels in osteoblast-enriched cultures (McCarthy *et al.*, 1989a), and the increase noted in organ culture medium therefore probably results from matrix release. Studies with cloned osteosarcoma or bone-derived cell cultures indicate that 1,25OH$_2$D$_3$ and estradiol can each augment TGF-β levels in the culture medium (Petkovich *et al.*, 1987; Komm *et al.*, 1988). In osteoblast-enriched cultures from fetal rat bone, PTH attenuates the biochemical effects of TGF-β on DNA and collagen synthesis and on alkaline phosphatase activity. These findings may be related to the additional observation that PTH alters TGF-β binding, an effect which occurs primarily at low affinity receptor sites (Centrella *et al.*, 1988a). In total, these studies indicate that TGF-β activity, at least in bone, can be regulated by systemic hormones and growth factors and suggest that certain osteotropic hormones may function in part by regulating the local activity of this important bone growth factor.

Molecules with varying degrees of sequence homology to human platelet TGF-β can be found in a variety of tissues. Of these, several have been isolated from bone matrix and will be discussed later in this chapter.

Insulin-Like Growth Factors (IGF I and IGF II)

IGF I was originally determined as an insulin-like serum component that could not be suppressed by anti-insulin antibody preparations, and later studies revealed that it was the homologue of the sulfation-inducing factor termed somatomedin C. Early work revealed that serum levels of IGF I varied directly with those of growth hormone (GH), that GH enhanced production of IGF I by the liver, and suggested that liver-derived IGF I was likely to be the direct mediator of the potent anabolic effect of GH on longitudinal bone growth (Froesch et al., 1985; Isaksson et al., 1987). Initial studies on bone cultures indicated the presence of immunoreactive somatomedin C in culture medium conditioned by intact fetal rat bone explants (Canalis et al., 1980). More recently, results from several laboratories now demonstrate that osteoblast-enriched cultures contain IGF I polypeptide and IGF I mRNA (Ernst and Froesch, 1988; McCarthy et al., 1989a); locally produced IGF I may therefore have a more immediate and direct role than liver-derived IGF I in regulating bone formation.

IGF I is a single-chain polypeptide of M_r 7,500; it has about 40% sequence homology to insulin and about 60% homology to IGF II (discussed below); a variety of other polypeptides with IGF I-like sequences may also occur, but IGF I and IGF II are the most well characterized (Froesch et al., 1985). In intact bone explant cultures, IGF I enhances both cell replication and type I collagen synthesis. Histological studies reveal that the mitogenic effect of IGF I is primarily in a periosteal pre-osteoblastic zone of cells within the tissue, indicating that it enhances production of a cell pool that may be necessary for persistent bone growth. In contrast, the stimulatory effect of IGF I on type I collagen production is coincident with an increase in bone matrix apposition (this effect occurs primarily in the endosteum) and is partially independent of the stimulatory influence of IGF I on cell replication (Hock et al., 1988b). On the molecular level, IGF I enhances the amount of type I collagen mRNA in osteoblast-enriched cultures from fetal rat bone. In addition to its ability to stimulate collagen synthesis directly, IGF I decreases the rate of collagen degradation in intact bone organ cultures (McCarthy et al., 1989b), thereby indirectly enhancing type I collagen accumulation.

Osteoblast-enriched cultures contain a complex pattern of receptors for IGF I; ligand/receptor complexes can be distinguished at M_r 260,000, 240,000, and 130,000. Binding of radioactive IGF I at all sites can be displaced by unlabeled IGF I, whereas insulin displacement occurs essentially at M_r 260,000 and 130,000. IGF II displaces IGF I binding with high affinity at the M_r 240,000 receptor and with lesser affinity at the other two sites; antibody blocking studies indicate that the M_r 240,000 site is the primary IGF II receptor (Centrella et al., 1990).

At least two IGF-binding proteins have been detected in bone culture medium (Canalis et al., 1989a), and they may be similar to some of those reported in serum (Baxter and Martin, 1989). The function of these molecules in serum or in bone cultures is unknown; they may have a protective role to guard IGF I from protease activity, they may regulate its biological activity, or they help to deliver IGF I to its target cell.

As with its effect in the liver, GH has now been shown to enhance IGF I production by bone cells (Ernst and Froesch, 1988; McCarthy et al., 1989b); this suggests an even more direct influence by GH on bone formation and further demonstrates that systemic factors may modify local growth factor activity within bone. Furthermore, in addition to the better known effects of PTH on bone resorption, this hormone also enhances bone formation in vivo and in vitro. While the mechanism by which this occurs has long been unclear, it may in part be linked to changes in local IGF I activity. Recent studies indicate that PTH increases IGF I mRNA and polypeptide production in osteoblast-enriched cultures and that anti-IGF I antibody blocks the increase in collagen synthesis induced by pulsatile treatment of intact bone cultures with PTH (McCarthy et al., 1989a; Canalis et al., 1989b).

One of the factors described in some early studies suggesting the presence of local bone growth regulators was an agent termed skeletal growth factor (SGF). It is now apparent that many of the initial preparations that exhibited bone growth promoting activity contained multiple stimulatory agents. Nevertheless, recent studies propose that the active material in SGF preparations was IGF II, and IGF II has been independently isolated from bone matrix (Mohan et al., 1988; Frolik et al., 1988). As indicated above, IGF II is similar in amino acid sequence to IGF I. Like IGF I, IGF II enhances cell replication and collagen synthesis and decreases collagen turnover in intact bone organ cultures, but approximately sevenfold more IGF II is needed to produce similar results. In contrast, while the meaning of this finding is unclear, Northern blot studies indicate that IGF II is somewhat more effective than IGF I at enhancing type I collagen mRNA in osteoblast-enriched cultures (McCarthy et al., 1989b; Canalis et al., 1989a). This may in part relate to the observation that IGF I and IGF II preferentially bind to their own cognate receptors, and each biochemical effect may be induced to various degrees by the level of specific receptor occupancy. More work is therefore necessary to determine whether the effects of IGF I and IGF II are mediated at single or multiple receptor sites.

Beta$_2$ Microglobulin (β_2m)

Initial studies with culture medium conditioned by intact bone explants revealed at least three stimulatory activities for secondary bone cultures (Canalis et al., 1980). Further characterization showed that two of these could be accounted for by TGF-β and IGF-I, as described earlier. Amino acid sequence studies indicated that the third element, first termed BDGF II, is the rat homologue of β_2m, a polypeptide of M_r 11,800 that is a component of the cell surface major histocompatibility (HLA) complex in man (Canalis et al., 1987). In addition to its expression on the surface of lymphocytes and its presumed structural role within the HLA complex, β_2m has been shown to regulate mitogen-induced replication in lymphocyte and reticuloendothelial cell cultures and to be over- or under-expressed in several pathological conditions (Messner, 1984; Gorevic *et al.*, 1986), but its physiological function remains unclear.

In rat bone organ and cell cultures, both rat and human β_2m enhance DNA and collagen synthesis, although the mechanism by which this occurs is not certain (Canalis and Centrella, 1986; Canalis *et al.*, 1987a). Since β_2m does not appear to bind directly to a cognate receptor, its effects are likely to be indirect and may involve other local growth regulators in bone. Studies with anti-HLA antibodies in lymphocyte and monocyte cultures demonstrate that β_2m associates noncovalently with the insulin receptor and thereby may change the ability of insulin to recognize its own receptor and produce its biological effects (Due *et al.*, 1986). Given the structural homology between the insulin and the IGF I receptor complexes (Goldfine, 1987), β_2m could also regulate local IGF I binding and function in bone tissue. β_2m enhances IGF I binding in rat bone cell cultures and appears to shift interactions among various ligand binding sites. Therefore, part of the effect of β_2m may result from changes in the relative level of occupancy at the IGF I and IGF II receptors. Furthermore, β_2m enhances IGF I mRNA and polypeptide levels in osteoblast-enriched cultures, suggesting multiple levels of biological activity (Centrella *et al.*, 1989a). More recent studies have further shown that β_2m, or a closely related protein, isolated from synovial cell culture medium, increases collagenase activity in fibroblast cultures (Brinckerhoff *et al.*, 1989), suggesting a diverse function for this protein in bone physiology.

Very little is known about the regulation of β_2m synthesis. Among a large variety of osteotropic hormones and growth factors that have been examined, only β_2m itself appears to increase β_2m transcript levels appreciably in osteoblast-enriched cultures (T.L. McCarthy, unpublished results). The meaning of auto-stimulation, and the limitations that must eventually be imposed on such an effect, are presently uncertain. In rabbit synovial cell cultures, β_2m synthesis is stimulated by the tumor promoter phorbol myristate acetate (Brinckerhoff *et al.*, 1989), suggesting involvement of protein kinase C activation (Nishizuka, 1984). Further studies are needed to resolve the enigma of β_2m within bone and to determine whether it has a physiological function in normal bone remodeling.

Platelet-Derived Growth Factor (PDGF)

PDGF was initially described as a growth-promoting factor in serum-supplemented cell culture medium and later was identified as the product of blood platelets. Human PDGF, of M_r 28,000 to 31,000 (due to differences in glycosylation), contains two polypeptide chains designated as A and B. PDGF may exist in the organism as a heterodimer (PDGF-AB), homodimers of PDGF-AA or PDGF-BB chains, or some combination of the three; several normal and neoplastic cell lines appear to express only the PDGF-A chain or the PDGF-B chain (Deuel, 1987). Expression of either PDGF-A or PDGF-B chain transcripts and/or polypeptides has been reported in osteosarcoma cultures (Graves *et al.*, 1984; Heldin *et al.*, 1986), whereas culture medium conditioned by primary tissue explants of fetal rat bones contains undetectable levels of PDGF (Centrella and Canalis, 1985). PDGF production by bone cells may therefore be limited to a particular and highly differentiated cell population or may require the influence of a stimulatory agent absent in fetal bone cultures; alternately, PDGF synthesis by osteosarcoma cells may be related to the induction or maintenance of the neoplastic state.

Highly purified recombinant PDGF-BB enhances cell replication in intact calvariae; however, similar studies in cell cultures isolated from fetal rat parietal bone indicate that the effects are not specific to an osteoblastic cell population. PDGF may therefore increase replication by cells at both earlier and later stages of differentiation within bone, and this may be important to provide an immediate and generalized healing response in fracture repair. The mitotic response to PDGF by cells within osteoblast-enriched cultures occurs in the absence of other growth promoters. This is in contrast to results reported for rodent fibroblasts, in which the stimulatory effects of PDGF and IGF I on cell replication are interdependent (Pledger *et al.*, 1978). PDGF also enhances collagen synthesis in bone and bone cell cultures, and this effect is essentially contingent on an increase in cell replication (Canalis *et al.*, 1989c; Centrella *et al.*, 1989b). When all three PDGF isoforms have been examined directly in the same trial, PDGF-BB is the most stimulatory in osteoblast-enriched cultures from fetal rat bone (M. Centrella, unpublished results).

In addition to its growth-promoting influence in bone cultures, PDGF stimulates resorption in neonatal mouse calvariae, and this increase is blocked by inhibitors of cyclo-oxygenase activity which prevent *de novo* prostaglandin production (Tashjian *et al.*, 1982). Since there is no clear evidence to indicate that PDGF has a direct effect on the osteoclast, the increase in bone resorption likely occurs by way of some other cellular intermediate(s) in bone. Other agents (described later in this chapter) that induce resorption appear to require the presence of osteoblasts, or some osteoblast-derived factor, in agreement with the hypothesis proposed by Rodan and Martin (1981). While prostaglandin synthesis appears necessary for increased resorption in mouse calvariae, an additional intermediary also must be involved, since prostaglandins do not directly stimulate the osteoclast (Chambers *et al.*, 1985); the precise nature of this second intermediary is still uncertain and may not be the same in all situations.

Two distinct types of cell surface PDGF receptors have been reported on fibroblasts; the first type binds all three isoforms of PDGF, whereas the second is slightly greater in M_r and has a much higher affinity for PDGF-BB and PDGF-AB than for PDGF-AA (Heldin *et al.*, 1988; Hart et al., 1988). In contrast, osteoblast-enriched cultures appear to contain only a single class of receptors for PDGF-BB (Centrella *et al.*, 1989b). Further studies are necessary to determine whether these cultures also contain a distinct and non-cross-reactive receptor that binds PDGF-A chains.

Regulation of PDGF synthesis by bone cells has not been reported, whereas studies in mouse embryo-derived fibroblasts indicate that TGF-β enhances the transcript (c-*sis*) levels for the PDGF-B chain (Leof *et al.*, 1986). Since fetal rat bone culture medium contains high levels of TGF-β, but undetectable levels of PDGF, regulation of its production by bone cells is likely to be somewhat more complex than in fibroblast cultures.

Colony Stimulating Factors (CSFs)

The CSFs are polypeptide factors that are either necessary or responsible for blood cell precursor activation and replication. They were first identified as the products of activated lymphocytes or monocytes and by their general or specific roles in regulating hematopoiesis. The nomenclature for these agents can be accounted for in part by an apparent hierarchy in CSF activity. For instance, the number of differentiated blood cells ultimately influenced by multi-CSF (IL-3) is larger than that by granulocyte-macrophage CSF (GM-CSF), which itself is larger than that for either granulocyte CSF (G-CSF) or macrophage CSF (M-CSF) (Dinarello and Mier, 1987; Nathan, 1987; Sieff, 1987). Primary and osteosarcoma-derived bone cell cultures appear capable of synthesizing some of the CSFs. Bone cell CSF production is not detectable unless it is induced by agents such as PTH, which increase bone resorption, or bacterial products such as lipopolysaccharides (LPS), which are involved in the inflammatory process. Of the CSFs that have been examined, none has been reported to have potent or reproducible direct effects on nonneoplastic bone-forming cells. Therefore, CSF production in bone may represent a complementary relationship between the osteological and hematological systems, in which cells within each of these tissue systems may produce factors that support the growth or activity of cells within the other. Part of this restriction between bone and blood may be related to the lack of expression of appropriate receptors for the reciprocally exclusive factors in each tissue compartment.

Communication between these two tissue compartments may be complex. For example, the blood cell population could be augmented by bone cell-derived CSFs, and the larger pool size of blood cells could then provide an increased supply of blood cell-derived factors that directly influences osteoblastic cell activity and bone formation. Alternately, since the osteoclast is thought to derive from a common progenitor cell that also supplies myeloid blood cells, the CSFs produced by bone cells could increase the level of bone-resorbing osteoclasts; therefore, the CSFs could enhance osteoclast development and in this way limit bone formation. Consequently, the CSFs may have multiple profound but indirect effects on bone growth and repair.

The CSFs thought to regulate osteoclast precursor development include M-CSF (also termed CSF-1; M_r 70,000), GM-CSF (M_r 22,000), and multi-CSF (IL-3; M_r 20,000–26,000). In general, they are relatively small glycoproteins; different levels of glycosylation and oligomerization are likely to account for some of the size disparities reported in the early descriptions of these agents (Sieff, 1987). The CSFs have a limited through broad host range on myelopoiesis, but all appear functional in osteoclast development (MacDonald et al., 1986; Lorenzo et al., 1987). This suggests that the progenitor cell for the osteoclast is likely to be one at a fairly primitive stage within blood cell ontogeny. Also, each of these CSFs has been demonstrated, although to varying degrees, in bone or bone cell culture medium after appropriate stimulation. In primary or clonal osteoblast-like cell cultures, the principal and therefore perhaps the most important CSF induced by PTH or LPS is GM-CSF, or a very closely related factor. This is based both on biological evidence using responder cell cultures with restricted abilities to respond to specific lymphokines and monokines and on neutralization studies with anti-GM-CSF antibody (Felix et al., 1988; Horowitz et al., 1989; Weir et al., 1989). Similarly, the bone resorption stimulators IL-1 and tumor necrosis factor-α (TNF-α) enhance M-CSF production by clonal osteoblast-like cell cultures (Felix et al., 1989).

The effects of the CSFs appear to be limited to an early stage in osteoclast precursor differentiation since they require other agents, such as $1,25OH_2D_3$, to induce osteoclast multinucleation and do not themselves increase bone resorption (MacDonald et al., 1986; Lorenzo et al., 1987). Therefore, like the bone-resorbing agents known to induce CSF production, the CSFs themselves are not directly responsible for resorption, and a second intermediary still remains to be identified.

As described earlier, there is yet no strong evidence for a direct effect of the CSFs on osteoblastic cells, although a recent study has shown that GM-CSF increases proliferation in some human osteosarcoma cultures (Dedhar et al., 1988). Consequently, bone cell receptors for these agents have not yet been described, nor have the interacting effects of the CSFs with other bone growth regulators. However, GM-CSF has been reported to increase endothelial cell proliferation and activity, suggesting a direct positive effect on neovascularization (Bussolino et al., 1989). By increasing the blood supply to the fracture site, GM-CSF may potentiate nutrient, growth factor, and oxygen supply to the damaged tissue and indirectly enhance bone repair. The complex role this agent may have in both osteoclastic bone resorption and, indirectly, in bone formation is an example of the fine control that must exist between the interacting effects of multiple growth regulators at different sites and on different biological processes within bone. Nevertheless, further work remains to establish a definite direct role for the CSFs in bone formation.

Growth Factors and Cytokines Produced by Hematological Cells

Platelet-Derived Factors

In addition to TGF-β and PDGF, platelet extracts contain a protein that competes for receptor binding and produces biological effects identical to mouse submaxillary gland-derived epidermal growth factor (EGF; Assoian *et al.*, 1984). Earlier studies suggested that analogous EGF-like material isolated from tumors might be responsible for inducing or maintaining the transformed (that is, the neoplastic) cell state (Keski-Oja *et al.*, 1987), and this agent was initially termed TGF alpha (TGF-α). The importance of TGF-β and PDGF on bone formation has been described earlier in this chapter and consequently will not be considered further here. Unlike TGF-β and PDGF, TGF-α is not detected in culture medium from primary rat bone cultures (Centrella and Canalis, 1985) or in bone matrix extracts (M. Centrella, unpublished results). Therefore, it is unlikely that TGF-α has a primary local function in normal bone growth or *de novo* bone formation; nevertheless, its release from platelets at the fracture site may have a significant impact on bone repair or remodeling. TGF-α is also produced by activated macrophages (Madtes *et al.*, 1988), and alterations in the integrity of bone tissue at inflammation sites may be associated with release of TGF-α (among other factors) during infection or trauma. Furthermore, a number of tumors associated with the paraneoplastic syndrome of hypercalcemia produce TGF-α or closely related factors, and these agents may contribute to the biochemical abnormalities connected with this disease (Mundy, 1988). While there is no physiological evidence to support a role for submaxillary gland-derived EGF on bone formation, *in vitro* studies with EGF have provided results analogous to those with TGF-α and are likely to predict the function of platelet- or macrophage-derived TGF-α in bone.

TGF-α is a polypeptide of M_r 5,600 with approximately 35% amino acid sequence homology to EGF (Carpenter and Zendegui, 1986). Both factors stimulate DNA synthesis in cloned osteoblast-like cells and in primary cultures of intact bone and osteoblast-enriched fetal rat bone cells (Canalis and Raisz, 1979; Centrella *et al.*, 1987c, Lorenzo *et al.*, 1988). These findings are clearly not osteoblast specific since effects of similar magnitude occur in fibroblast, osteoblast-poor, and osteoblast-enriched cell cultures from rat fetuses (Centrella and Canalis, 1985; Centrella *et al.*, 1987c). Both factors also inhibit bone collagen synthesis and alkaline phosphatase activity (Canalis and Raisz, 1979; Ibbotson *et al.*, 1986), and these effects predict a decrease in new bone matrix formation.

In addition to their influence on macromolecular synthesis, TGF-α and EGF enhance bone resorption in fetal rat long bone and neonatal mouse calvariae (Raisz *et al.*, 1980; Stern *et al.*, 1985; Tashjian *et al.*, 1985, 1986; Ibbotson *et al.*, 1986). In mouse calvariae, both factors increase prostaglandin synthesis, and agents that inhibit prostaglandin production mitigate their stimulatory effect on bone resorption (Tashjian et al., 1986). In contrast, in fetal rat long bone, the influence of TGF-α or EGF on resorption is prostaglandin independent (Lorenzo et al., 1988). Continual bone resorption induced by constitutive production of TGF-α by a variety of tumors may contribute, at least in part, to the malignancy-associated hypercalcemic state. The mechanisms by which TGF-α or EGF induce resorption are not known with certainty; however, more recent studies indicate that these factors directly enhance osteoclast precursor development and that this effect is inhibited by TGF-β (Chenu et al., 1988).

TGF-α/EGF receptors have been detected in primary osteoblast-enriched and cloned osteosarcoma cell cultures (Ng et al., 1983); cross-linking and autoradiographic studies have demonstrated a receptor-ligand complex of M_r 175,000 (M. Centrella, unpublished results), similar to that found in a large number of cells and tissues (Carpenter and Zendegui, 1986). Very short term in vivo labeling studies with radioactive EGF suggest that the bone cells with high affinity binding sites for EGF are neither fully differentiated osteoblasts nor osteoclasts. Morphologically, these EGF-binding (and therefore likely EGF-responsive) cells appear to be earlier or perhaps precursor cells within both cell lineages (Martineau-Doize et al., 1988). Further studies may be necessary in order to determine if more differentiated bone cells retain fewer or have lower affinity receptors, which may still permit a functional biological response to EGF/TGF-α.

Although TGF-α does not appear to be synthesized by bone cells, or to accumulate in the bone matrix, it may be produced within bone in pathological conditions (such as osteosarcoma) or under the influence of other growth regulators. However, except for TGF-α production by activated macrophages, no other information is yet available to indicate the control of its synthesis or its release by integral cells within bone.

The Interleukins (ILs)

A large number of monocyte- and lymphocyte-derived proteins are known to regulate a complex interchange of information among the variety of cell types involved in the immunological response. Of these, we have previously addressed the CSFs, which appear to be synthesized by bone cells as well as by hematological cells. Also within this group are the interleukins, and among this family of growth regulators, only IL-1 appears to induce important direct effects on bone-forming cell activity.

IL-1 is a polypeptide of M_r 17,000 to 18,000 and is produced by mitogen- or antigen-activated monocytes, although it can also be synthesized by cells from a large variety of tissues. In general, IL-1 production is nearly always associated with inflammation, trauma, or an acute-phase response. Early studies indicated an essential role for IL-1 in T lymphocyte activation (therefore its initial descriptive designation as lymphocyte activating factor, or LAF activity). There are two isoforms of IL-1 (IL-1α and IL-1β) which differ in isoelectric point, but have identical biological function and appear to bind the same high affinity receptor on target cells (Dower *et al.*, 1986).

IL-1 enhances DNA synthesis in cultures of intact bone and in isolated osteoblast-enriched or osteoblast-like cells (Canalis, 1986; Lorenzo *et al.*, 1988). At low concentrations IL-1 also increases type I collagen synthesis in bone cultures, but higher concentrations or sustained exposure to IL-1 inhibits collagen production (Canalis, 1986). The decrease in collagen synthesis may in part be related to a stimulatory effect on collagenase activity, as recently demonstrated with cartilage cells (Stephenson *et al.*, 1987) and osteoblast-enriched primary bone cell cultures (Shen *et al.*, 1988). Some of the effects of IL-1 on macromolecular synthesis may be associated with an increase in prostaglandin production; for example, prostaglandin synthesis inhibitors block the acute effect of IL-1 on collagen production, but do not influence DNA synthesis (Canalis, 1986).

Bone resorption is enhanced by IL-1, but the mechanism by which this occurs is unclear, and similar to a number of other bone-resorbing agents described in this chapter, IL-1 has no direct effects on the osteoclast (Thomson *et al.*, 1986). Part of the signal for resorption may be related to the synergistic effect between IL-1 and TGF-α on prostaglandin production, which has been demonstrated in intact bone and isolated bone cell cultures (Lorenzo *et al.*, 1988). However, prostaglandin itself cannot be wholly responsible since, as mentioned earlier, it does not appear to stimulate osteoclast activity (Chambers *et al.*, 1985).

The bone cell receptor for IL-1 has not been fully characterized, and more work remains to clarify the role of this agent in bone remodeling.

Tumor Necrosis Factors (TNF-α and TNF-β)

TNF-α is an M_r 17,000 polypeptide produced by activated mononuclear phagocytes, and experimental evidence indicates that it may be the agent responsible for hemorrhagic necrosis and tissue degeneration seen in certain chronic infections, neoplastic diseases, or endotoxin-induced shock (Old, 1985; Beutler and Cerami, 1986). TNF-α also regulates cell replication and the expression of differentiated cell function in a number of nonneoplastic tissue systems, and its effects can be modulated by other growth regulators (Peetre *et al.*, 1986; Kronke *et al.*, 1987; Sugarman *et al.*, 1987). Similar to the situation with many blood cell-derived factors, cells that produce TNF-α can accumulate in bone during inflammation, trauma, or metabolic disease. In these pathophysiological situations, several of these agents may impinge on the normally orderly processes of bone growth, remodeling, or repair. In intact bone organ cultures, short term exposure to TNF-α increases the number of cells that produce type I collagen; however, sustained treatment with TNF-α decreases collagen synthesis and alkaline phosphatase activity and enhances the rate of collagen degradation (Canalis, 1987; Smith et al., 1987). In osteoblast-enriched bone cell cultures, TNF-α also has a small but significant stimulatory effect on cell replication and decreases alkaline phosphatase activity and type I collagen synthesis (Centrella et al., 1988c). The mitogenic effect of TNF-α is additive to that of submaximal TGF-β levels in osteoblast-enriched cultures. Nevertheless, at maximal TGF-β concentrations, TNF-α inhibits TGF-β-induced DNA synthesis (Centrella et al., 1987c). The inhibitory effect of TNF-α on collagen polypeptide production does not appear to correlate with the total level of type I collagen mRNA transcripts, as determined by slot blot analysis (Centrella et al., 1988c). Changes in mRNA processing may account for this dichotomy, but this has not yet been determined.

In intact fetal rat bone cultures, TNF-α increases bone resorption and enhances collagenolysis (Bertolini et al., 1986; Canalis, 1987). In contrast to its effect in intact bone, TNF-α does not modify collagen turnover in osteoblast-enriched cultures (Centrella et al., 1988c). This suggests that the increase in collagen turnover noted in intact bone cultures may be due to an increase in proteolytic activity within a non-osteoblastic cell population or that additional conditions, such as the presence of a calcified matrix, may be required to observe TNF-α-induced tissue wasting within bone.

In addition to its direct effects on bone cells, TNF-α, like GM-CSF, potentiates angiogenesis (Leibovich et al., 1987). Again, it is uncertain whether this apparently beneficial aspect of TNF-α activity is coincident with or subjugated to its anti-anabolic and catabolic effects in bone. All may be necessary, at discrete times, to provide a concerted response for proper bone remodeling during fracture repair.

TNF-β (also termed lymphotoxin; M_r 18,600) is a product of activated lymphocytes, has approximately 30% amino acid sequence homology to TNF-α, and is likely related to TNF-α by a primitive tandem gene duplication. The genes for TNF-α and TNF-β are proximally located on the same chromosome in man, and their expression may be coordinately regulated (Beutler and Cerami, 1986). TNF-β also has cytotoxic effects for neoplastic cells, and its biological effects in bone appear identical to those of TNF-α. For example, TNF-β inhibits collagen synthesis and stimulates DNA synthesis in calvarial cultures, and it enhances bone resorption (Bertolini et al., 1986; Smith et al., 1987).

The receptor(s) for TNF-α and TNF-β have not yet been described in bone cultures. Except for the interacting effects of TNF with TGF-β (described above) or with interferon gamma (described below), little else is known about either the direct or indirect influence of these agents on bone formation.

Interferon Gamma (INF-γ)

The last of the hematological cell-derived growth regulators that will be addressed in this chapter is INF-γ. The INFs were initially described in the supernatants of cells infected with particular viruses and were so named based on their ability to interfere with or prevent the spread of infection within the culture. This terminology now also encompasses factors that can be induced by inflammation-related prokaryotic products, such as bacterial cell wall-derived LPS. Of the INFs, the only member with marked effects on bone cells appears to be INF-γ (M_r 34,000), which appears to be produced exclusively by activated T lymphocytes. The cascade of events in INF-γ induction is thought to proceed from LPS induction of IL-1 and IL-2, to IL-1 induction of IL-2 receptors on appropriate T cells, through IL-2 induction of INF-γ (Morrison and Ryan, 1987).

In contrast to the mitogenic effects of the other inflammation-related cytokines, IL-1 and the TNFs, INF-γ inhibits DNA synthesis in intact bone cultures; however, like IL-1 and the TNFs, INF-γ inhibits collagen synthesis and amplifies the inhibitory effects of the TNFs on this process (Smith *et al.*, 1987). These results suggest a direct inhibitory effect by INF-γ on osteoblasts, reminiscent of those in lymphocyte cultures, where the INF-γ can have potent anti-proliferative and immunosuppressive activity (Dinarello and Mier, 1987). In further contrast to IL-1 and the TNFs, which induce bone resorption *in vitro*, INF-γ inhibits osteoclastic activity induced by these agents (Gowen and Mundy, 1986).

The receptor for INF-γ on the osteoblast has not been reported, and further work remains to determine if INF-γ modifies the effects of other bone growth regulators. Nevertheless, since INF-γ appears to be produced only under very limited conditions, its role in normal bone physiology is probably minimal.

Bone Matrix-Derived Growth Factors

Growth factors derived from the bone matrix have attracted considerable attention in the last several years since, on the basis of tissue mass, bone is likely to be the largest reservoir of growth factor activity in the organism. Some of the matrix-derived factors have been characterized by their biochemical or biophysical relationship to well-described factors from other tissues (Hauschka *et al.*, 1986) or to factors found in culture medium conditioned by bone explants (Canalis *et al.*, 1988b). It is still unclear how these agents are released from the matrix and made available in a biologically active form to bone cells, and there is no evidence to indicate that bone-derived factors function in other peripheral tissues. Nevertheless, the abundance of these molecules in the bone matrix has strengthened the notion that they play an important regulatory role in increasing or maintaining bone mass. Of the factors well established to be found in bone matrix, we have already addressed TGF-β, IGF I and IGF II, β₂m, and PDGF. In addition, it appears that bone also stores several other molecules which produce potent effects on bone cells *in vitro*.

Fibroblast Growth Factors (FGFs)

FGFs were originally isolated from neural tissue extracts, but have since been detected in a large number of normal and neoplastic tissues. There are two well-characterized classes of FGF that can be distinguished based on isoelectric point differences. The prototype of the proteins within the anionic class is termed acidic FGF (aFGF) and is now known to be a processed form of endothelial cell growth factor (ECGF). Members of the cationic or basic class of FGFs (bFGF) seem to have a broader tissue distribution and also to be proteolytically processed variations of a single primary translation product distinct from that for aFGF. aFGF and bFGF each have M_r of approximately 17,000 and share 55% sequence homology; they are encoded on different chromosomes in the human genome and are likely to have evolved from a primitive gene duplication and translocation. Both classes of FGFs produce analogous biochemical and biological effects and associate with similar cell surface receptors. Quantitative differences between these agents may perhaps be accounted for by differential affinities of each factor for particular cognate receptors (Gospodarowicz *et al.*, 1986; Folkman and Klagsbrun, 1987).

The FGFs or FGF-like proteins have been reported in bone matrix extracts (Hauschka *et al.*, 1986), and a recent study suggests that cultured bone cells may produce FGFs and store these factors in their extracellular matrix (Globus *et al.*, 1989). The latter studies were performed with serially passaged bovine bone cells cultured in medium supplemented with relatively high serum concentrations. Consequently, although it is likely that the extracellular matrix in bone, much like that in other tissues, stores FGFs (Gospodarowicz *et al.*, 1986), autologous FGF production by primary bone cells in the absence of external stimulation has not yet been demonstrated.

aFGF and bFGF each enhance DNA synthesis in intact calvariae (Canalis *et al.*, 1987b; Canalis *et al.*, 1988a) and in cell cultures prepared from fetal rat (Centrella *et al.*, 1987c; McCarthy *et al.*, 1989b; Rodan *et al.*, 1987) and bovine bone (Globus *et al.*, 1988). Mitotic responses are detected in both the endosteum and periosteum and in osteoblast- and fibroblast-enriched bone cell cultures. In fetal rat bone cells, the FGFs have a relatively greater influence in the fibroblast-enriched cell population, and on a molar basis, bFGF is more potent than aFGF (McCarthy *et al.*, 1989b). Some of these studies were performed with either low (Rodan *et al.*, 1987) or relatively high (Globus *et al.*, 1988) serum concentrations, but acute mitogenic effects can be observed in the absence of serum factors (McCarthy *et al.*, 1989b).

Both FGFs induce a proportionally greater increase in noncollagen protein synthesis, thereby reducing the relative percent of collagen synthesized by bone cells, but neither factor enhances collagen turnover in intact bone or isolated bone cell cultures (Canalis et al., 1987b; Canalis et al., 1988a; McCarthy et al., 1989b). Similarly, aFGF (ECGF) does not increase bone resorption in fetal rat long bone cultures (Canalis et al., 1987b). Furthermore, since both aFGF and bFGF also decrease bone alkaline phosphatase activity (McCarthy et al., 1989b) and bFGF reduces the effect of PTH on cyclic AMP production in isolated bone cells (Globus et al., 1988), these agents appear to limit the expression of the osteoblast phenotype.

FGF receptors have been reported in a number of tissue systems; whereas some cells appear to have two distinct but cross-reactive receptors for aFGF and bFGF, others express only a single receptor type (Gospodarowicz et al., 1986; Folkman and Klagsbrun, 1987). Detailed studies have not been reported for bone cells, and it remains to be determined if the quantitatively different effects of aFGF and bFGF in bone can be accounted for by competition for a single FGF receptor class.

In serum-free fetal rat bone cell cultures, the combined effects of submaximal levels of bFGF and TGF-β on the rate of DNA synthesis are simply additive; however, at maximally stimulatory TGF-β concentrations, bFGF produces a dose-dependent decrease in DNA synthesis (Centrella et al., 1987c). In contrast, in fetal bovine bone cultures grown and treated in relatively high serum, the effect of chronic exposure to both agents is synergistic (Globus et al., 1988). It is therefore likely that each of these factors produces a complex spectrum of effects that can be regulated in different ways by the presence of individual or multiple growth regulators.

In addition to their ability to influence bone cells directly, the FGFs may participate in bone formation indirectly by way of their potent angiogenic activity (Folkman and Klagsbrun, 1987). Similar to the effects described earlier for GM-CSF and TNF-α, increased neovascularization would augment the supply of nutrients and other growth factors delivered to growing or damaged bone tissue and consequently could accelerate the processes of bone growth or fracture repair.

Osteoinductive Factors

A unique agent that can specifically induce bone growth has been proposed and sought for many years. Early studies to characterize such a factor utilized an *in vivo* model of bone formation that consisted of bone extracts reimplanted into muscle cavities within a living rodent. After an appropriately long incubation period, tissue at the ectopic implantation site was shown histologically to contain newly forming endochondral bone. The protein presumably responsible for this activity was termed bone morphogenetic protein (BMP; Urist et al., 1984) or osteogenin (Sampath et al., 1987), but the identity of this factor remained elusive.

Several research groups interested in isolating the active principle in bone matrix obtained a number of biologically active proteins from matrix extracts. For example, the bovine bone matrix-derived proteins initially termed cartilage inducing factors (CIF) A and B are now known to be the homologues of TGF-β types 1 and 2 found in porcine platelet extracts. There appear to be some differences in the ability of particular TGF-β receptors on bone cells to bind TGF-β 1 and TGF-β 2, but no dissimilarity in biochemical or biological activities has been found between these two factors in bone cell cultures (reviewed in Centrella et al., 1988d; M. Centrella, unpublished results). By itself TGF-β appears incapable of osteoinduction (Sampath et al., 1987). However, other matrix proteins with somewhat less, but still highly significant, sequence homology to TGF-β recently have been reported, and some of these factors may account for BMP and/or osteogenin. Of the three native (purified from bone matrix) or synthetic (recombinant) BMPs recently described, BMP-1 appears to be a unique polypeptide, while BMP-2A and BMP-3 are members of the TGF-β-related protein family. Each of these factors seems independently capable of cartilage induction in the ectopic bone formation assay in vivo (Wang et al., 1988; Wozney et al., 1988). In addition to the BMPs, another, and presumably unique, bone matrix-derived factor has also been reported. This molecule, termed osteoinductive factor, may be related to osteogenin (Bentz et al., 1989), but much work still remains to determine the relationship among all of these newly emerging candidates for specific bone-inducing factors. It is still unclear whether these factors will be able to proceed to induce bone from newly synthesized cartilage, and if they can, whether they will be able to do so in the absence of other local or systemic growth promoters. Further studies clearly are needed to determine at what stage these TGF-β-related and unrelated osteoinductive proteins may function in bone growth.

Conclusion

As we have seen in this chapter, data from a large number of studies strongly support the contention that growth factors and cytokines have integral roles in the local regulation of bone growth and repair. These agents function both to increase and to decrease net bone formation in vitro. In many physiological situations, the combined influence of several of these factors on both processes may be necessary to maintain adequate bone mass and appropriate bone shape. In pathological situations, the effects of these factors may be absent or unregulated and thereby lead to insufficient or unrestricted bone growth. Accordingly, a fragile equilibrium must be maintained between induction and suppression of both the synthesis and the activity of a large number of locally active agents in this tissue.

We have seen that many of the important local growth factors in bone are

Table 2.

Regulatory Effects of Growth Factors and Cytokines on Processes Related to Increasing or Maintaining Bone Mass

	Anabolic Effects		Catabolic Effects	
Factors	Replication	Matrix Protein	Resorption	Matrix Turnover
TGF-β	+, 0, −	+	+, −	−
IGFs	+	+	?	−
β₂m	+	+	?	?
PDGF	+	+	+	+
CFSs	0	?	+	?
TGF-α	+	−	+	?
ILs	+	+, −	+	?
TNFs	+	+, −	+	+, 0
INF-γ	−	−	−	?
FGFs	+	+	0	0
BMP/OIF	+	+	?	?

The effects of the factors are indicated by: (+), stimulation; (−), inhibition; (0), no effect; and (?), presently unknown. When more than one symbol is shown, different effects have been demonstrated in either normal or neoplastic cultures, during acute or chronic exposure to the factor, and/or with high or low dosage administration.

the same as those found in other tissues. Recent studies have shown that some of the well-known calcium-regulating hormones may control the synthesis or activity of several of these agents. Consequently, these hormones may provide one of the mechanisms by which local, tissue-nonspecific factors can be controlled in a tissue-specific fashion within bone. However, several of these hormones appear to affect the activity of more than a single local bone growth factor. Therefore, many important questions still remain regarding the fine control of the simultaneous synthesis and interactions of several local bone growth regulators.

New information regarding the isolation of the long postulated osteoinductive agents has reopened the question of bone-specific growth factors. The surprising discovery of a high degree of sequence homology between several of these molecules with TGF-β offers an opportunity to determine whether some of the various TGF-β receptors may be primary receptors for other agents. At what stage of bone formation does each of these factors operate, and on what cell populations? Are other agents required to induce their synthesis? This should be an active area of research in the near future.

Literature describing the control of bone formation by local and systemic growth factors and cytokines continues to accumulate at an ever-accelerating rate. Nonetheless, while much has been accomplished in the last several years, considerable gaps in our understanding of bone formation still remain. Table 2 summarizes our current concept of the effects of many of these agents on both the anabolic and catabolic phases of bone formation and indicates where information is still lacking. As new results become available, we may be able to continue to unravel these complicated interactions between and among specific and nonspecific bone growth factors, calcium regulating hormones, and the various cell populations which function in synergy to regulate bone formation.

References

Assoian, R. K., Grotendorst, G. R., Miller, D. M., and Sporn, M. B. (1984). Cellular transformation by three peptide growth factors from human platelets. *Nature (London)*, **309**: 804.

Baxter, R. C. and Martin, J. L. (1989). Binding proteins for the insulin-like growth factors: structure, regulation and function. *Progress Growth Factor Res.*, **1**: 49.

Bentz, H., Nathan, R., Rosen, D., Armstrong, R., Thompson, A., Segarini, P., Matthews, M., Dasch, J., Piez, K., and Seyedin, S. (1989). Purification of an osteoinductive factor from bovine demineralized bone. *J. Cell Biol.*, **107**: 162a (abstract).

Bertolini, D. R., Nedwin, G., Bringman, D., Smith, D., and Mundy, G. R. (1986). Stimulation of bone resorption and inhibition of bone formation by human tumour necrosis factors. *Nature (London)*, **319**: 516.

Beutler, B. and Cerami, A. (1986). Cachectin and tumour necrosis factor as two sides of the same biological coin. *Nature (London)*, **320**: 584.

Brinckerhoff, C. E., Mitchell, T. I., Karmilowicz, M. J., Kluve-Beckerman, B., and Benson, M. D. (1989). Autocrine induction of collagenase by serum amyloid α-like and β_2-microglobulin-like proteins. *Science*, **243**: 655.

Bussolino, F., Wang, J. M., DiFilippi, P., Turrini, F. Sanavio, F., Edgell, C.-J. S., Aglietta, M., Arese, P., and Montovani, A. (1989). Granulocyte and granulocyte-macrophage-colony stimulating factors induce human endothelial cells to migrate and proliferate. *Nature (London)*, **337**: 471.

Canalis, E. (1986). Interleukin-1 has independent effects on deoxyribonucleic acid and collagen synthesis in cultures of rat calvariae. *Endocrinology*, **118**: 74.

Canalis, E. (1987). Effects of tumor necrosis factor on bone formation in vitro. *Endocrinology*, **121**: 1596.

Canalis, E. and Centrella, M. (1986). Isolation of a nontransforming bone-derived growth factor from medium conditioned by fetal rat calvariae. *Endocrinology*, **118**: 202.

Canalis, E., Centrella, M., and McCarthy, T. L. (1988). Effects of basic fibroblast growth factor on bone formation in vitro. *J. Clin. Invest.*, **81**: 1572.

Canalis, E., Centrella, M., and McCarthy, T. L. (1989a). Role of insulin-like growth factor I and II on skeletal remodeling. In: *Molecular and Cellular Aspects of Insulin-Like Growth Factors and Their Receptors*, D. Le Roith and Raizada, M. K., Eds., Plenum, New York, 459–466.

Canalis, E., Centrella, M., and McCarthy, T. L. (1989b). Insulin-like growth factor I mediates selective anabolic effects of parathyroid hormone in bone cultures. *J. Clin. Invest.*, **83**: 60.

Canalis, E., McCarthy, T., and Centrella, M. (1987a). A bone-derived growth factor isolated from rat calvariae is $\beta_2$microglobulin. *Endocrinology*, **121**: 1198.

Canalis, E., Lorenzo, J., Burgess, W. H., and Maciag, T. (1987b). Effects of endothelial cell growth factor on bone remodeling in vitro. *J. Clin. Invest.*, **79**: 52.

Canalis, E., McCarthy, T. L., and Centrella, M. (1988b). Isolation of growth factors from adult bovine bone matrix. *Calcif. Tissue Int.*, **43**: 346.

Canalis, E., McCarthy, T. L., and Centrella, M. (1989). Effects of platelet-derived growth factor on bone formation in vitro. *J. Cell. Physiol.*, **140**: 530.

Canalis, E., Peck, W. A., and Raisz, L. G. (1980). Stimulation of DNA and collagen synthesis by autologous growth factor in cultured fetal rat calvaria. *Science*, **210**: 1021.

Canalis, E. and Raisz, L. G. (1979). Effect of epidermal growth factor on bone formation in vitro. *Endocrinology*, **104**: 862.

Carpenter, G. and Zendegui, J. G., (1986). Epidermal growth factor, its receptor, and related proteins. *Exp. Cell Res.*, **164**: 1.

Centrella, M. and Canalis, E. (1985). Transforming and nontransforming growth factors are present in culture medium conditioned by fetal rat calvariae. *Proc. Natl. Acad. Sci. U.S.A.*, **82**: 7335.

Centrella, M. and Canalis, E. (1987a). Isolation of EGF-dependent transforming growth factor (TGFβ-like) activity from culture medium conditioned by fetal rat calvariae. *J. Bone Min. Res.*, **2**: 29.

Centrella, M., Massague, J., and Canalis, E. (1986). Human platelet-derived transforming growth factor-β stimulates parameters of bone growth in fetal rat calvariae. *Endocrinology*, **119**: 2306.

Centrella, M., McCarthy, T. L., and Canalis, E. (1987b). Transforming growth factor β is a bifunctional regulator of replication and collagen synthesis in osteoblast-enriched cultures from fetal rat bone. *J. Biol. Chem.*, **262**: 2869.

Centrella, M., McCarthy, T. L., and Canalis, E. (1987c). Mitogenesis in fetal rat bone cells simultaneously exposed to type β transforming growth factor and other growth regulators. *FASEB J.* **1**: 312.

Centrella, M., McCarthy, T. L., and Canalis, E. (1988a). Parathyroid hormone modulates transforming growth factor β activity and binding in osteoblast-enriched cell cultures from fetal rat parietal bone. *Proc. Natl. Acad. Sci. U.S.A.*, **85**: 5889.

Centrella, M., McCarthy, T. L., and Canalis, E. (1989a). β_2 microglobulin (β_2m) enhances insulin-like growth factor I binding and synthesis in bone cell cultures. *J. Biol. Chem.*, **264**: 18268.

Centrella, M., McCarthy, T. L., and Canalis, E. (1989b). Platelet-derived growth factor enhances deoxyribonucleic acid and collagen synthesis in osteoblast-enriched cultures from fetal rat parietal bone. *Endocrinology*, **125**: 13.

Centrella, M., McCarthy, T. L., and Canalis, E. (1988c). Tumor necrosis factor-α inhibits collagen synthesis and alkaline phosphatase activity independently of its effect on deoxyribonucleic acid synthesis in osteoblast-enriched bone cell cultures. *Endocrinology*, **123**: 1442.

Centrella, M., McCarthy, T. L., and Canalis, E. (1988d). Skeletal tissue and transforming growth factor β. *FASEB J.*, **2**: 3066.

Centrella, M., McCarthy, T. L., and Canalis, E. (1990). Receptors for insulin-like growth factors I and II in osteoblast-enriched cultures from fetal rat bone. *Endocrinology*, **126**: 39.

Chambers, T. J., McSheehy, P. M. J., Thomson, B. M., and Fuller, K. (1985). The effect of calcium-regulating hormones and prostaglandins on bone resorption by osteoclasts disaggregated from neonatal rabbit bones. *Endocrinology*, **116**: 342.

Chenu, C., Pfeilschifter, J., Mundy, G. R., and Roodman, G. D. (1988). Transforming growth factor-β inhibits formation of osteoclast-like cells in long term human marrow cultures. *Proc. Natl. Acad. Sci. U.S.A.*, **85**: 5683.

Dedhar, S., Gaboury, L., Galloway, P., and Eaves, C. (1988). Human granulocyte-macrophage colony-stimulating factor is a growth factor acting on a variety of cell types of nonhemopoietic origin. *Proc. Natl. Acad. Sci. U.S.A.*, **85**: 9253.

Deuel, T. F. (1987). Polypeptide growth factors: roles in normal and abnormal cell growth. *Ann. Rev. Cell Biol.*, **3**: 443.

Dinarello, C. A. and Mier, J. W. (1987). Current concepts: lymphokines. *N. Engl. J. Med.*, **317**: 940.

Dower, S. K., Kronheim, S. R., Hopp, T. P., Cantrell, M., Deely, M., Gillis, S., Henney, C. S., and Urdal, D. L. (1986). The cell surface receptors for interleukin-1 alpha and interleukin-1 beta are identical. *Nature (London)*, **324**: 266.

Due, C., Simonsen, M., and Olsson, L. (1986). The major histocompatibility complex class I heavy chain as a structural subunit of the human membrane insulin receptor: implications for the range of biological functions of histocompatibility antigens. *Proc. Natl. Acad. Sci. U.S.A.*, **83**: 6007.

Ernst, M. and Froesch, E. R. (1988). Growth hormone dependent stimulation of osteoblast-like cells in serum-free cultures via local synthesis of insulin-like growth factor I. *Biochem. Biophys. Res. Commun.*, **151**: 142.

Felix, R., Elford, P. R., Stoerckle, C., Cecchini, M., Wetterwald, A., Trechsel, U., Fleisch, H., and Stadler, B. M. (1986). Production of hemopoietic growth factors by bone tissue and bone cells in culture. *J. Bone Min. Res.* **1**: 27.

Felix, R., Fleisch, H., and Elford, P. R. (1989). Bone-resorbing cytokines enhance release of macrophage colony-stimulating activity by the osteoblastic cell line MC3T3-E1. *Calcif. Tissue Int.*, **44**: 356.

Folkman, J. and Klagsbrun, M. (1987). Angiogenic factors. *Science*, **235**: 442.

Froesch, E. R., Schmid, C., Schwander, J., and Zapf, J. (1985). Actions of insulin-like growth factors. *Annu. Rev. Physiol.*, **47**: 443.

Frolik, C. A., Ellis, L. F., and Williams, D. C. (1988). Isolation and characterization of insulin-like growth factor II from human bone. *Biochem. Biophys. Res. Commun.*, **151**: 1011.

Gehron Robey, P., Young, M. F., Flanders, K. C., Roche, N. S., Kondaiah, P., Reddi, A. H., Termine, J. D., Sporn, M. B., and Roberts, A. B. (1987). Osteoblasts synthesize and respond to transforming growth factor type β (TGF-β) in vitro. *J. Cell Biol.*, **105**: 457.

Globus, R. K., Patterson-Buckendahl, P., and Gospodarowicz, D. (1988). Regulation of bovine bone cell proliferation by fibroblast growth factor and transforming growth factor β. *Endocrinology*, **123**: 98.

Globus, R. K., Plouet, J., and Gospodarowicz, D. (1989). Cultured bovine bone cells synthesize basic fibroblast growth factor and store it in their extracellular matrix. *Endocrinology*, **124**: 1539.

Goldfine, I. D. (1987). The insulin receptor: molecular biology and transmembrane signaling. *Endocrinol. Rev.*, **8**: 235.

Gorevic, P. D., Munoz, P. C., Casey, T. T., DiRaimondo, C. R., Stone, W. J., Prelli, F. C., Rodrigues, M. M., Poulik, M. D., and Frangione, B. (1986). Polymerization of intact β$_2$-microglobulin in tissue causes amyloidosis in patients on chronic hemodialysis. *Proc. Natl. Acad. Sci. U.S.A.*, **83**: 7908.

Gospodarowicz, D., Neufeld, G., and Schweigerer, L. (1986). Fibroblast growth factor. *Mol. Cell. Endocrinol.*, **46**: 187.

Gowen, M. and Mundy, G. R. (1986). Actions of recombinant interleukin 1, interleukin 2, and interferon gamma on bone resorption in vitro. *J. Immunol.*, **136**: 2478.

Graves, D. T., Owen, A. J., Barth, R. K., Tempst, P., Winoto, A., Fors, L., and Hood, L. E. (1984). Detection of c-sis transcripts and synthesis of PDGF-like proteins by human osteosarcoma cells. *Science*, **226**: 972.

Hart, C. H., Forstrom, J. W., Kelly, J. D., Seifert, R. A., Smith, R. A., Ross, R., Murray, M. J., and Bowen-Pope, D. F. (1988). Two classes of PDGF receptor recognize different isoforms of PDGF. *Science*, **240**: 1529.

Hauschka, P. V., Mavrakos, A. E, Iafrati, M. D., Doleman, S. E., and Klagsbrun, M. (1986). Growth factors in bone matrix. Isolation of multiple types by affinity chromatography on heparin sepharose. *J. Biol. Chem.*, **261**: 12665.

Heldin, C.-H., Johnsson, A., Wennergren, S., Wernstedt, C., Betsholtz, C., and Westermark, B. (1986). A human osteosarcoma cell line secretes a growth factor structurally related to a homodimer of PDGF A chains. *Nature (London)*, **319**: 511.

Heldin, C.-H., Backstrom, G., Ostman, A., Hammacher, A., Ronnstrand, L., Rubin, K., Nister, M., and Westermark, B. (1988). Binding of different dimeric forms of PDGF to human fibroblasts: evidence for two separate receptor types. *EMBO J.*, **7**: 1387.

Hock, J. M., Centrella, M., and Canalis, E. (1988a). Transforming growth factor beta (TGF-beta-1) stimulates bone matrix apposition and bone cell replication in cultured rat calvaria. *Calc. Tissue Int.*, **42**: A32 (abstract).

Hock, J. M., Centrella, M., and Canalis, E. (1988b). Insulin-like growth factor has independent effects on bone matrix formation and cell replication. *Endocrinology*, **122**: 254.

Horowitz, M. C., Coleman, D. L., Flood, P. M., Kupper, T. S., and Jilka, R. L. (1989). Parathyroid hormone and lipopolysaccharide induce murine osteoblast-like cells to secrete a cytokine indistinguishable from granulocyte-macrophage colony-stimulating factor. *J. Clin. Invest.*, **83**: 149.

Ibbotson, K. J., Harrod, J., Gown, M., D'Souza, S., Smith, D. D., Winkler, M. E., Derynck, R., and Mundy, G. R. (1986). Human recombinant transforming growth factor α stimulates bone resorption and inhibits bone formation in vitro. *Proc. Natl. Acad. Sci. U.S.A.*, **83**: 2228.

Isaksson, O. G. P., Lindahl, A., Nilsson, A., and Isgaard, J. (1987). Mechanism of the stimulatory effect of growth hormone on longitudinal bone growth. *Endocrinol. Rev.*, **8**: 426.

Keski-Oja, J., Leof, E. B., Lyons, R. M., Coffey, Jr., R. J., and Moses, H. L., (1987). Transforming growth factors and control of neoplastic cell growth. *J. Cell. Biochem.*, **33**: 95.

Koma, B. S., Terpening, C. M., Benz, D. J., Graeme, K. A., Gallegos, A., Korc, M., Greene, G. L., O'Malley, B. W., and Haussler, M. R. (1988). Estrogen binding receptor mRNA, and biologic response in osteoblast-like osteosarcoma cells. *Science*, **241**: 81.

Kronke, M., Schluter, C., and Pfizenmaier, K. (1987). Tumor necrosis factor inhibits myc expression in HL-60 cells at the level of mRNA transcription. *Proc. Natl. Acad. Sci. U.S.A.*, **84**: 469.

Leibovich, S. J., Polverini, P. J., Shepard, H. M., Wiseman, D. M., Shively, V., and Nuseir, N. (1987). Macrophage-induced angiogenesis is mediated by tumour necrosis factor-α. *Nature (London)*, **329**: 630.

Leof, E. B., Proper, J. A., Goustin, A. S., Shipley, G. D., DiCorleto, P. E., and Moses, H. L. (1986). Induction of c-sis mRNA and activity similar to platelet-derived growth factor by transforming growth factor β: a proposed model for indirect mitogenesis involving autocrine activity. *Proc. Natl. Acad. Sci. U.S.A.*, **83**: 2453.

Lorenzo, J. A., Sousa, S. L., Fonseca, J. M., Hock, J. M., and Medlock, E. S. (1987). Colony-stimulating factors regulate the development of multinucleated osteoclasts from recently replicated cells in vitro. *J. Clin. Invest.*, **80**: 160.

Lorenzo, J. L., Sousa, S. L., and Centrella, M. (1988). Interleukin-1 in combination with transforming growth factor-α produces enhanced bone resorption in vitro. *Endocrinology*, **123**: 2194.

MacDonald, B. R., Mundy, G. R., Clark, S., Wang, E. A., Kuehl, T. J., Stanley, E. R., and Roodman, G. D. (1986). Effects of recombinant CSF-GM and highly purified CSF-1 on the formation of multinucleated cells with osteoclast characteristics in long-term bone marrow cultures. *J. Bone Min. Res.*, **1**: 227.

Madtes, D. K., Raines, E. W., Sakariassen, K. S., Assoian, R. K., Sporn, M. B., Bell, G. I., and Ross, R. (1988). Induction of transforming growth factor alpha in activated human alveolar macrophages. *Cell*, **53**: 285.

Martineau-Doize, B., Lai, W. H., Warshawsky, H., and Bergeron, J. J. M. (1988). In vivo demonstration of cell types in bone that harbor epidermal growth factor receptors. *Endocrinology*, **123**: 841

Massague, J. (1984). Type β transforming growth factor from feline sarcoma virus-transformed cells: isolation and biological properties. *J. Biol. Chem.*, **259**: 9756.

McCarthy, T. L., Centrella, M., and Canalis, E. (1989a). Parathyroid hormone enhances the transcript and polypeptide levels of insulin-like growth factor I in osteoblast-enriched cultures from fetal rat bone. *Endocrinology*, **124**: 1247.

McCarthy, T. L., Centrella, M., and Canalis, E. (1989b). Effects of fibroblast growth factors on deoxyribonucleic acid and collagen synthesis in rat parietal bone cells. *Endocrinology*, **125**: 2118.

McCarthy, T. L., Centrella, M., and Canalis, E. (1989b). Regulatory effects of insulin-like growth factor I and II on bone collagen synthesis in rat calvarial cultures. *Endocrinology*, **124**: 301.

Messner, R. P. (1984). β$_2$-microglobulin: an old molecule assumes a new look. *J. Lab. Clin. Med.*, **104**: 141.

Miyazono, K., Hellman, V., Wernstedt, C., and Heldin, C.-H. (1988). Latent high molecular weight complex of transforming growth factor β1. Purification from human platelets and structural characterization. *J. Biol. Chem.*, **263**: 6407.

Mohan, S., Jennings, J. C, Linkhart, T. A., and Baylink, D. J. (1988). Primary structure of human skeletal growth factor: homology with insulin-like growth factor II. *Biochim. Biophys. Acta*, **966**: 44.

Morrison, D. C. and Ryan, J. L. (1987). Endotoxins and disease mechanisms. *Annu. Rev. Med.*, **38**: 417.

Mundy, G. R. (1988). Hypercalcemia of malignancy revisited. *J. Clin. Invest.*, **82**: 1.

Nathan, C. F. (1987). Secretory products of macrophages. *J. Clin. Invest.*, **79**: 319.

Ng, K. W., Partridge, N. C., Niall, M., and Martin, T. J. (1983). Epidermal growth factor receptors in clonal lines of a rat osteogenic sarcoma and osteoblast-rich bone cells. *Calcif. Tissue Int.*, **35**: 298.

Nishizuka, Y. (1984). The role of protein kinase C in cell surface signal transduction and tumour promotion. *Nature (London)*, **308**: 693.

Noda, M. (1989). Transcriptional regulation of osteocalcin production by transforming growth factor-β in rat osteoblast-like cells. *Endocrinology*, **124**: 612.

Noda, M. and Rodan, G. A. (1986). Type β transforming growth factor inhibits proliferation and expression of alkaline phosphatase in murine osteoblast-like cells. *Biochem. Biophys. Res. Commun.*, **140**: 56.

Noda, M. and Rodan, G. A. (1987). Type-beta transforming growth factor (TGF-beta) regulation of alkaline phosphatase expression and other phenotype-related messenger-RNAs in osteoblastic rat osteosarcoma cells. *J. Cell. Physiol.*, **133**: 426.

Noda, M., Yoon, K, Prince, C. W., Butler, W. T., and Rodan, G. A. (1988). Transcriptional regulation of osteopontin production in rat osteosarcoma cells by type β transforming growth factor. *J. Biol. Chem.*, **263**: 13916.

Old, L. J. (1985). Tumor necrosis factor (TNF). *Science*, **230**: 630.

Peetre, C., Gullberg, U., Nilsson, E., and Olsson, I. (1986). Effects of recombinant tumor necrosis factor on proliferation and differentiation of leukemic and normal hemopoietic cells in vitro. *J. Clin. Invest.*, **78**: 1694.

Petkovich, P. M., Wrana, J. L., Grigoriadis, A. E., Heersche, J. N. M., and Sodek, J. (1987). 1,25 Dihydroxyvitamin D_3 increases epidermal growth factor receptors and transforming growth factor β-like activity in a bone-derived cell line. *J. Biol. Chem.*, **262**: 13424.

Pfeilschifter, J., D'Souza, S. M., Mundy, G. R. (1987). Effects of transforming growth factor-β on osteoblastic osteosarcoma cells. *Endocrinology*, **121**: 212.

Pfeilschifter, J. and Mundy, G. R. (1987). Modulation of type β transforming growth factor activity in bone cultures by osteotropic hormones. *Proc. Natl. Acad. Sci. U.S.A.*, **84**: 2024

Pfeilschifter, J., Seyedin, S. M., and Mundy, G. R. (1988). Transforming growth factor beta inhibits bone resorption in fetal rat long bone cultures. *J. Clin. Invest.*, **82**: 680.

Pledger, W. J., Stiles, C. D., Antoniades, H. N., and Scher, C. D. (1978). An ordered sequence of events is required before BALB/c-3T3 cells become committed to DNA synthesis. *Proc. Natl. Acad. Sci. U.S.A.*, **75**: 2839.

Raisz, L. G., Simmons, H. A., Sandberg, A. L., and Canalis, E. (1980). Direct stimulation of bone resorption by epidermal growth factor. *Endocrinology*, **107**: 270.

Rodan, G. A. and Martin, T. J. (1981). Role of osteoblasts in hormonal control of bone resorption — a hypothesis. *Calcif. Tissue Int.*, **33**: 349.

Rodan, S. B., Wesolowski, G., Thomas, K., and Rodan, G. A. (1987). Growth stimulation of rat calvaria osteoblastic cells by acid fibroblast growth factor. *Endocrinology*, **121**: 1917.

Rosen, D. M., Stempien, S. A., Thompson, A. Y., and Seyedin, S. M. (1988). Transforming growth factor β modulates the expression of osteoblast and chondroblast phenotypes in vitro. *J. Cell. Physiol.*, **134**: 337.

Rossi, P., Karsenty, G., Roberts, A. B., Roche, N. S., Sporn, M. B., and DeCrombrugghe, B. (1988). A nuclear factor 1 binding site mediates the transcriptional activation of type I collagen promoter by transforming growth factor-β. *Cell*, **52**: 405.

Sampath, T. K., Muthukumaran, N., and Reddi, A. H. (1987). Isolation of osteogenin, an extracellular matrix-associated bone-inductive protein, by heparin affinity chromatography. *Proc. Natl. Acad. Sci. U.S.A.*, **84**: 7109.

Shen, V., Kohler, G., Jeffrey, J. J., and Peck, W. A. (1988). Bone-resorbing agents promote and interferon-γ inhibits bone cell collagenase production. *J. Bone Mineral Res.*, **3**: 657.

Sieff, C. A. (1987). Hemopoietic growth factors. *J. Clin. Invest.*, **79**: 1549.

Smith, D. D., Gowen, M., and Mundy, G. R. (1987). Effects of interferon-γ and other cytokines on collagen synthesis in fetal rat bone cultures. *Endocrinology*, **120**: 2494.

Sporn, M. B., Roberts, A. B., Wakefield, L. M., and DeCrombrugghe, B. (1987). Some recent advances in the chemistry and biology of transforming growth factor-beta. *J. Cell Biol.*, **105**: 1039.

Stephenson, M. L., Goldring, M. B., Birkhead, J. R., Krane, S. M., Rahmsdorf, H. J., and Angel, P. (1987). Stimulation of procollagenase synthesis parallels increases in cellular procollagenase mRNA in human articular chondrocytes exposed to recombinant interleukin 1 beta or phorbol ester. *Biochem. Biophys. Res. Commun.*, **144**: 583.

Stern, P. H., Krieger, N. S., Nissenson, R. A., Williams, R. D., Winker, M. E., Derynck, R., and Strewler, G. J. (1985). Human transforming growth factor alpha stimulates bone resorption in vitro. *J. Clin. Invest.*, **76**: 2016.

Sugarman, B. J., Lewis, G. D., Eessalu, T. E., Aggarwal, B. B., and Shepard, H. M. (1987). Effects of growth factors on the antiproliferative activity of tumor necrosis factors. *Cancer Res.*, **47**: 780.

Tashjian, A. H., Hohman, E. L., Antoniades, H. N., and Levine, L. (1982). Platelet-derived growth factor stimulates bone resorption via a prostaglandin mediated mechanism. *Endocrinology*, **111**: 118.

Tashjian, A. H., Voelkel, E. F., Lazzaro, M., Singer, F. R., Roberts, A. B., Derynck, R., Winkler, M. E., and Levine, L. (1985). α and β human transforming growth factors stimulate prostaglandin production and bone resorption in cultured mouse calvaria. *Proc. Natl. Acad. Sci. U.S.A.*, **82**: 4535.

Tashjian, Jr., A. H., Voelkel, E. F., Lloyd, W., Derynck, R., Winkler, M. E., and Levine, L. (1986). Action of growth factors on plasma calcium. Epidermal growth factor and human transforming growth factor-alpha cause elevation of plasma calcium in mice. *J. Clin. Invest.*, **78**: 1405.

Thomson, B. M., Saklatvala, J., and Chambers, T. J. (1986). Osteoblasts mediate interleukin 1 stimulation of bone resorption by rat osteoclasts. *J. Exp. Med.*, **164**: 104.

Urist, M. R., Juo, Y.-K., Brownell, A. G., Hohl, W. M., Buyske, J., Lietze, A., Tempst, P., Hunkapillar, M., and DeLange, R. J. (1984). Purification of bone morphogenetic protein by hydroxyapatite chromatography. *Proc. Natl. Acad. Sci. U.S.A.*, **81**: 371.

Wang, E. A., Rosen, V., Cordes, P., Hewick, R. M., Kriz, M. J., Luxenberg, D. P., Sibley, B. S., and Wozney, J. M. (1988). Purification and characterization of other distinct bone-inducing factors. *Proc. Natl. Acad. Sci. U.S.A.*, **85**: 9484.

Weir, E. C., Insogna, K. L., and Horowitz, M. C. (1989). Osteoblast-like cells secrete granulocyte-macrophage colony-stimulating factor in response to parathyroid hormone and lipopolysaccharide. *Endocrinology*, **124**: 899.

Wozney, J. M., Rosen, V., Celeste, A. J., Mitsock, L. M., Whitters, M. J., Kriz, R. W., Hewick, R. M., and Wang, E. A. (1988). Novel regulators of bone formation: molecular clones and activities. *Science*, **242**: 1528.

4

Calcium Metabolism and Bone Mineralization

BENEDETTO DE BERNARD

Dipartimento Biochimica
Biofisica e Chimica delle Macromolecole
Università di Trieste
Italy

Introduction
Bone cells and other structural components
Intracellular calcium homeostasis
Ca^{2+} fluxes and metabolism of phosphatidylinositol phosphates
Bone and plasma calcium homeostasis
Bone blood equilibrium
Role of protons in the mineral phase of bone
Role of noncollagenous bone proteins
Calcium supply
PTH regulation of calcium metabolism
General conclusions
References

Introduction

Bone in higher organisms represents a sink for most of the Ca^{2+} immobilized as hydroxyapatite $(Ca_{10}(PO_4)_6(OH)_2)$. Only a few grams out of a total of about 1250 circulates in the extracellular and intracellular fluids. In the extracellular fluid (plasma) about half of the total Ca^{2+} is ionized (free Ca^{2+}), whereas only 0.1% or less of the total Ca^{2+} is ionized within cells. The concentration of free Ca^{2+} in plasma reflects the movements of the ion to and from the bone deposits; the set point is fixed at about 3 mM. This concentration is very high compared to the sub μM concentration of free Ca^{2+} inside the cell; the consequence is that a large electrochemical force on the ion favors its role as an intracellular messenger. Indeed, even minor changes in the permeability of cell membranes to the ion, produced by physiological stimuli, will cause important variations in its cytosolic concentration.

From the facts cited on the previous page, this chapter was set up to consider:

(a) The cells of bone which are involved in the minute-to-minute regulation of calcium ion concentrations of the extracellular fluid
(b) The mechanism of intracellular calcium homeostasis
(c) Ca^{2+} fluxes and the metabolism of phosphatidyl-inositol phosphate
(d) Bone and plasma calcium homeostasis
(e) Equilibrium between blood and bone
(f) The possible role of protons in the mineral phase of bone
(g) The possible role of noncollagenous bone proteins
(h) Calcium supply
(i) The role of PTH

Data concerning bone mineralization are organized in the context of overall calcium metabolism, tissue-specific reactions and possible new lines of research.

Bone Cells and Other Structural Components

Four types of cells are identified in bone: osteoblasts, osteocytes, bone lining cells and osteoclasts.

Osteoblasts derive from mesenchymal cells located in the deep layer of the periosteum and in the reticular stroma of the bone marrow (Hall, 1987; see also Chapter 1 in Volume 1). During mineralization some osteoblasts are included in the bone tissue to become osteocytes. Those osteoblasts which are not trapped in the bone at the end of the osteogenetic activity assume a flattened shape and become bone lining cells (Marotti, 1988).

Multinucleated osteoclasts are the primary bone-resorbing cells. There is strong evidence that osteoclasts form by fusion of mononuclear precursors; the best candidate for such a precursor seems to be a stem cell of the monocyte-macrophage family (Mundy and Roodman, 1987).

Osteoblasts are located on the periosteal and endosteal vascular surfaces of bone during active osteogenesis. Osteoblasts are also present in Haversian canals. The plasma membrane of these cells protrudes in numerous and short cytoplasmic processes which allow contact with not only osteoblasts, but also with preosteocytes and osteocytes.

Mineralizing vesicles (Bonucci, 1971), where the early mineral crystals are detectable, derive from the processes of osteoblasts and preosteocytes which radiate towards the calcification front.

Osteocytes lay immersed in the bone fluid compartment which also bathes the thin processes, typical of these cells, present in the canalicular network.

Bone lining cells cover the vascular surfaces of inactive bone. They look like flat endothelial cells, showing an ultrastructure of cells in a dormant state. As they lie close to the blood vessels, lining cells are directly supplied with nutrients by the extracellular fluid.

Consequently, lining cells appear to separate the bone liquid compartment from the extracellular fluid (Matthews *et al.*, 1977). Since the chemical composition of the two liquid phases seems to differ (higher content of potassium and lower content of Ca^{2+} in the bone fluid compartment than in the extracellular fluid, Talmage, 1970), lining cells appear to be directly involved in control of the traffic of mineral ions (Norimatsu *et al.*, 1978; Matthews *et al.*, 1980).

Osteoclasts, like osteoblasts, are located on the vascular surfaces, but only during resorption activity of bone. The mechanism of osteoclast action is still under investigation; the success in preparing pure osteoclasts and in cultivating them *in vitro* is rather recent, and new interesting data from the current studies are expected (Zambonin Zallone *et al.*, 1982; Teti and Zallone, 1987; see also Chapter 4 in Volume 2). It seems likely that mineral is released initially and that degradation of the matrix follows thereafter. The former event appears to be related to hydrogen ion production, and different hypotheses have been suggested about the mechanism of proton delivery to the immediate extracellular environment (Vaes, 1988). Lysosomal enzymes are related to matrix degradation and an interplay between proteolytic activity and natural inhibitors is suggested on the basis of some recent investigations (Elzanowski *et al.*, 1988).

Intracellular Calcium Homeostasis

It is impossible to study the relationship between intra- and extracellular calcium concentrations if one does not know the mechanisms which allow the cells to protect intracellular space from excess of the cation and also the mechanism which controls the influx and efflux of Ca^{2+} in specific cells. Eukaryotic cells contain Ca^{2+} transporting systems in the plasma membrane, in mitochondria and in endoplasmic reticulum (ER) (Carafoli, 1987; Carafoli and Sottocasa, 1984). Comprehensive reviews on intracellular calcium homeostasis have appeared and may be consulted for detailed information (Carafoli, 1987).

In general, plasma membranes contain three systems: a specific ATPase, a Ca^{2+} channel and a Na^{+}/Ca^{2+} exchanger. Not all cells contain these three systems; there is evidence that the latter system is present in neither chondrocytes (Zanetti *et al.*, 1982) nor in bone cells (Nijweide and Van der Plas, 1979). On the contrary, a Ca^{2+}-ATPase in bone cells has been recently shown by a cytochemical method (Akisaka *et al.*, 1988).

Mitochondria contain an electrophoretic uniporter that is used exclusively for the uptake of Ca^{2+}. This transport is driven by the potential (about 180 mV, negative inside) set up across the inner mitochondrial membrane as the consequence of H^{+} extrusion by the respiratory chain. Ca^{2+} uptake can be inhibited by ruthenium red; a carrier-mediated process was suggested which was necessarily supposed to be endowed with Ca^{2+} binding activity and to be ruthenium red sensitive. The best characterized is the protein isolated by Sottocasa *et al.* (1971) named calvectin. This mediator appears to be involved in the mitochondria Ca^{2+} efflux pathway (Panfili *et al.*, 1980).

A Na^{+}/Ca^{2+} exchanger different from that of plasma membrane is the predominant mechanism involved in the release of Ca^{2+} from mitochondria to the cytosol.

It is worthwhile mentioning that mitochondria are not profoundly disturbed by the deposition of Ca^{2+} and phosphate unless high levels of loading are reached. Matrix loading of mitochondria with Ca^{2+} and phosphate appears as a safety device that gives to mitochondria the role of a buffer system for the extra Ca^{2+} above the physiological concentration of cytosol (McCormack and Denton, 1986).

The deposits inside mitochondria do not show the X-ray diffraction pattern of crystalline hydroxyapatite. This phenomenon suggests that in mitochondria, compounds may exist that prevent the crystalline transformation of hydroxyapatite. Phosphocitrate has been recently proposed as the possible substance capable of exerting such an inhibitory effect (Williams and Sallis, 1979). In any case, thanks to this high buffering system, mitochondria protect the cell from high waves of calcium increase until the excess of the ion in the cytosol subsides again.

The concept that mitochondria act as long-term Ca^{2+} sinks, able to store high amounts of Ca^{2+}, implies that this condition is compatible with their biochemical activity. In fact, bone cells which are situated in an unusually high Ca^{2+} traffic across the cytoplasm have mitochondria loaded with Ca^{2+}, but are still able to function adequately (Krieger and Tashjian Jr., 1980).

It is always possible for cells which are involved in the process of bone mineralization that mitochondria not only store Ca^{2+} and phosphate, but also export the mineral deposits, as suggested by Lehninger (1970).

The idea that preformed calcium phosphate minerals may be exported as micropackets by crossing the different cell membranes will be examined in another section. Also, ER contains a specific ATPase for Ca^{2+} uptake, and an unknown system is used for the release of Ca^{2+} to cytoplasm.

Evidence is rapidly accumulating which indicates that ER is much more involved than mitochondria in intracellular Ca^{2+} homeostasis. This shift of role from mitochondria to ER is, at least partially, due to the recent discovery that the intracellular messenger inositol triphosphate (Ins P_3) releases Ca^{2+} from the intracellular stores of ER more than from mitochondria.

Of special interest in this regard is a protein recently isolated from non-muscle cells, similar to calsequestrin of muscle (MacLennan *et al.*, 1983) and endowed with Ca binding properties (high capacity and moderate affinity, Volpe *et al.*, 1988). The protein appears to be surrounded by membrane, forming an intracellular organelle called a "calciosome". The total Ca^{2+} capacity of the calciosome pool is estimated to be around 0.2 to 0.4 mmol/

liter of cell volume. This amount of Ca^{2+} would adequately represent the Ca^{2+} store to be rapidly exchanged when the cell is activated by agonists, an activation that is coupled to the generation of Ins P_3. The intracellular target of Ins P_3 in nonmuscle cells would be calciosome (see next section).

A new series of proteins capable of aggregating phospholipid vesicles in a Ca^{2+}-dependent manner has been recently identified (Geisow and Walker, 1986); their role appears to be exerted between intracellular Ca^{2+} homeostasis, phospholipid metabolism and cell signaling pathways.

Ca^{2+} Fluxes and Metabolism of Phosphatidylinositol Phosphates

As has been considered before, a minimal amount of cell calcium is free in the cytoplasm, whereas the largest proportion is stored in internal districts, predominantly in the ER. Upon the effect of a calcium mobilizing stimulus, some of this stored calcium is released to the cytosol and later some calcium will enter the cell across the plasma membrane.

It is known that osteoblasts respond to the hormones which regulate calcium homeostasis; it is then conceivable that the intracellular Ca^{2+} may fluctuate under their stimuli (see the following sections).

Since 1975 Mitchell noted that agonists which use calcium as an intracellular messenger also stimulate the hydrolysis of inositol lipids of plasma membranes. Inositol phosphates, water-soluble products of lipid hydrolysis, appear to regulate calcium signaling (Berridge, 1984; Berridge and Irvine, 1984). Very recently Kawase and Suzuki (1988) reported that phosphatidic acid, a metabolite of phosphatidylinositol (PtdIns) turnover, produces in osteoblasts a transient increase in the cytosolic free Ca^{2+} concentration.

It seems, therefore, useful to briefly describe inositol phosphate metabolism in order to understand the mechanism of intracellular Ca^{2+} fluctuations as a response to hormonal stimuli.

There is also a second reason to consider membrane lipid metabolism. Although the role is still highly debated, alkaline phosphatase (AP) is generally considered an important factor in the mechanism of bone mineralization. Now, AP can be classified as an integral membrane protein, anchored to the plasma membrane by a phosphatidylinositol-glycan (PLG) moiety (Howard et al., 1987). During the process of mineralization, however, the molecule is found in extracellular matrix vesicles (de Bernard et al., 1986) or possibly released during hydrolysis of the phosphoinositides of the chondrocytes or osteoblast membranes. A review on synthesis and degradation of inositol phosphates which recently appeared (Majerus et al., 1988) may be useful for the reader who wishes to consider the question in detail.

Different phosphorylated forms of (PtdIns) are found in equilibrium in vertebrate cells thanks to the activities of specific kinases and phosphatases:

$$PtdIns \rightleftharpoons PtdIns_4P \rightleftharpoons PtdIns4,5P_2$$

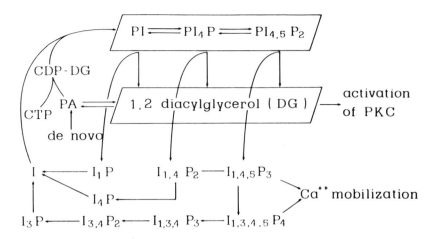

Fig. 1 Pathway for inositol phosphate metabolism. The three compounds, phosphatidyl inositol (PI), phosphatidyl inositol 4-phosphate (PI_4P), and phosphatidyl inositol 4,5-bisphosphate ($PI_{4,5}P_2$), are cleaved by phospholipase C. Various inositol phosphates are produced: inositol 1-phosphate (I_1P), inositol 1,4-bisphosphate ($I_{1,4}P_2$), inositol 1,4,5-trisphosphate ($I_{1,4,5}P_3$), and 1,2-diacylglycerol (DG). The latter compound activates the enzyme protein kinase C (PKC), whereas inositol 1,4,5-trisphosphate ($I_{1,4,5}P_3$) is capable of mobilizing calcium from intracellular stores. A 5-phosphomonoesterase degrades inositol 1,4,5-trisphosphate ($I_{1,4,5}P_3$) to inositol 1,4-bisphosphate ($I_{1,4}P_2$), and a kinase is capable of phosphorylating the compound to inositol 1,3,4,5-tetrakisphosphate ($I_{1,3,4,5}P_4$), which seems to be able to stimulate Ca^{2+} entry from the extracellular environment. The 5-phosphomonoesterase also catalyzes the hydrolysis of the inositol tetrakisphosphate to yield inositol 1,3,4-trisphosphate ($I_{1,3,4}P_3$), which is then converted to inositol 3,4-bisphosphate ($I_{3,4}P_2$) by an inositol polyphosphate-1-phosphomonoesterase. This enzyme is also responsible for the hydrolysis of inositol 1,4-bisphosphate ($I_{1,4}P_2$) to inositol 4-phosphate (I_4P). The 4-phosphomonoesterase converts inositol 3,4-bisphosphate ($I_{3,4}P_2$) to inositol 3-phosphate (I_3P). The compounds inositol monophosphate (I_1P), inositol 4-phosphate (I_4P), and inositol 3-phosphate (I_3P) are further degraded by an enzyme named inositol monophosphatase, and free inositol (I) is produced. The latter molecule may be incorporated into a newly synthesized phosphatidic acid (PA) to again form phosphatidyl inositol (PI) with the intervention of cytidine triphosphate (CTP). An intermediate compound, cytidine diphosphate diacylglycerol (CDP-DG), is the acceptor of the free inositol for the production of phosphatidyl inositol (PI). [From Majerus *et al.* (1988) modified.]

The initial reaction of the metabolism of membrane inositols involves a phospholipase C (phosphoinositidase), which cleaves the membrane PtdIns4,5 P_2 into inositol 1,4,5 P_3 and 1,2-diacylglycerol (Fig. 1).

It is the inositol 1,4,5 P_3 which has the property of mobilizing Ca^{2+} from the intracellular stores (Berridge, 1984; Berridge and Irvine, 1984). The main function of Ins 1,4,5 P_3 is in stimulating the passive release of calcium, probably by binding to a specific receptor, followed by the opening of a channel through which calcium flows out from ER to cytosol. Concomitantly, a parallel influx of potassium is observed to neutralize the outflow of the positive charges of calcium (Muallem *et al.*, 1985).

It is known that diacylglycerol (DG) activates protein kinase C (Nishizuka, 1986) and that during PtdIns metabolism it may be phosphorylated back to phosphatidic acid (PA).

The latter metabolite was suspected to function as a calcium ionophore (Putney et al., 1980) responsible, therefore, for the entry of calcium across the plasma membrane. The studies by Kawase and Suzuki (1988) seem to exclude this role and rather to suggest the function of a calcium mobilizing agent, as admitted also by Moolenar and co-workers (1986).

A new series of inositol polyphosphates has been recently discovered: the 1,3,4,5-tetrakisphosphate (Batty et al., 1985) and its dephosphorylated derivative the Ins 1,3,4 P_3 (see Fig. 1). According to Putney (1986), the permeability of plasma membrane to the external Ca^{2+} is affected by these inositol polyphosphates, derived from the Ins 1,4,5 P_3, the Ca^{2+} mobilizer from ER. The intracellular Ca^{2+} discharge would then produce a different flow of reactions in the metabolism of inositol phosphates towards the formation of inositol polyphosphates, which in turn would favor the inflow of calcium from the extracellular environment. ER is then responsible for the modification of the membrane permeability to Ca^{2+} as a function of the level of the cation stored in it.

Another control of Ca^{2+} homeostasis is exerted by the DG-protein kinase C pathway, which seems to function as a negative feedback regulator of the enhancement of cytosolic Ca^{2+}. In fact, phosphorylation of the agonist receptors curtails the hydrolysis of PtdIns 4,5 P_2 (Leeb-Lundberg et al., 1985).

In conclusion, the information we receive from these studies is that whenever the membrane of a cell is stimulated by an agonist (hormone, for example), the physiological response is mediated by a cascade of reactions related to the accelerated metabolism of the lipids of the membrane itself. The production of phosphatidylinositol, the increment of $(Ca^{2+})i$, the synthesis of cyclic nucleotides and of protein kinases and the phosphorylation of specific proteins are the early signs of the response of the cell to the stimulus. The response to the perturbed membrane includes increase of Ca^{2+} movements in and out of the cell and, probably, the release in the extracellular space of proteins anchored to the membrane, like AP of chondrocytes and osteoblasts.

Bone and Plasma Calcium Homeostasis

For the presentation of the following sections it may be useful to visualize a schema of calcium metabolism in an adult man on an average calcium intake and in zero balance (Nordin, 1976, Fig. 2, Table 1). In this example, calcium pool is in equilibrium with total absorbed intestinal calcium and with the urinary and digestive juice calcium. Since the subject is in zero balance and the rate of bone formation is equal to that of bone resorption, the net amount of Ca^{2+} absorbed (Ca^{2+} intake − Ca^{2+} fecal) is equivalent to the amount of Ca^{2+} lost with urine.

The information we obtain from this example is that plasma Ca^{2+} homeostasis reflects the rate of intestinal Ca^{2+} absorption, the rate of urinary Ca^{2+} excretion and that of Ca^{2+} exchange between blood and bone.

CALCIUM METABOLISM

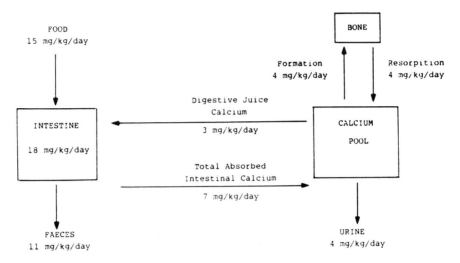

Fig. 2 Schema of calcium metabolism for the normal human adult on an average calcium intake and in zero balance. [From Nordin, B. E. C. (1976). *Calcium, Phosphate, and Magnesium Metabolism*, Churchill Livingstone, Edinburgh, 41. With permission.] The amount of net Ca^{2+} absorbed by the gastrointestinal tract is represented by the difference between calcium intake and fecal calcium. The endogenous fecal calcium (E.F.C.) is that portion of the digestive juice calcium which is eliminated with the feces. The digestive juice calcium is Ca^{2+} secreted with the digestive juices. Net calcium absorption is about 25 to 30% of the dietary intake, equal to approximately 4 mg/kg/day, which is equivalent to Ca^{2+} intake minus fecal calcium: $15 - 11 = 4$ mg/kg/day; equivalent to total absorbed intestinal Ca^{2+} minus digestive juice Ca^{2+}: $7 - 3 = 4$; equivalent to Ca^{2+} excreted with urine, in a subject who is in zero balance.

Table 1.

Chemical Disequilibrium between Blood and Bone

Condition	$Ca^{2+}\ HPO_4$ ion product $(mmol/l)^2$
Precipitation of amorphous calcium phosphate at pH 7.4	2.0 (1.6–2.4)
Normal adult human plasma	0.9 (0.7–1.1)
Growth of hydroxyapatite crystals of pH 7.4	0.6 (0.5–0.7)

Note: If exposed directly to normal human plasma, amorphous calcium phosphate would dissolve and hydroxyapatite crystals would grow.

From Parfitt, A. M. (1981). In: *Osteoporosis — Recent Advances in Pathogenesis and Treatment*, Deluca, H. F., Frost, H., Jee, W., Johnston, C., and Parfitt, M., Eds., University Park Press, Baltimore, 115–126. Reproduced with permission.

As the only organ which acts as either a source or sink for calcium, bone plays an important role in the constant regulation of calcium ion concentration in the extracellular fluid.

The idea that a cellular envelope isolates the fluid compartment of bone from that of the extracellular fluids is increasingly gaining favor among scientists. Since bone salts have a low solubility and since a supersaturation of the relative ions in the extracellular fluids exists, the idea that calcium and phosphate ions diffuse passively into the bone fluid compartment seems logical.

Considering the opposite pathway, the hypothesis was put forward that calcium ions are pumped actively from the latter compartment back into the circulating extracellular fluids. The pump was supposed to be active at the "membrane" or surface lining cells, but was never identified.

More recently, three theories were proposed to explain plasma calcium homeostasis (Parfitt, 1987). According to the first theory, plasma calcium concentration would be determined by the rate of osteoclastic bone resorption. This theory confounds regulation of mineral homeostasis with the regulation of bone mass. The latter control maintains bone form according to the laws of biomechanics and not the set point for plasma calcium.

Only in special cases where intestinal Ca^{2+} absorption is not sufficient to replace Ca^{2+} losses, the remodeling activity may cover the difference by sacrificing bone tissue.

Furthermore, calcium fluxes are of much greater magnitude than those produced by bone remodeling (Parfitt, 1979; Talmage et al., 1983), and Ca^{2+} homeostasis needs too rapid adjustments of the set point to be adequately protected by hormonal regulation, as explained also by Hurvitz et al. (1983).

Indeed, the idea of separating bone remodeling from calcium homeostatic mechanisms was first emphasized by Amprino (1946) who proposed that only structural remodeling at the microscopic level may be involved in Ca^{2+} homeostasis.

According to the second theory, the plasma Ca^{2+} set point would be determined by the threshold for renal tubular resorption of calcium (Nordin, 1976). For many physiological and pathophysiological considerations, this theory is also not satisfactory. It does not provide unambiguous explanations in conditions where the set point of plasma calcium should correlate with renal tubular reabsorption.

With the third theory, attention is shifted to a completely different mechanism which would operate in the lining cells. In the adult skeleton about 80% of all free bone surfaces are reported to be quiescent and covered by lining cells which may be considered as osteoblasts transformed to thin flat cells at the end of every phase of bone formation (Parfitt, 1987). The existence of a blood-bone equilibrium received strong support from the comparison of autoradiographs and micrographs of trabecular bone of an animal receiving $^{45}Ca^{2+}$. Intense calcium uptake was found at sites of bone formation but also over all other parts of the trabecular surfaces regardless of the state of remodeling activity (Parfitt, 1979). Since no addition of bone to the surface occurs, equivalent amounts of unlabeled calcium ions must be released. Inward movements of calcium at nongrowing bone sites must be in balance with equal outward calcium fluxes. According to this new way of considering the problem, the exchanges of Ca^{2+} between plasma and bone are not related to the process of bone formation and resorption.

Lining cells are in contact with osteocytes (see specific section) and contribute to form a special volume of the extracellular fluid, the bone fluid compartment (Talmage et al., 1983).

This theory has the important feature of explaining the property of bone to release calcium when necessary without the intervention of other mechanisms. In plasma calcium homeostasis it would represent the gross short-term mechanism of adjustment, while a finer regulation of the plasma calcium set point would be modulated by specific calcium hormones. The circadian rhythm of ionized calcium concentration in human blood provides a physiological basis for understanding the interaction between bone salts and the activity of hormones which regulate calcium metabolism (Markowitz et al., 1981). In fact, lining cells have receptors for parathyroid hormone (PTH), as do the osteoblasts from which they derive (Wong, 1986), and their shapes and ultrastructure are deeply affected by the hormone. This interesting hypothesis is then buttressed by several lines of evidence.

Osteocytes which derive from osteoblasts, such as the lining cells, may also participate in the homeostatic mechanism since they make contact through gap junctions with surface lining cells (the lining cell-osteocyte unit).

Osteocytes which are endowed with contractile cytoskeletons (Holtrop and Weinger, 1975) may help fluid circulate through the lacunar canalicular system and percolate through the submicroscopic channels of bone, transporting Ca^{2+} with great efficiency.

It is reported that osteocytes do not resorb bone by enlarging their lacunae (Boyde, 1981), but perilacunar mineral is probably a site for loss or gain of calcium and phosphate without affecting bone matrix.

Indirect support of the third theory derives from the observation that in young, rapidly growing animals, put on a low calcium diet (who have a large demand for calcium and in whom most free bone surfaces undergo either resorption or formation with practically no quiescent bone surface), hypocalcemia and secondary hyperparathyroidism are observed (Parfitt, 1984; Drivdahl et al., 1984).

In this and other similar situations, plasma calcium homeostasis is clearly impaired. According to Anast et al. (1989), the lack of quiescent bone surface would explain why children are generally more prone to hypocalcemia than adults.

Bone Blood Equilibrium

On the basis of what has been discussed in the previous section, it is clear that blood and bone must be in physicochemical equilibrium.

Unfortunately there is a paradox concerning equilibration of the skeleton with the extracellular fluid (ECF).

Hydroxyapatite is relatively insoluble and cannot be in equilibrium with any calcium phosphate ion product to be found in ECF *in vivo* (Neuman and Neuman, 1958; Neuman, 1982). Body fluids are supersaturated with respect to the hydroxyapatite of bone mineral (Levinskas and Neuman, 1985). On the other hand, they are undersaturated with respect to the first calcium phosphate precipitate formed from body fluids (see Table 1).

Brushite ($CaHPO_4$, $2H_2O$) was considered as a possible salt of the initial precipitate: its ion product is equivalent to a Ca^{2+} × Pi product of 4.2 × 10^{-3} M in body fluids. Once formed, brushite is unstable and at physiological pH, it redissolves before its autocatalytic conversion to hydroxyapatite (Neuman *et al.*, 1982), passing through different stages: amorphous calcium phosphate and octacalcium phosphate ($Ca_8H_2(PO_4)_6.5H_2O$).

The situation therefore appears as follows: on the formation side, the soluble brushite (or an equivalent salt), unstable at neutral pH, and on the dissolution side, the stable insoluble apatite. Blood Ca^{2+} × PO_4^{3-} product is in the middle of this region of ions.

Fortunately, after a long period of research, brushite has been found in young bones (Neuman and Bareham, 1975). Physicochemical measurements with X-rays, electron diffraction and ^{31}P-NMR have shown that brushite or similar mineral is the major component of recently formed bone mineral.

If brushite is the salt in equilibrium with blood calcium and phosphate, the transformation of brushite to hydroxyapatite should be regulated. In fact, this reaction may be inhibited (Neuman, 1982) and brushite may be stabilized by an acid environment, by several noncollagenous proteins and by pyrophosphate (Parfitt and Kleerekoper, 1980; Russell and Fleisch, 1976).

Even small changes in pH may affect the solubility of brushite, a fact of physiological significance (Neuman *et al.*, 1982). The overall pH of bone fluid is only about 0.1 units lower than that of the ECF (Neuman and Neuman, 1980); however, a considerable solubility increase of brushite (expressed as the ion activity products) was observed when pH was 7.3 as compared to 7.4 (Neuman *et al.*, 1982).

Noncollagenous bone proteins prepared from cortical sections of long bones also have the ability to delay or prevent the hydrolysis of brushite in apatite (Neuman *et al.*, 1982). There is an apparent difficulty: sooner or later all the metastable forms of mineral, brushite or amorphous calcium phosphate or octacalcium phosphate, will turn to hydroxyapatite and the mineral phase in equilibrium with bood ions will disappear. However, a certain amount of new bone is always present in the skeleton as part of the remodeling activities. A small fraction of unstable mineral should always then be available to the processes of stabilization with proteins and to the buffering mechanism of general calcium homeostasis.

The leading opinion at this moment is that the brushite-apatite system appears to be adequate for the process of calcium homeostasis.

The existence of nonapatite mineral at the bone surface could be related to the electron-dense material identified beneath the lining cells after feeding (VanderWiel and Talmage, 1981) and related to calcitonin secretion (Talmage *et al.*, 1983). It is considered a provisional storage form which may participate in the circadian changes in calcium balance.

A final question must be considered in order to complete the overall picture. How can brushite form in the ECF since the ion product, $Ca^{2+} \times PO_4^{3-}$ is less than one third that required for spontaneous solid formation?

The role of cells, therefore, becomes essential. In fact, the ion product, $Ca^{2+} \times HPO_4^{2\pm}$ in bone fluids is not markedly different from that of circulating fluids of the body (Neuman *et al.*, 1980); calcium and phosphate ions are not excreted by bone cells out to the ECF, but into the mineralizing districts in order to exceed the Ksp of brushite. Consequently brushite formation must be highly localized where osteoblasts or lining cells transfer Ca^{2+} ions by either extruding special complexes or by membrane vesicles, as demonstrated in the chorioallantoic membrane (Terepka *et al.*, 1976).

The conclusion is that on the supply side, Ca^{2+} must be extruded by bone cells to provide $Ca^{2+} \times HPO_4^{2-}$ ion product for brushite precipitation. On the demand side, blood is in equilibrium with bone fluid, which is in equilibrium with a mineral more soluble than apatite.

Studies on Ca^{2+} movements across periosteal and endosteal membranes of embryo chick calvaria indicate that Ca^{2+} movements in and out of bone are passive (Scarpace and Neuman, 1973).

From the general description of the studies concerning bone and calcium homeostasis, the following points must be considered in detail:

(1) Proton production, essential to keeping a metastable mineral form (in fact, during the transformation of brushite to apatite, protons are released)
(2) The role of the noncollagenous bone proteins
(3) Ca^{2+} of bone-circulating fluid to be pumped in across bone cells to exceed the Ksp for brushite formation
(4) Regulation by PTH

Role of Protons in the Mineral Phase of Bone

The presence of a metastable calcium phosphate phase and its partial stabilization by cellular production of protons provides a fundamental mechanism for regulation of calcium uptake and release from bone (Neuman and Bareham, 1975). Protons are released during the formation of calcium phosphate precipitates (Fueredi-Milhofer *et al.*, 1971):

$$xCa^{2+} + nHPO^{2-} + mH_2PO_4^- + zH_2O \rightleftharpoons Ca\,(HPO_4)u(PO_4)vOHz \\ + (n+2m+z-u)H^+$$

In dead bone, the phase undergoes spontaneous transformation to a higher Ca/Pi ratio. In viable bone, the soluble phase is stabilized by the production of acid metabolites such as lactate.

Since the buffering capacity of bone fluid is limited, it is possible that temporary local decreases in pH occur as protons are released by cells.

The extrusion of protons from cells is a phenomenon which is related to the Na^+ pump. Different types of cells use a plasma membrane Na^+-H^+ antiporter to maintain intracellular pH (Seifter and Aronson, 1986; Ives and Rector Jr., 1984; Madshus, 1988; Siffert and Akkerman, 1988a).

Since cells have a large inside negative membrane potential, a passive influx of H^+ across the plasma membrane would produce an acid intracellular pHi not compatible with cell functions. The equilibrium relation between membrane potential (Vm) and internal and external H^+ concentrations is illustrated by the Nernst expression (Madshus, 1988):

$$Vm = 1000 \ (RxT/F) \ \ln \ ((H^+)o/(H^+)i)$$

where R and F are the gas and Faraday constants, respectively, and Vm is membrane potential expressed in mV.

When the latter is -59 mV, at 22°C, calculations give a cytosolic pH of 6.4 if the extracellular pH is 7.4 This cytosolic pH is clearly not compatible with cell functions and is different from that actually determined.

Special mechanisms must exist for the uphill extrusion of H^+ in the ECF to guarantee the optimal pH for many cell processes; in a general view, with increasing cytosolic pH, the metabolic machinery of cells works faster. Cytosolic alkalinization is reported to accelerate many fundamental cellular functions including glycolysis.

The electrochemical Na^+-H^+ countertransport appears to be the most diffused mechanism operating in cells. The thermodynamic driven force for proton extrusion in the coupled Na^+/H^+ exchange is the energy of the inwardly directed electrochemical gradient. The Na^+ concentration in the cells is maintained below that of ECF by the active removal of the cation through Na^+-K^+-ATPase. One of the properties of the Na^+-H^+ exchange is reversible inhibition by the pyrazine diuretic amiloride (Kinsella and Aronson, 1981).

The amiloride-sensitive Na^+/H^+ exchange appears to be involved in hormonal stimulation of cell growth. As an example, the polypeptide epidermal growth factor (EGF) stimulates amiloride-sensitive Na^+ uptake and produces cytosolic alkalinization followed by an increase in DNA synthesis in many cells (Seifter and Aronson, 1986).

Platelet-derived growth factor (PDGF) causes an increase in pH of cultured fibroblasts; other mitogenic peptides which stimulate Na^+-H^+ exchange are known, such as angiotensin (Smith and Brock, 1983), lys-bradykinin (Owen and Villereal, 1983) and vasopressin (Mendoza et al., 1980). Insulin is reported to increase Na^+-H^+ countertransport in skeletal muscle cells (Moore,

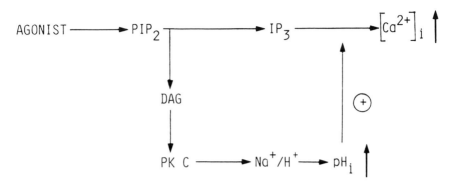

Fig. 3 Role of protein kinase C in Ca^{2+} mobilization and cell alkalinization. [From Siffert and Akkerman (1988b) modified.] Following binding of an agonist to its receptor, the hydrolysis of phosphatidyl inositol 4,5-bisphosphate (PIP_2) takes place with the formation of 1,2-diacylglycerol (DAG) and inositol 1,4,5-trisphosphate (IP_3). While DAG activates protein kinase C, IP_3 induces the mobilization of Ca^{2+} from the intracellular stores. The activation of protein kinase C induces the activation of the Na^+/H^+ exchange and consequently an increase in intracellular pH is observed, which may enhance the effect of IP_3.

1979). Thrombin activation of platelets is related to their increase of Na^+ uptake (Greenberg-Sepersky and Simons, 1984).

The existence of a Na^+-H^+ exchanger was demonstrated in osteoblasts by Redhead and Baker (1988); of great interest is the fact that osteoblasts exposed to PTH show an intracellular acidification.

It is however, not correct to think in terms of activation of Na^+/H^+ exchange only as the consequence of cell stimulation by agonists. Continuous removal of protons, produced by the metabolic activity of the cells in order to maintain the correct intracellular pH, is operating. At pH higher than 7.1, the Na^+/H^+ exchanger is almost nil. In the range between pH 7.1 to 6.5, proton extrusion follows sigmoidal kinetics with respect to the cytosolic H^+ concentration. It is then proposed that the classical Michaelis-Menten kinetics is followed in the exchange of H^+i with Na^+o, but that H^+ may also act as the allosteric activator of the exchanger when a sudden intracellular increase of protons occurs (Siffert and Akkerman, 1988b).

The sequence of biochemical steps mediating the hormone-induced rise in pH is not fully elucidated. Changes in intracellular pH and in cytosolic Ca^{2+} are often associated phenomena, e.g., activators of phospholipase C produce independent pHi variations and $Ca^{2+}i$ oscillations which are linked to inositol 1,4,5-triphosphate and DG (Frelin et al., 1988).

Protein kinase C is considered one of the best candidates for a transducer role of the agonist mediated activation of the Na^+/H^+ antiporter (Siffert and Akkerman, 1988b) (Fig. 3).

The most recent opinion (Siffert and Akkerman, 1988b) would predict hydrolysis of PIP_2 with formation of DAG and IP_3 (see the special section on phosphatidylinositol metabolism). DAG activates protein kinase, which induces an acceleration of Na^+-H^+ antiporter and increase in pH. Concurrently, IP_3 induces the mobilization of Ca^{2+} from intracellular stores (see Fig. 3).

Activation of the antiporter by agonists may be mediated by other mechanisms such as those operating in the reactions activated by Ca^{2+}-calmodulin or GTP-binding proteins.

The main goal of this section was to demonstrate that there are at least two possible ways to acidify the extracellular space and therefore maintain in solution the calcium phosphate metastable phase: production of acid metabolites (lactate) and proton extrusion by activated and nonactivated bone cells.

Role of Noncollagenous Bone Proteins

Noncollagenous bone proteins (NCBP) at 1 mg/ml are capable of preventing or delaying *in vitro* the transformation of brushite in apatite mixture (Neuman *et al.*, 1982). Among the proteins which were assayed, only phosvitin at the concentration of 1 mg/ml was as inhibitory as NCBP. Only at high concentrations do albumin and fetal calf serum proteins exhibit inhibitory activity.

The problem is whether the stabilizing proteins are present in bone in sufficient amounts to be efficient. By considering that most of the apatite mineral in bone is buried within collagen fibers (Neuman *et al.*, 1982), only a small amount, about 1% of the mineral, is available for the phenomenon of exchange and dissolution. On the basis of this consideration, the ratio NCBP/mineral is 1 mg/0.5 mg apatite, which is the ratio used for the *in vitro* experiments (Neuman *et al.*, 1982).

A legitimate question at this point concerns the chemical nature of the NCBP, which may have the important role of stabilizing the brushite phase of calcium phosphate deposits. The spectrum of composition of NCBP has been studied in detail by Termine (1983). From this study the following components have been identified: proteoglycans, phosphoproteins, sialoproteins and glycoproteins, osteonectin and osteocalcin. A new role has been recently ascribed to HS-glycoprotein, which has been found in bone since 1976 (Triffitt *et al.*, 1976), that of inhibiting the activity of endogenous proteases (Elzanowski *et al.*, 1988). All the other compounds may very well be inhibitors of the transformation of soluble minerals to hydroxyapatite as shown also *in vitro* (Termine *et al.*, 1970; Stagni *et al.*, 1976).

An analysis of osteons at different degrees of calcification (Pugliarello *et al.*, 1970) has shown that at 70% of mineralization they contain more NCBP than osteons fully mineralized.

In either case, would hydrogen ions or NCBP inhibit the formation of the stable hydroxyapatite, only bone cells play the role of regulating the amount of calcium available to the homeostasis process. This is a fundamental aspect since it is well known that calcium homeostasis is finely adjusted by the interplay of specific hormones and this tuning can be operated only by cells sensitive to hormones.

Calcium Supply

Studies by Neuman *et al.* (1982) on the fluxes of ions to and from bone have demonstrated that there is not the tight compartmentalization of electrolytes that was assumed for years and that the ion product Ca^{2+} × HPO_4^{2-} in bone fluid is not significantly different from that in the general circulating fluids.

As stated in the previous section, bone circulating fluid must cross bone cells to exceed the Ksp for brushite formation. Consequently, the osteoblasts and the lining cells must catalyze a transmembrane transport of Ca^{2+} in critical sites. Bone cells have been reported to contain high amounts of calcium (Aaron, 1978) and to form "calcium complexes" in the vicinity of their plasma membrane (Remagen *et al.*, 1969; Kashiva, 1970 and 1971; Weisbrode *et al.*, 1974; Talmage *et al.*, 1975; Gay and Schraer, 1975; Aaron, 1978; Appleton and Morris, 1979).

The Lehninger hypothesis (1970) of Ca^{2+} transport across osteoblasts in the form of calcium-containing micropackets seems to find experimental support even in the most recent literature. Doughtery (1983) reports ultrastructural evidence that membrane-associated amorphous-appearing deposits are visible in chondrocytes and matrix vesicles of epiphyseal plates. Extracellular vesicles are considered loci of early mineralization in matarix of cartilage and bone (Bonucci, 1971; Bonucci and Silvestrini, 1984).

A living model to understand the mechanism of calcium transport through cell membranes is provided by the chorioallantoic membrane which is an extraembryonic cellular membrane surrounding the avian embryo and lining the internal surface of the porous cellular shell membrane adjacent to the eggshell (Tuan *et al.*, 1978; Tuan, 1980). This membrane is the only barrier which separates the calcium source, the eggshell, from the circulating fluids of the embryo. Terepka *et al.* (1976) have shown that the membrane is responsible for an active unidirectional transcellular transport of calcium from the eggshell to the embryonic tissues.

A calcium-binding protein (CaBP) has been purified from the membrane, a basic protein of about 100,000 daltons, composed of four subunits of identical MW. It shows ten high Ca^{2+} affinity sites, with a Ka of 2.35×10^{-7} M^{-1} and 100 to 120 low-affinity sites with a Ka of $2.00 \times 10^{-5} M^{-1}$. Although the protein contains some γ-Glu residues, the high affinity for Ca^{2+} cannot rely upon these ligands (Tuan *et al.*, 1978). The expression of the protein is strictly dependent on embryo development.

A study by Tuan (1980) showed that the chorioallantoic CaBP is translocated and segregated within microsomal vesicles; this fact would indicate that intracellular CaBP is packaged for export to the cellular surface.

This mechanism of Ca^{2+} transfer from inside the cell to the extracellular matrix is also invoked to explain the AP activity present in Bonucci's matrix vesicles. This enzyme has a high Ca^{2+} affinity, is an integral membrane protein of chondrocytes and osteoblasts and is present in calcified areas as shown by immunogold techniques, although here the molecule becomes inert from the catalytic point of view (de Bernard *et al.*, 1986). The transfer of Ca^{2+} bound to protein is then a transmural mechanism frequently found in nature.

The preparation of the matrix to be calcified would consist therefore of an accumulation of proteins capable of forming a crystal template so that Ca^{2+} is bound at sites along the structure with a spacing which would almost match the spacing of calcium in the lattice of the forming crystal (Wheeler *et al.*, 1987). It is the epitaxy mechanism which is proposed by some investigators (Weiner and Hood, 1975; Weiner and Traub, 1984).

A similar mechanism is also proposed in teeth calcification where a highly phosphorylated protein represents a sort of negative membrane, capable of trapping Ca^{2+} and phosphate ions and fixing them in a nucleating complex to which other Ca^{2+} and phosphate ions may be added (Zanetti *et al.*, 1981; Cooksan *et al.*, 1980).

PTH Regulation of Calcium Metabolism

Literature on bone physiology was in the past rather meager of data concerning cell metabolic activity since biochemical studies with isolated bone cells were not available.

As reported in the previous sections, the situation is rapidly changing. Even the response of bone to mechanical stress is explained in terms of biochemical reactions, i.e., in the phosphatidylinositol metabolism of cell membrane, as the consequence of the activated phospholipase C (PLC) (Jones and Scholuebbers, 1987).

In line with this point of view, the regulation of Ca^{2+} homeostasis, operated by PTH, a major bone-active hormone, may be presented according to the biochemical mechanisms illustrated in the preceding sections. The role of PTH appears fundamental when the short-term movements of calcium are not sufficient to maintain serum Ca^{2+} homeostasis.

From the physiology and endocrinology of PTH we learn that the hormone has many functions, certainly related to the numerous target tissues, to the different circulating fragments of the "greater PTH" and the related receptors (Potts *et al.*, 1982; Wong, 1986).

In bone, the osteoblast is the only cell type which has receptors for the hormone, and since an increment of Ca^{2+} efflux from the tissue results from parathyroid stimulation, the mechanism of action should be explained by the cascade of events occurring in the stimulated osteoblasts.

One of the oldest observations is that as a consequence of PTH stimulation, an increment of cAMP is observed (Herrmann-Erlee and Konijn, 1970). The possibility of measuring with accuracy changes in free cytosolic calcium concentration by using fluorescent probes has shown that PTH causes a dose-related increase in $(Ca^{2+})i$ in the osteoblast-like cell line UMR-106 (Loewik *et al.*, 1985).

As the response, one or more factors would be released which stimulate osteoclast activity (early effect) and their number (late effect). The early effect should be regulated by cAMP and the late effect of PTH on bone resorption would be regulated by the intracellular Ca^{2+} concentration (Hermann-Erlee et al., 1988).

A biphasic regulation of bone metabolism by PTH was also found in the medullary bone of laying hens on a calcium-depleted diet (de Bernard et al., 1980).

It has been proposed that osteoblasts possess two different receptors for PTH (Loewik et al., 1985); one receptor would control the activity of the adenylate cyclase (cAMP production) and the other the influx of Ca^{2+} in the osteoblasts (Yamaguchi et al., 1987). The former receptor is presumably activated by the first two amino acids of the NH_2 terminus of PTH and the latter by the domain of the hormone sequence between amino acids 3 and 34 (Loewik et al., 1988).

Evidence has recently been obtained that activation of the type I receptor pathways causes an increase in differentiation and function of cells, whereas stimulation of the type II receptor produces an increase in mitosis and cell growth (Ratan and Shelanski, 1986; Hesch et al., 1988). Both type I and type II receptors have recently been described in various tissues (Hruska et al., 1986; Hruska et al., 1987).

Recent studies with UMR-106 osteosarcoma cells have shown that PTH produces release of inositol phosphate (Dewhirst et al., 1988) and activation of protein kinase C (Iida-Klein et al., 1988). Direct stimulation of PLC by PTH in ROS 17/2.8 cells is reported by Cosman et al. (1988); PLC appears to be a guanine nucleotide and calcium-dependent enzyme.

Such a result is paralleled by the observation of Babich et al. (1988) who have found in the same cells that GTP activates polyphosphoinositide-specific PLC and relate therefore the raise of intracellular Ca^{2+} in osteoblasts to the activation of PLC, mediated by a G-protein.

PTH produces accumulation of inositol phosphates and cAMP in murine osteoblast cultures (Farndale et al., 1988) and in the same type of cells phosphatidic acid induces calcium mobilization from intracellular stores (Kawase and Suzuki, 1988).

The following picture (Fig. 4), which illustrates the mechanisms by which Ca^{2+}-mobilizing agonists, in general, exert their effects (Mayr, 1988), seems to illustrate fairly well the effects of PTH, as so far identified in osteoblasts (see also Exton, 1988).

In fact, PTH bound to the receptor(s) on the outer surface of the osteoblast promotes the activation of specific types of G-proteins. The activated G-proteins then stimulate a PiP_2-specific PLC, generating IP_3; this compound causes the release of internal Ca^{2+} from intracellular stores. The control of the Ca^{2+} channels would also be controlled by G-proteins.

Finally, according to Redhead and Baker (1988), PTH causes an intracellular acidification in osteoblasts; the regulation of intracellular pH could influence the extracellular pH in the immediate vicinity of the cells and thus could affect bone calcium mobilization.

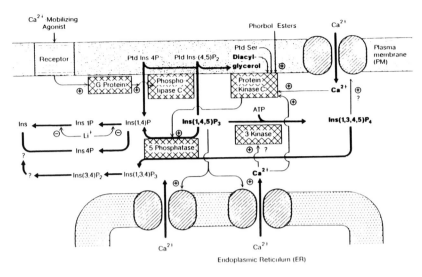

Fig. 4 Model of the cellular effects of calcium-mobilizing agonists. [From Mayr, G. W. (1988). *Topics in Biochemistry*, Boehringer, Mannheim, 1–18. With permission.] The binding of calcium-mobilizing agonists to their membrane receptors activates GTP-binding proteins, causing the activation of phospholipase C. This enzyme cleaves inositol phosphates from plasma membrane phosphoinositides. The phosphoinositide cascade, like the adenylate cyclase cascade, transduces extracellular signals into intracellular events. In the cytoplasmic districts close to the plasma membrane, an increase in the concentration of inositol 1,4,5-trisphosphate, $Ins(1,4,5)P_3$; inositol 1,4-bisphosphate, $Ins(1,4)P_2$; and inositol monophosphate, $(Ins\ 1P)$ is observed. Concomitantly, the concentration of diacylglycerol increases in the plasma membrane. $Ins(1,4,5)P_3$ binds to specific receptors of the endoplasmic reticulum causing calcium mobilization from it, probably as the consequence of an opening of $Ins(1,4,5)P_3$-dependent Ca^{2+} channels. Ca^{2+} channels may be opened also in plasma membrane during this phosphoinositide cascade, causing Ca^{2+} influx from the extracellular environment. The enhancement of cytosolic Ca^{2+} concentration triggers other cellular reactions. Several calcium-dependent protein kinases are activated, in particular protein kinase C, which is activated also by diacylglycerol. This enzyme therefore represents the pivot system of the phosphoinositides-degrading agonists. Like other second messengers, diacylglycerol and $Ins(1,4,5)P_3$ must be removed from the sites of influence. A diacylglycerol lipase will cleave one of the two fatty acids (preferentially arachidonic acid) or diacylglycerol may be recycled to phosphatidic acid. For the metabolism of phosphoinositides see also Figure 1. The abbreviations used are: ATP, adenosin-triphosphate; Ins, inositol; Ins 1P, inositol monophosphate; Ins 4P, inositol 4-monophosphate; $Ins(1,4)P_2$, inositol 1,4-bisphosphate; $Ins(3,4)P_2$, inositol 3,4-bisphosphate; $Ins(1,3,4)P_3$, inositol 1,3,4-trisphosphate; $Ins(1,4,5)P_3$, inositol 1,4,5-trisphosphate; $Ins(1,3,4,5)P_4$, inositol 1,3,4,5-tetrakisphosphate; Ptd-Ins-4P, phosphatidyl inositol 4-phosphate; Ptd-Ins-$(4,5)P_2$, phosphatidyl inositol 4,5-bisphosphate; Ptd-Ser, phosphatidyl serine.

Like ACTH, PTH also controls a steroid synthesis pathway, i.e., the synthesis of $1,25\ (OH)_2D_3$.

In conclusion, it appears that osteoclast activation during the skeletal response to PTH occurs through PTH stimulation of the osteoblast which acts as the intermediary cell. Activation of osteoblasts would induce Ca^{2+}-dependent synthesis of factors (e.g., PGE_2) able to activate bone remodeling or resorption, accompanied by mineral release.

General Conclusions

Bone participates with all of its cells in the metabolism of calcium in the organism. However, this contribution is carried out not by macroscopic bone remodeling, responsible for skeletal homeostasis, but by microscopic or structural remodeling, i.e., by bone turnover. This latter process is performed by the combined actions, in the same sites, of the osteoblasts and osteoclasts, the so-called coupled resorption-formation phenomenon.

The homeostatic mechanism which regulates plasma calcium concentration does not depend only upon the remodeling activity of bone. The minute-to-minute regulation of plasma calcium is maintained by the rates of intestinal Ca^{2+} absorption and of renal tubular Ca^{2+} reabsorption, but in primis by the equilibrium between blood and bone fluid.

Bone salts therefore should be in equilibrium with the bathing fluids; since neither amorphous calcium phosphate nor crystalline hydroxyapatite is in equilibrium with the relative plasma ions, local means for the modification of mineral solubility are invoked.

The site appears to be the lining cell-osteocyte unit which can participate in Ca^{2+} homeostasis thanks to the large surface area it forms, in contact with bone interstitial fluid, ideally situated to mediate the short-term movements of Ca^{2+} from and to bone.

By proton extrusion or by NCBP, cells are able to maintain the solubility of these salts, by controlling the rate of their transformation in crystalline hydroxyapatite. This mechanism of short-term storage and release of Ca^{2+} does not involve structural changes in bone.

To satisfy a Ca^{2+} need which lasts longer than a few hours or days, an increase in bone turnover is observed, accompanied by a reversible minimal deficit and characterized by remodeling space, osteoid tissue formation and partially calcified bone. No permanent loss of bone volume is observed in these conditions.

If Ca^{2+} need exceeds about 1500 mmol or lasts longer than a year, irreversible bone loss is predicted as the result of the difference between the volume of new bone and that of the cavities of resorption (Parfitt, 1981).

Recent studies on the mechanism by which bone cells control calcium metabolism and mineralization open new insight into the function of cell membranes.

Plasma membranes are not only the target for some hormones but also produce intracellular messengers such as inositol phosphates or cAMP. Variations of intracellular Ca^{2+} concentrations, usually maintained at very low levels, are amplified to create intracellular signals of extraordinary efficiency.

Bone cells, as cells of other tissues, strictly control the inflow and efflux of Ca^{2+}. Being, however, in the middle of an intense Ca^{2+} traffic, osteoblasts have acquired the capacity to store high amounts of Ca^{2+} and Pi under various forms, such as reversible precipitates (stabilized in colloidal form by organic compounds), membrane-surrounded enclosures or membrane vesicles.

The extrusion of this mineral material in the matrix seems to be preceded or accompanied by the export of organic substances; the presence of crystal-associated organic material in the matrix appears to be specific to calcified tissues. The chemical composition of the organic phase (crystal ghosts, Bonucci *et al.*, 1988) is not yet known, although the presence of proteoglycans and glycoproteins, both endowed with Ca^{2+} affinity, appears reasonably well documented.

References

Aaron, J. E. (1978). Histological aspects of the relationship between vitamin D and bone. In: *Vitamin D*, Lawson, D. E. M., Ed., Academic Press, New York.

Akisaka, T., Yamamoto, T., and Gay, C. V. (1988). Ultracytochemical investigation of calcium-activated adenosine triphosphatase (Ca^{2+}-ATPase) in chick tibia. *J. Bone Min. Res.*, **3**: 19–25.

Amprino, R. (1946). Fattori che regolano il rimaneggiamento strutturale delle ossa. *Arch. Scienze Biol.*, **31**: 208–224.

Anast, C. S., Carpenter, T. O., and Key Jr., L. (1989). Metabolic bone diseases in children. In: *Metabolic Bone Diseases*, 2nd ed., Avioli, L. V. and Krane, S. M., Eds., Grune and Stratton, New York, in press.

Appleton, J. and Morris, D. C. (1979). An ultrastructural investigation of the role of the odontoblast in matrix calcification using the potassium pyroantimoniate osmium method for calcium localisation. *Arch. Oral. Biol.*, **24**: 467–475.

Babich, M., King, K. L., and Nissenson, R. A. (1988). Role of a GTP-binding protein in activation of poly-phosphoinositide-specific phospholipase C in UMR-106 cells. *J. Bone Min. Res.*, 3 S. Abstr. **606**: 220.

Batty, I. R., Nahorski, S. R., and Irvine, R. F. (1985). Rapid formation of inositol 1,3,4,5-tetrakisphosphate following muscarinic receptor stimulation of rat cerebral cortical slices. *Biochem. J.*, **232**: 211–215.

de Bernard, B., Bianco, P., Bonucci, E., Costantini, M., Lunazzi, G. C., Martinuzzi, P., Modricky, C., Moro, L., Panfili, E., Pollesello, P., Stagni, N., and Vittur, F. (1986). Biochemical and immuno-histochemical evidence that in cartilage an alkaline phosphatase is a Ca^{2+}-binding glycoprotein. *J. Cell Biol.*, **103**: 1615–1623.

de Bernard, B., Stagni, N., Camerotto, R., Vittur, F., Zanetti, M., Zambonin Zallone, A., and Teti, A. (1980). Influence of calcium depletion on medullary bone of laying hens. *Calcif. Tissue Int.*, **32**: 221–228.

Berridge, M. J. (1984). Inositol triphosphate and diacylglycerol as second messengers. *Biochem. J.*, **220**: 345–360.

Berridge, M. J. and Irvine, R. F. (1984). Inositol triphosphate, a novel second messenger in cellular signal transduction. *Nature (London)*, **312**: 305–321.

Bonucci, E. (1971). The locus of initial calcification in cartilage and bone. *Clin. Orthop.*, **78**: 108–139.

Bonucci, E. and Silvestrini, G. (1984). Electron microscope investigations on the origin of matrix vesicles in bone. In: *Endocrine Control of Bone and Calcium Metabolism*, Vol. 8B, Cohn, D. V., Potts Jr., J. J., and Fujita, A. T., Eds., Elsevier, Amsterdam, 414–417.

Bonucci, E., Silvestrini, G., and Di Grezia, R. (1988). The ultrastructure of the organic phase associated with the inorganic substance in calcified tissues. *Clin. Orthop. Rel. Res.*, **233**: 243–261.

Boyde, A. (1981). Evidence against "osteocytic osteolysis". In: *Bone Histomorphometry*, III Int. Workshop; Jee, W. S. S. and Parfitt, M., Eds., Armour-Montagu, Paris, 239–255.

Carafoli, E. (1987). Intracellular calcium homeostasis. *Annu. Rev. Biochem.*, **56**: 395–433.

Carafoli, E. and Sottocasa, G. L. (1984). The uptake and the release of calcium by mitochondria. In: *Bioenergetics*, Ernster, L., Ed., Elsevier, Amsterdam, 269–289.

Cookson, D. J., Levine, B. A., Williams, R. J. P., Jontell, M., Linde, A., and de Bernard, B. (1980). Cation binding by rat-incisor-dentine phosphoprotein. A spectroscopic investigation. *Eur. J. Biochem.*, **110**: 273–278.

Cosman, F., Morrow, B. S., Kopal, M. A., and Bilezikian, J. P. (1988). Control of phospholipase C activity in ROS cells homogenates by GTP and Calcium. *J. Bone Min. Res.*, 3 S, Abstr., **164**: 109.

Dewhirst, F. E., Ago, J. M. and Stashenko, P. (1988). Phosphoinositide metabolism stimulated by PTH and Il-1 in UMR-106 osteoblast cell line. *J. Bone Min. Res.*, 3 S, Abstr., **167**: 110.

Dougherty, W. J. (1983). Ca-enriched amorphous mineral deposits associated with the plasma membranes of chondrocytes and matrix vesicles of rat epiphyseal cartilage. *Calcif. Tissue Int.*, **35**: 486–495.

Drivdahl, R. H., Liu, C-C., Baylink, D. J. (1984). Regulation of bone repletion in rats subjected to varying low-calcium stress. *Am. J. Physiol.*, **246R**: 190–196.

Elzanowski, A., Barker, W. C., Hunt, L. T., and Seibel-Ross, E. (1988). Cystatin domains alpha-2-HS-glycoprotein and fetuin. *FEBS Lett.*, **227**: 167–170.

Exton, J. H. (1988). Mechanisms of action of calcium-mobilizing agonists: some variations on a young theme. *FASEB J.*, **2**: 2670–2676.

Farndale, R. W., Sandy, J. R., Atkinson, S., Pennington, S. R., Meghji, S., and Meikle, M. C. (1988). Parathyroid hormone and prostaglandin E2 stimulate both inositol phosphates and cyclic AMP accumulation in mouse osteoblast cultures. *Biochem. J.*, **252**: 263–268.

Frelin, C., Vigne, R., Ladoux, A., and Lazdunski, M. (1988). The regulation of the intracellular pH in cells from vertebrates. *Eur. J. Biochem.*, **174**: 3–14.

Fueredi-Milhofer, H., Purgaric', B., Brecevic', Lj., and Pavkovic', N. (1971). Precipitation of calcium phosphates from electrolyte solutions. *Calcif. Tissue Res.*, **8**: 142–153.

Gay, C. V. and Schraer, H. (1975). Frozen thin-sections of rapidly forming bone: bone cell ultrastructure. *Calcif. Tissue Res.*, **19**: 39–49.

Geisow, M. J. and Walker, J. H. (1986). New proteins involved in cell regulation by Ca^{2+} and phospholipids. *TIBS*, **11**: 420–423.

Greenberg-Sepersky, S. M. and Simons, R. E. (1984). Cation gradient dependence of the steps in thrombin stimulation of human platelets. *J. Biol. Chem.*, **259**: 1502–1508.

Hall, B. K. (1987). Earliest evidence of cartilage and bone development in embryonic life. *Clin. Orthop. Rel. Res.*, **225**: 255–272.

Hermann-Erlee, M. P. M. and Konijn, T. M. (1970). Effect of parathyroid extract on cyclic AMP content of embryonic mouse calvaria. *Nature*, **227**: 177–178.

Hermann-Erlee, M. P. M., Van der Meer, J. M., Loewik, C. W. G. M., Van Leeuwen, J. P. T. M., and Boonekamp, P. M. (1988). Different roles for calcium and cyclic AMP in the action of PTH: studies in bone explants and isolated bone cells. *Bone*, **9**: 93–100.

Hesch, R. D., Brabant, G., Rittinghaus, E. F., Atkinson, M. J., and Harms, H. (1988). Pulsatile secretion of parathyroid hormone and its action on a Type I and Type II PTH receptor: a hypothesis for understanding osteoporosis. *Calcif. Tissue Int.*, **42**: 341–344.

Holtrop, M. E. and Weinger, J. M. (1975). Ultrastructural evidence for a transport system in bone. In: *Calcium, Parathyroid Hormone and the Calcitonins*, Excerpta Medica, Amsterdam, 365–374.

Howard, A. D., Berger, J., Gerber, L., Familletti, P., and Udenfriend, S. (1987). Characterisation of the phosphatidyl inositol-glycan membrane anchor of human placental alkaline phosphatase. *Proc. Natl. Acad. Sci. U.S.A.*, **84**: 6055–6059.

Hruska, K. A., Goligorsky, M., Scoble, J., Tsutsumi, M. T., West-book, S., and Moskowitz, D. (1986). Effects of parathyroid hormone on cytosolic calcium in renal proximal tubular primary cultures. *Am. J. Physiol.*, **251**: F188–F198.

Hruska, K. A., Moskowitz, D., Esbrit, P., Civitelli, R., and Huskey, M. (1987). Stimulation of inositol triphosphate and diacylglycerol production in renal tubular cells by parathyroid hormone. *J. Clin. Invest.*, **78**: 230–239.

Hurvitz, S., Fishman, S., Bar, A., Pines, M., Riesenfeld, G., and Talpaz, H. (1983). Simulation of calcium homeostasis: modeling and parameter estimation. *Am. J. Physiol.*, **245**: R664–R672.

Iida-Klein, A., Varlotta, V., and Hahn, TY. J. (1988). The effects of parathyroid hormone and insulin on protein kinase C in UMR-106 osteosarcoma cells. *J. Bone Min. Res.,* 3 S, Abstr., **165**: 110.

Ives, H. E. and Rector Jr., F. C. (1984). Proton transport and cell function. *J. Clin. Invest.,* **73**: 285–290.

Jones, D. B. and Scholuebbers, G. (1987). Evidence that phospholipase C mediates mechanical stress response in bone. *Calcif. Tissue Int.,* 41 S. Abstr. Workshop on biology and regulation of bone metabolism: clinical significance. 93.

Kashiva, H. K. (1970). Calcium phosphate in osteogenic cells. *Clin. Orthop.,* **70**: 200–211.

Kashiva, H. K. (1971). Mineralized spherules in the cells and matrix of calcifying cartilage from developing bone. *Anat. Rec.,* **170**: 119–127.

Kawase, T. and Suzuki, A. (1988). Phosphatidic acid induced Ca^{2+} mobilisation in osteoblasts. *J. Biochem.,* **103**: 581–582.

Kinsella, J. L. and Aronson, P. S. (1981). Interaction of NH^+ and Li^+ with the renal microvillus membrane Na^+-H^{4+} exchanger. *Am. J. Physiol.,* **241**: C220–C226.

Krieger, N. S. and Tashjian, Jr., A. H. (1980). PTH stimulates bone resorption via a Na^+-Ca^{2+} exchange mechanism. *Nature,* **287**: 843–845.

Leeb-Lundberg, L. M. F., Cotecchia, S., Lomasney, J. W., DeBernardis, J. F., Lefkowitz, R. J., and Caron, M. G. (1985). Phorbol esters promote alpha 1-adrenergic receptor phosphorylation and receptor uncoupling from inositol phospholipid metabolism. *Proc. Natl. Acad. Sci. U.S.A.,* **82**: 5651–5655.

Lehninger, A. L. (1970). Mitochondria and calcium ion transport. *Biochem. J.,* **119**: 129–138.

Levinskas, G. J. and Neuman, W. F. (1985). The solubility of bone mineral. I. Solubility studies of synthetic hydroxyapatite. *J. Phys. Chem.,* **59**: 164–168.

Loewik, C. W. G. M., Olthof, A. A., van Leeuwen, J. P. T. M., van Zeeland, J. K., and Hermann-Erlee, M. P. M. (1988). Induction of ornithine decarboxylase activity in isolated chicken osteoblasts by PTH: the role of cAMP and calcium. *Calcif. Tissue Int.,* **43**: 7–18.

Loewik, C. W. G. M., van Leeuwen, J. P. T. M., van der Meer, J. M., van Zeeland, J. K., Scheven, B. A. A., and Hermann-Erlee, M. P. M. (1985). A two-receptor model for the action of parathyroid hormone on osteoblasts: a role for intracellular free calcium and cAMP. *Cell Calcium,* **6**: 311–326.

MacLennan, D. H., Cambell, K. P., and Reithmeyer, R. A. F. (1983). In: *Calcium and Cell Function,* Vol. IV, Cheung, W. Y., Ed., Academic Press, New York, 151–173.

Madshus, I. H. (1988). Regulation of intracellular pH in eukaryotic cells. *Biochem. J.,* **250**: 1–8.

Majerus, P. W., Connolly, T. M., Bansal, V. S., Inhorn, R. C., Ross, T. S. and Lips, D. L. (1988). Inositol phosphates: synthesis and degradation. *J. Biol. Chem.,* **263**: 3051–3054.

Markowitz, M., Rotkin, L., and Rosen, J. F. (1981). Circadian rhythms of blood minerals in humans. *Science,* **213**: 672–674.

Marotti, G. (1988). Ruolo delle cellule ossee nella regolazione dell'omeostasi fosfocalcica. *Giornale Clin. Med.,* **68**: 243–261.

Matthews, J. L., Talmage, R. V., and Doppelt, R. (1980). Responses of osteocyte lining cell complex, the bone cell unit, to calcitonin. *Metab. Bone Dis. Rel. Res.,* **2**: 113–122.

Matthews, J. L., Talmage, R. V., Martin, J. H., and Davis, W. L. (1977). Osteoblasts, bone lining cells and the bone fluid compartment. *Bone Histomorphometry,* Armour-Montagu, Paris, 239–247.

Mayr, G. W. (1988). Inositol phosphates: structural components, regulators and signal transducers of the cell — a review. *Topics in Biochemistry,* Boehringer, Mannheim, 1–18.

McCormack, J. C. and Denton, R. M. (1986). Ca^{2+} as a second messenger within mitochondria. *TIBS,* **11**: 258–262.

Mendoza, S. A., Wigglesworth, N. M., and Rozengurt, E. (1980). Vasopressin rapidly stimulates Na^+ entry and Na-K pump activity in quiescent cultures of mouse 3T3 cells. *J. Cell Physiol.,* **105**: 153–162.

Michell, R. H. (1975). Inositol phospholipids and cell surface receptor function. *Biochim. Biophys. Acta,* **415**: 81–147.

Moolenar, W. H. Kruijer, W., Tilly, B. C., Verlaan, I., Bierman, A. J., and de Laat, S. W. (1986). Growth factor-like action of phosphatidic acid. *Nature (London)*, **323**: 171–173.

Moore, R. D. (1979). Elevation of intracellular pH by insulin in frog skeletal muscle. *Biochem. Biophys. Res. Commun.*, **91**: 900–904.

Muallem, S., Schoeffield, M., Pandol, S., and Sachs, G. (1985). Inositol triphosphate modification of ion transport in rough endoplasmic reticulum. *Proc. Natl. Acad. Sci. U.S.A.*, **82**: 4433–4437.

Mundy, G. R. and Roodman, G. (1987). Osteoclast ontogeny and function. In: *Bone and Mineral Research*, Vol. V, Peck, W. A., Ed., Elsevier, Amsterdam, 209–279.

Neuman, M. W. and Neuman, W. F. (1980). On the measurement of water compartments, pH and gradient in calvaria. *Calcif. Tissue Int.*, **31**: 135–145.

Neuman, W. F. (1982). Blood:bone equilibrium. *Calcif. Tissue Int.*, **34**: 117–120.

Neuman, W. F. and Bareham, B. J. (1975). Evidence for the presence of secondary calcium phosphate in bone and its stabilisation by acid production. *Calcif. Tissue Res.*, **18**: 161–172.

Neuman, W. F., Diamond, A. G., and Neuman, M. W. (1980). Blood/bone disequilibrium. IV. Reciprocal effect of calcium and phosphate concentrations on ion fluxes. *Calcif. Tissue Int.*, **32**: 229–236.

Neuman, W. F. and Neuman, M. W. (1958). *The Chemical Dynamics of Bone Mineral*, University of Chicago Press, Chicago.

Neuman, W. F., Neuman, M. W., Diamond, A. G., Menanteau, J. and Gibbons, W. S. (1982). Blood:bone disequilibrium. VI. Studies of the solubility characteristics of brushite:apatite mixtures and their stabilisation by noncollagenous proteins of bone. *Calcif. Tissue Int.*, **34**: 149–157.

Nijweide, P. J. and Van der Plas, A. (1979). Regulation of calcium transport in isolated periosteal cells, effects of hormones and metabolic inhibitors. *Calcif. Tissue Int.*, **29**: 155–161.

Nishizuka, Y. (1986). Studies and perspectives of protein kinase C. *Science*, **233**: 305–312.

Nordin, B. E. C. (1976). *Calcium, Phosphate and Magnesium Metabolism*, Churchill Livingstone, Edinburgh, 41.

Norimatsu, H. C., VanderWiel, C. J., and Talmage, R. V. (1978). Morphological support of a role for cell lining bone surfaces in maintenance of plasma calcium concentration. *Clin. Orthop. Rel. Res.*, **138**: 254–262.

Owen, N. E. and Villereal, M. L. (1983). Lys-bradykinin stimulates Na^+ influx and DNA synthesis in cultured human fibroblasts. *Cell*, **32**: 979–985.

Panfili, E., Sottocasa, G. L., Sandri, G., and Liut, G. (1980). The Ca^{2+}-binding glycoprotein as the site of metabolic regulation of mitochondrial Ca^{2+} movements. *Eur. J. Biochem.*, **105**: 205–210.

Parfitt, A. M. (1979). Equilibrium and disequilibrium hypercalcemia: new light on an old concept. *Metab. Bone Dis. Rel. Res.*, **1**: 279–293.

Parfitt, A. M. (1981). The integration of skeletal and mineral homeostasis. In: *Osteoporosis — Recent Advances in Pathogenesis and Treatment*, DeLuca, H. F., Frost, H., Jee, W., Johnston, C., and Parfitt, M., Eds., University Park Press, Baltimore, 115–126.

Parfitt, A.M. (1984). The cellular basis of bone remodeling. The quantum concept reexamined in light of recent advances in cell biology of bone. *Calcif. Tissue Int.*, **36**: S37–S45.

Parfitt, A. M. (1987). Bone and plasma calcium homeostasis. *Bone*, **8**: S1–S8.

Parfitt, A. M. and Kleerekoper, M. (1980). The divalent ion homeostatic system. Physiology and metabolism of calcium, phosphorus, magnesium and bone. In: *Clinical Disorders of Fluid and Electrolyte Metabolism*, 3rd ed. Maxwell, M. and Kleeman, C. R., Eds., McGraw-Hill, New York, 269–398.

Potts, Jr., J. T., Kronenberg, H. K., and Rosenblatt, M. (1982). Parathyroid hormone: chemistry, biosynthesis and mode of action. *Adv. Protein Chem.*, **35**: 323–396.

Pugliarello, M. C., Vittur, F., de Bernard, B., Bonucci, E., and Ascenzi, A. (1970). Chemical modifications in osteones during calcification. *Calcif. Tissue Res.*, **5**: 108–114.

Putney, Jr., J. W. (1986). A model for receptor-regulated calcium entry. *Cell Calcium*, **7:** 1–12.

Putney, Jr., J. W., Weiss, S. J., Van De Walle, C. M., and Haddas, R. A. (1980). Is phosphatidic acid a calcium ionophore under neurohumoral control? *Nature (London)*, **284**: 345–347.

Ratan, R. R. and Shelanski, M. L. (1986). Calcium and the regulation of mitotic events. *TIBS*, **11**: 456–459.

Redhead, C. R. and Baker, P. F. (1988). Control of intracellular pH in rat calvarial osteoblasts: coexistence of both chloride-bicarbonate and sodium-hydrogen exchange. *Calcif. Tissue Int.*, **42**: 237–242.

Remagen, W., Hoehling, H. J., Hall,, T. A., and Caesar, R. (1969). Electron microscopical and microprobe observation on the cell sheath of stimulated osteocytes. *Calcif. Tissue Res.*, **4**: 60–68.

Russell, R. G. G. and Fleisch, H. (1976). Pyrophosphate and diphosphonates. The biochemistry and physiology of bone. In *Calcification and Physiology*, Vol. IV, Bourne, G. H., Ed., Academic Press, New York, 61–104.

Scarpace, P. J. and Neuman, W. F. (1973). Quantitation of Ca^{2+} fluxes in chick calvaria. *Biochim. Biophys. Acta*, **323**: 267–275.

Seifter, J. L. and Aronson, P. S. (1986). Properties and physiological roles of the plasma membrane sodium-hydrogen exchanger. *J. Clin. Invest.*, **78**: 859–864.

Shen, V., Kohler, G., and Peck, W. A. (1983). A high affinity, calmodulin-responsive (Ca^{2+} + Mg^{2+})-ATPase in isolated bone cells. *Biochim. Biophys. Acta*, **727**: 230–238.

Siffert, W. and Akkerman, J. W. (1988a). Na^+/H^+ exchange as a modulator of platelet activation. *TIBS*, **13**: 148–151.

Siffert, W. and Akkerman, J. W. (1988b). Protein kinase C enhances Ca^{2+} mobilisation in human platelets by activating Na^+/H^+ exchange. *J. Biol. Chem.*, **263**: 4223–4227.

Smith, J. B. and Brock, T. A. (1983). Analysis of angiotensin-stimulated sodium transport in cultured smooth muscle cells from rat aorta. *J. Cell Physiol.*, **114**: 284–290.

Sottocasa, G. L., Sandri, G., Panfili, E., and de Bernard, B. (1971). A glycoprotein located in the intermembrane space of rat liver mitochondria. *FEBS Lett.*, **17**: 100–105.

Stagni, N., Furlan, G., Carli, F., Vittur, F., and de Bernard, B. (1976). Influence of the cartilage Ca^{2+}-binding glycoprotein on precipitation of calcium phosphate "in vitro". Symp. CEMO-I. Exploration morphologique et fonctionelle du squelette. *Geneve. Ed. Med. et Hygiene*, 194–199.

Talmage, R. V. (1970). Morphological and physiological considerations in a new concept of calcium transport in bone. *Am. J. Anat.*, **129**: 467–476.

Talmage, R. V., Cooper, C. W., and Toverud, S. U. (1983). The physiological significance of calcitonin. In: *Bone and Mineral Research/1*, Peck, W. A., Ed., Excerpta Medica, Amsterdam, 74–143.

Talmage, R. V., Matthews, J. L., Martin, J. H., Kennedy, J. W., Davis, W. L. and Roycroft, Jr., J. H. (1975). Calcitonin, phosphate, and the osteocyte-osteoblast bone cell unit. In: *Calcium Regulating Hormones*, Talmage, R. V., Owen, M., and Parsons, J. A., Eds., Elsevier, New York, 284–296.

Terepka, A. R., Colemn, J. R., Ambrecht, H. J. and Gunter, T. E. (1976). Transcellular transport of calcium. *Calcium in Biological Systems*, Symposia of the Society for Experimental Biology, Cambridge University Press, 117–140.

Termine, J. D. (1983). Osteonectin and other newly described proteins in developing bone. In: *Bone and Mineral Research/1*, Peck, W. A., Ed., Excerpta Medica, Amsterdam, 144–156.

Termine, J. D., Peckauskas, R. A., and Posner, A. S. (1970). Calcium phosphate formation in vitro. II. Effects of environment on amorphous-crystalline transformation. *Arch. Biochem. Biophys.*, **140**: 318–325.

Teti, A. and Zambonin Zallone, A. (1987). A working hypothesis: calcium concentration controls directly osteoclast activity in calcium regulation and bone metabolism. In: *Basic and Clinical Aspects*, Cohen, D. V., Martin, T. J., and Meunier, P. J., Eds., Excerpta Medica, Amsterdam, 358–363.

Triffitt, T. T., Gebauer, U., Ashton, B. A., Owen, M. E., and Reynolds, T. T. (1976). Origin of plasma alpha HS-glycoprotein and its accumulation in bone. *Nature (London)*, **262**: 226–227.

Tuan, R. S. (1980). Biosynthesis of calcium-binding protein of chick embryonic chorioallonoic membrane: in vitro organ culture and cell-free translation. *Cell Calcium*, **1**: 411–429.

Tuan, R. S., Scott, W. A., and Cohn, Z. W. (1978). Purification and characterisation of calcium binding protein from chick chorioallantoic membrane. *J. Biol. Chem.*, **253**: 1011–1016.

Vaes, G. (1988). Cellular biology and biochemical mechanism of bone resorption. *Clin. Orthop.*, **231**: 239–271.

VanderWiel, C. J. and Talmage, R. V. (1981). Ultrastructural and physiological evidence for calcitonin-induced postprandial calcium storage in bone of rats. *Calcif. Tissue Int.*, **33**: 417–424.

Volpe, P., Krause, K. H., Hashimoto, S., Zorzato, F., Pozzan, T., Meldolesi, J., and Lew, D. P. (1988). "Calciosome", a cytoplasmic organelle: the inositol 1,4,5,-triphosphate-sensitive Ca^{2+} store of nonmuscle cells? *Proc. Natl. Acad. Sci. U.S.A.*, **85**: 1091–1095.

Weiner, S. and Hood, H. L. (1975). Soluble protein of the organic matrix of mollusk shells: a potential template for shell. *Science,* **190**: 987–989.

Weiner, S. and Traub, W. (1984). Macromolecules in mollusk shells and their functions in biomineralisation. *Philos. Trans. R. Soc. London,* **304B**: 425–434.

Weisbrode, S. E., Capen, C. C., and Nagode, L. A. (1974). Influence of parathyroid hormone on ultrastructural and enzymatic changes induced by vitamin D in bone of thyroparathyroidectomized rats. *Lab. Invest.,* **30**: 768–794.

Wheeler, A. P., Rusenko, K. W., George, J. W., and Sikes, C. S. (1987). Evaluation of calcium binding by molluscan shell organ matrix and its relevance to biomineralization. *Comp. Biochem. Physiol.,* **87B**: 953–960.

Williams, G. and Sallis, J. D. (1979). Structure activity relationship of hydroxyapatite formation. *Biochem. J.,* **184**: 181–184.

Wong, G. L. (1986). Skeletal effects of PTH. In: *Bone and Mineral Research/4*, Peck, W. A., Ed., Excerpta Medica, Amsterdam, 103–130.

Yamaguchi, D. T., Hahn, T. J., Iida-Klein, A., Kleeman, C. R., and Muallem, S. (1987). Parathyroid hormone-activated calcium channels in an osteoblast-like clonal osteosarcoma cell line. *J. Biol. Chem.,* **262**: 7711–7718.

Zambonin Zallone, A., Teti, A., and Primavera, M. V. (1982). Isolated osteoclasts in primary culture: first observations on structure and survival in culture media. *Anat. Embryol.,* **165**: 405–413.

Zanetti, M., Camerotto, R., Romeo, D., and de Bernard, B. (1982). Active extrusion of Ca^{2+} from epiphyseal chondrocytes of normal and rachitic chickens. *Biochem. J.,* **202**: 303–307.

Zanetti, M., de Bernard, B., Jontell, M., and Linde, A. (1981). Ca^{2+}-binding studies of the phosphoprotein from rat-incisor dentine. *Eur. J. Biochem.,* **113**: 541–545.

5

Energy Metabolism in Bone

IRVING M. SHAPIRO and JOHN C. HASELGROVE
Department of Biochemistry
School of Dental Medicine
University of Pennsylvania
Philadelphia, Pennsylvania

Introduction

The focus of this chapter is to examine energy metabolism by the cells of bone. We will examine the energy requirements of hard tissue cells in terms of "housekeeping" as well as specific biosynthetic functions. A priori, it should be noted that much of the metabolic energy that is generated by bone cells is utilized for the formation and maintenance of the extracellular matrix. Numerous studies have demonstrated that biosynthesis of matrix proteins and glycosoaminoglycans is dependent on a supply of energy-rich molecules. Nucleoside triphosphates are required for early transcriptional and translational events as well as serving as a requirement for the translocation of molecules across cellular membranes. Energy-rich compounds are needed for posttranslational modifications of synthesized macromolecules. Details of these requirements are described elsewhere in the book (see Chapter 3 in Volumes 1 and 2). A high percentage of the total energy generated by the cell is required for the maintenance of the functional state of the plasma membrane and the internal membranes of the cell. The cell conserves much of the energy required for transport by coupling together the movement of many permeant species. For example, 30 to 40% of the total energy generated by a red blood cell is used to maintain the concentration of the major intracellular electrolytes.

Common Indices of Energy Metabolism in Bone

In thermodynamic terms, energy is measured by the free energy change $(-\Delta G)$ of a system. Frequently, however, when dealing with multicompartment biological systems, it is more convenient to use a less rigorous approach in which the energy status is related to the number of molecules containing an energy-rich bond. Hydrolysis (or cleavage) of these bonds releases the available free energy that can then be used for a variety of metabolic purposes. Table 1 provides a partial list of common high energy molecules, while Fig. 1 outlines some of the pathways by which these molecules are generated.

In this review we refer to ATP as the major energy-rich molecule of the cell. With very few exceptions, cellular energy demands are met by hydrolysis (or phosphorolysis) of ATP to ADP and inorganic phosphate (Pi):

$$ATP + H_2O = ADP + PO + H$$

ATP is utilized in the cytoplasm, the endoplasmic reticulum and the nucleus to drive a wide range of endothermic reactions.

ATP can be regenerated in a number of ways. It can be rapidly synthesized from creatine phosphate (PCr) using the enzyme creatine phosphokinase.

$$ADP + PCr = ATP + Cr$$

Somjen and her colleagues (Somjen $et\ al.$, 1984, 1985, 1987) have documented

Table 1.
High-Energy Molecules

Energy-Rich Metabolites of Bone	
Compound (reaction)	$-\Delta G$ (kcal/mol)
ATP ($\rightarrow$ ADP)	-7.3
ADP ($\rightarrow$ AMP)	-7.3
NADH ($\rightarrow$ NAD)	-52.7
Acetyl CoA ($\rightarrow$ OAA)	-7.7
PEP ($\rightarrow$ pyruvate)	-14.3
Creatine P ($\rightarrow$ creatine)	-10.3

Commonly Used Indices of Energy Status	
ATP + ADP + AMP	(adenine nucleotide content)
ATP/ADP.Pi	(phosphorylation potential)
ATP + 0.5ADP/(ATP + ADP + AMP)	(energy charge ratio)
NAD/NADH	(redox ratio)
Oxygen uptake rate	

evidence of this system in bone cells. However, as there is only a limited supply of creatine phosphate in the cell and as ATP is required for its synthesis from creatine (Cr), this system is of limited importance as a long-term energy source. The major system for generating ATP in the aerobic cell is by oxidative phosphorylation reactions in the mitochondria (Fig. 1).

$$ADP + Pi + H = ATP + H_2O$$

It is important to note that the cell regulates the level of ATP very closely. Accordingly, when the energy needs of the cell increase, there is a concomitant elevation in the oxidative metabolic rate. An integral part of the control mechanism is that changes in the relative concentrations of ATP, ADP, AMP and the other nucleotides directly influence the rate of glycolysis, mitochondrial oxidative phosphorylation, fatty acid synthesis and oxidation, gluconeogenesis and urea synthesis and the activity of the pentose phosphate shunt.

Studies of a wide variety of tissues indicate that *in situ*, a major portion of the total energy needs of the cell can be generated by oxidative catabolism of carbohydrates, amino acids and lipids. Following metabolic processing by cytosolic enzymes, small carbon fragments of these primary nutrients are degraded by mitochondrial enzyme clusters in a series of linked dehydrogenation and decarboxylation reactions. As these compounds undergo dehydrogenation, co-enzymes such as NAD become reduced. The free energy of formation of this reduced pyridine nucleotide (NADH) can then be utilized to form ATP by oxidative phosphorylation. Since this process is dependent on the oxygen supply, measurement of the rate of oxygen uptake provides a useful guide to the energy demands of the cell (see Table 1).

Transport of ATP out of the mitochondria to the sites of use takes place

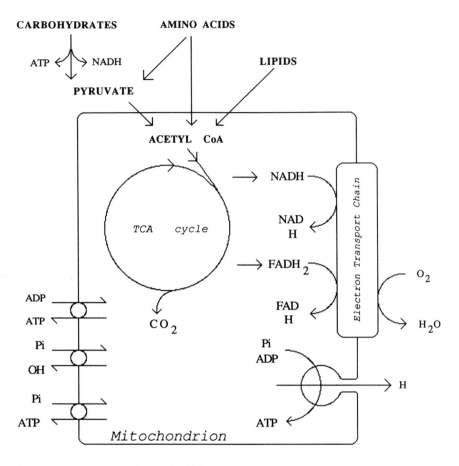

Fig. 1 Major pathways of the cell which produce the high-energy molecules NADH, FADH$_2$ and ATP. NADH and FADH$_2$ are used to produce ATP by oxygen-requiring steps in the mitochondrion. Degradation of carbohydrates in the cytosol does not require oxygen and produces only a small amount of ATP and NADH.

by an electrogenic exchange on a specific transporter protein complex (Klingenberg, 1989). Recently, another transporter system has been described that mediates the transfer of ATP-Mg and Pi (Aprille, 1988). The activity of this transporter and the direction of transport appears to be influenced by hormones and calcium ions. Even a modest increase in cell calcium has been shown to influence cellular oxidative activity and the energy status of the cell.

The cell can be viewed as a multicompartment system in which each organelle can exist at a different energetic state. Most authorities however, pay special attention to the metabolic status of the mitochondrion, as most of the cell's ATP is synthesized in this organelle. For this reason, a considerable number of studies have been devoted to determining the energetic state of the mitochondrion. In the laboratory, this is performed by measuring a number of different parameters. These include determination of the relative concentrations of selected energy-rich molecules such as the pyridine and adenine nucleotides as well as assessment of oxygen utilization (see Table 1).

Ion Translocation across Membranes

Cells participate in the mineralization process in a variety of ways, all of which require the expenditure of metabolic energy. Bone cells synthesize a specific organic matrix that favors and facilitates ion cluster formation and mineral development. Cells also remove circulating as well as resident inhibitors of mineral formation. Recent evidence indicates that hard tissue cells regulate mineral deposition by directing the transport of ions from the blood stream and extracellular fluid to selected sites in the matrix. Cells that have been identified with this latter process are osteoblasts, endothelial cells, perivascular cells and hypertrophic chondrocytes of the endochondral growth plate. As the transport of calcium ions to the calcification front is a major energy-requiring event in the mineralization process, we will begin this section of the chapter by reviewing cellular mechanisms for the accumulation and transport of calcium and consider relevant processes that may lead to ion release.

It may be argued that one of the most important functions of bone cells is to regulate the flow of calcium ions from the vascular system into bone and the transport of ions from bone into the systemic circulation. While it is likely that osteoblasts are active participants in both processes, other cells such as osteoclasts, osteocytes and lining cells may play a more important role in controlling calcium influx into bone. Recent work by Streeten et al., (1989) indicates that bone endothelial cells may function in this manner. Moreover, Rouleau et al., (1988) reported that there appears to be populations of cells in bone which are neither osteoblasts nor osteocytes, but which responded to calcium mobilizing signals of parathyroid hormone.

There are few details of the mechanisms utilized by the cells of bone to regulate calcium flow. It is necessary, therefore, to extrapolate to bone the results of investigations performed on a variety of soft tissues. This approach is not unreasonable as eukaryotic cells appear to share a number of common and evolutionary successful biochemical mechanisms. However, one important caveat exists: that is, in noncalcified tissues, cells do not function to produce a mineral phase — instead calcium ions are utilized at micromolar levels to modulate a wide range of activities that include gene transcription and enzyme function. In consequence, the total calcium flux is small. So, while studies of heart and skeletal muscle can be used to provide general information on transport processes and while hard and soft tissues may share common underlying mechanisms, it is likely that calcium transport in bone may depend on transport pathways that are either absent from soft tissue

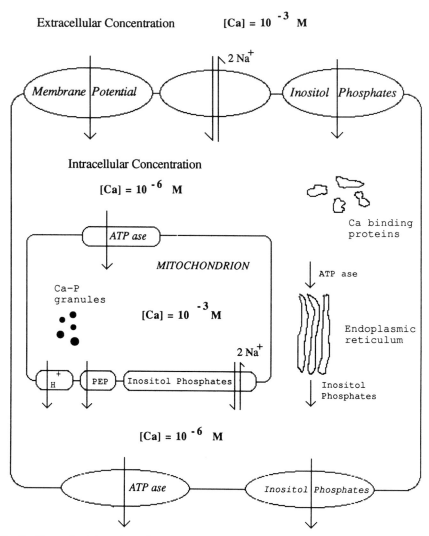

Extracellular Concentration $[Ca] = 10^{-3}$ M

Fig. 2 Flow of calcium through a cell. The diagram indicates the flow schematically as if calcium flows through the cell from top to bottom. Calcium levels in the cell are controlled by cell membrane, the endoplasmic reticulum, mitochondrion and calcium binding proteins. The factors controlling each step are indicated in italics beside the arrows. Unlabeled arrows indicate the flow of Ca^{2+} ions: coporters and antiporters are indicated specifically.

cells or of minor import. Fig. 2 shows schematically the major factors which influence the flow of calcium into, out of and within cells.

It is important to recognize that there are profound differences in the intra- and extracellular calcium concentration. In all tissues, the external calcium ion concentration is in the millimolar range, while the cytosolic free calcium concentration is maintained at micromolar levels. Accordingly, there is a thousandfold difference in the calcium ion concentration across the plasma membrane (Carafoli, 1987). That similar gradients exist in bone is supported by findings from a number of workers. Lieberherr (1987) used the same technique and found that the free calcium concentration of confluent osteoblast cultures was greater than 135 nM. This value was comparable to levels found in soft tissue cells and chondrocytes (100 to 250 nM) (Tsien, 1981, Star et al., 1987). Of considerable importance to the function of the bone cell was the observation that the calcium level was responsive to bone-resorbing factors (Lowik et al., 1985) and possibly to the extracellular potassium concentration (Boland et al., 1986).

Lieberherr (1987) showed that the cytosolic calcium concentration could be transiently increased by the metabolites of vitamin D. The transience occurred at physiological hormone concentrations and was rapid (less than 1 minute). Because the action was so fast, it is likely that the hormone action was at the level of the cell membrane and did not involve the genome. There is now intense interest in osteoblast membrane physiology: studies by Ypey et al., (1988) show that embryonic cultured osteoblasts have voltages activated calcium channels that exhibit short transient hyperpolarizing responses to hormones, while studies of ROS 17/2.8 cells indicate that there may also be a long hyperpolarizing response (Ferrier et al., 1985, 1986, 1987, 1988).

In many excitable tissues, gated channels that are specific for select divalent cations have been characterized. In most cases, the activity of the gates is regulated by the membrane potential. Channels of this sort have been described in bone by Chesnoy-Marchais and Fritsch (1988). An antiporter coupled sodium-calcium exchange system is present in bone and other nonexcitable tissues. The system is ATP-dependent and serves to transport calcium ions into the cell in exchange for sodium (Blaustein, 1977). The third type of transporter is a unidirectional plasma membrane calcium ATP-ase which pumps calcium out of the cell (Schatzmann and Vincenzi, 1969, Pershadsingh and McDonald, 1980). The transport system is active at cytosolic calcium levels (Km for calcium is below 1 μM) and according to Nijiweide and Van der Plas (1979), this system, or one that is similar to it, requires ATP for maximum activity. Akisaka et al., (1988) demonstrated histochemically the existence of an ATP-dependent enzyme system in the apical and lateral portions of the plasma membrane of osteoblasts. This observation was confirmed by Shen et al., (1983) using osteoblast-enriched cultures. In a later study of plasma membrane preparations of human and rat osteoblast cell lines, a high-affinity plasma membrane calcium magnesium ATP-ase that had a Km in the nanomolar range was chemically characterized (Shen et al., 1988).

While details of the function of the membrane ATP-ase are not fully understood, studies from other tissues provide some interesting information about this enzyme. The enzyme system is activated by a transient elevation of the cytosolic calcium ion concentration. Agonists that cause a transient change in intracellular calcium levels do so by activating the phosphatidyl-inositol pathway. It appears likely that inositol polyphosphates and diacyl-glycerol elevate the cytosolic calcium concentration by stimulating release of calcium ions from the endoplasmic reticulum and by increasing the rate of entry of calcium into the cell across the plasma membrane. The enzyme is stimulated by calmodulin (Carafoli, 1987). Treatment of bone cells with trifluoroperazine — a calmodulin inhibitor — produces a dose-dependent inhibition of ATP-ase activity.

Studies of calcium homeostasis in confluent calvarial osteoblast cultures indicate that the cytosolic calcium concentration is maintained through the combined activity of the plasma membrane calcium pump, the endoplasmic reticulum and the mitochondria. Lieberherr (1987) showed that prostaglan-din (PGE_2), parathyroid hormone and 1,25-dihydroxyvitamin D_3 caused a transient elevation in the cytosolic calcium level. The increase is due to an elevation in the rate of calcium influx into the cell from the extracellular fluid as well as release of calcium from the endoplasmic reticulum. Lieberherr considers that as the hormones mobilize calcium from the endoplasmic re-ticulum they "protect" calcium stored in the mitochondrion. These obser-vations are in line with current thinking concerning the importance of the endoplasmic reticulum in maintaining calcium homeostasis in the cell. The protective effect on the mitochondrion raises the question: does this organelle have a specific role to play in bone formation? Many workers in the field believe that mitochondria of hard tissue cells may help to initiate the cal-cification of bone.

Despite the regulatory systems described above, the calcium concentration of the cytosol is not constant. Oscillations, varying from 5 seconds to 1 minute, have been discerned in the cytosolic calcium levels (Prentki et al., 1988). Analysis of factors that control these transients indicates that within the cell there are complex feedback mechanisms that are driven by (a) hormones and other factors that bind to the plasma membrane and cause the formation of inositol 1,4,5-triphosphate and diacylglycerol and (b) the leakage of cal-cium into the cell from the extracellular fluid and on ATP-driven uptake of cytosolic calcium by the endoplasmic reticulum and the mitochondria. These latter membranes have both a high calcium sequestering activity and the ability to release calcium into the cytosol. For a review of mechanisms leading to calcium oscillations within the cell, the reader should consult Berridge and Galione (1988).

Intermediary Metabolism by Bone

Historical

Much of our current knowledge of bone cell metabolism is dependent on the results of studies performed by a limited number of investigators in a

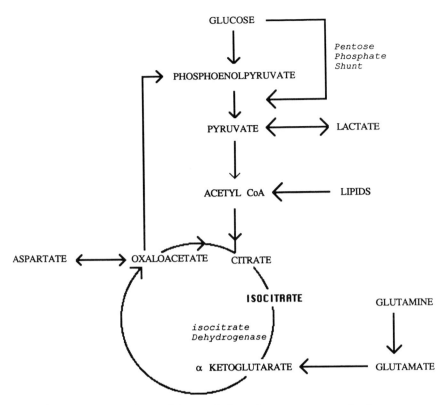

Fig. 3 Overview of some of the metabolic pathways common to all cell types.

five-year period ending in 1964. The aim of those studies was to elucidate the mechanism of energy production by bone cells and to use this knowledge to help explain the mechanism of parathyroid hormone-induced bone resorption. Surprisingly, despite extensive development of tissue and cell culture techniques and detailed knowledge of the mode of action of a number of calciotropic hormones, there have been few attempts since then to either confirm the results of the original studies or to extend current knowledge of bone cell energy metabolism.

The purpose of this section is to review some of the seminal concepts developed during that period and to describe the more recent studies of intermediary metabolism of cultured osteoblasts and embryonic bones. To help follow the ideas expressed in this section, the reader is advised to consult the reaction pathways shown in Fig. 3.

Early studies of bone were aimed at defining the relative importance of glycolytic and mitochondrial pathways of energy generation. In most cases, experiments were performed on endochondral bone chips and bone sections. Thus, the experimental cell populations were very poorly defined and, in retrospect, it is difficult to assess the relative contributions of osteoblasts and contaminating cartilage cells, marrow cells and vascular elements. Other problems with those studies included the use of media which were not optimized for bone cell metabolism, lack of purified hormone preparations, and the use of nonphysiological gas tensions. Nevertheless, those experiments established the following facts which still appear to be valid.

- Bone cells contain the enzyme systems required for anaerobic glycolysis. Bone metabolizes glucose to form lactate — the lactate anion is the major end-product of glucose degradation (Borle et al., 1960b; Cohn and Forscher, 1962).
- The rate of lactate formation is dependent on the medium pH, the lactate concentration and the glucose uptake rate. There is also evidence to indicate that the Pasteur effect might be operative in bone (Cohn and Forscher, 1962).
- Fetal and neonatal bone contain glycogen deposits and these deposits are rapidly depleted as the tissue matures. There is also some evidence to indicate that mature bone has an endogenous supply of glucose (Flanagan and Nichols, 1964).
- Bone cells metabolize glucose through the pentose phosphate shunt. The activity of this pathway, however, is limited. It was estimated that about 10 to 18% of total lactate is synthesized from glucose channeled through the shunt (Borle et al., 1960b).

Neuman et al. (1978), using carefully orientated cranial bones, confirmed many of the observations described above. In addition, they showed that there was a considerable outward flux of lactate from bone. It was speculated that the ion and pH gradient could serve to co-regulate the flow of calcium and phosphate ions to and from the skeleton. It was estimated that as the magnitude of the flux was very large, the skeleton was a major source of total body lactate.

While there has been little disagreement on the major aspects of glucose metabolism, there were conflicting views on the physiological importance of oxidative metabolism by bone cells. The conflict centered around the regulation of citrate formation and the importance of this anion in mediating bone resorption. Some experiments indicated that the effect of a resorptive signal, such as parathyroid hormone, was to increase oxidative activity of bone. It was argued that as the rate of citrate synthesis was elevated, the tricarboxylic acid would raise the blood calcium level by chelating bone calcium and transporting the bound ion into the vascular system (Dixon and Perkins, 1952).

Experiments conducted by Laskin and Engel (1956), Dixon and Perkins (1952) and then Hekkelman (1961) provided support for such a role for bone citrate. These workers claimed that citrate accumulated in bone due to the low activity of isocitrate dehydrogenase. As a result, citrate decarboxylation

Table 2.
Effect of Parathyroid Extract (PTE) on Carbohydrate and Oxidative Metabolism by Bone

	Lactate production	O_2 uptake	Glucose consumption	Citrate production
Control	2.6 ± 0.4	1.1 ± 0.2	1.5	0.04 ± 0.01
PTE-treated	3.4 ± 0.6	1.0 ± 0.2	1.5	0.04 ± 0.01

Note: Rates were measured as μm/hr/mg cell N_2.

From Borle, A. B., Nichols, N., and Nichols, G. (1960). *J. Biol. Chem.*, **235:** 1206–1214. With permission.

was blocked and the citrate anion accumulated. However, it was shown that bone contained the normal complement of mitochondrial oxidative enzymes (Dixon and Perkins, 1952, Laskin and Engel, 1956) and careful measurement of isocitrate dehydrogenase as well as aconitase activities in selected regions of bone did not support the idea that there was a block in the cycle (Van Reen, 1959). Indeed, preparations of bone cells exhibited normal respiration in the presence of Krebs cycle intermediates (Vaes and Nichols, 1961). Subsequently, support for the hypothesis waned as Neuman *et al.*, (1978) pointed out that most of the citrate was bound strongly to the bones' inorganic phase and it was probably synthesized in other tissues of the body.

A more profound area of dispute concerned the mode of action of parathyroid hormone. A number of investigators proposed that the action of the hormone on target tissues was due to stimulation of oxidative metabolism. However, Borle *et al.* (1960) showed that the hormone had a minimal effect on bone metabolism. Although they did report that there was a small increase in the rate of lactate synthesis, there was no appreciable stimulation of the oxygen consumption rate, citrate synthesis, or the rate of production of CO_2 from glucose (Table 2). In terms of energy production, Borle *et al.* (1960) and Cohn and Forscher (1962) clearly demonstrated that bone exhibited very low levels of oxidative activity. Studies by Wolinsky and Cohn (1969) and Chu *et al.* (1971) confirmed that the level of oxidative activity in bone was low. Indeed, they reported that parathyroid extract inhibited the production of CO_2 from glucose.

At this stage, it is worthwhile reporting results of later experiments on this topic performed by Cohn and his colleagues, as they have helped to clarify aspects of the dispute. Using suspensions of cells isolated from mouse calvaria, Wong *et al.* (1977) showed that citrate metabolism was inhibited not only by parathyroid hormone, but also by vitamin D. Moreover, the hormone stimulated the anaerobic glycolytic pathway in osteoblasts (the effect of parathyroid hormone on glycogen metabolism is discussed below). As these workers could separate the osteoblast-like cells from osteoclast-like cells, they were able to show that the hormone only affected the osteoblast-like cells of bone. It was noted that citrate formation as well as the accompanying inhibition in type I collagen synthesis provided a mechanism by which hormones can down-regulate bone formation and disturb the equilibrium between formation and resorption in favor of resorption. Use of the isolated cell system as well as cultured rat bones indicated that the effects described above were closely linked to the hormone-mediated mobilization of calcium from bone (Luben and Cohn, 1976). Finally, it was concluded that parathyroid hormone stimulated the release of free calcium ions, not calcium citrate chelates, from bone.

Glycogen and Glucose

Within the past few years there has been some renewed interest in bone carbohydrate metabolism. Three factors have stimulated this interest. First is the observation that pre-osteoblasts contain large glycogen deposits. Scott and Glimcher (1971) and Stewart et al. (1986) noted that as these cells matured, the glycogen granules decreased in size. The loss of glycogen was coupled with utilization of this complex polysaccharide for energy-requiring functions associated with the synthesis of matrix proteins and the formation of the extracellular mineral. Second, as discussed above, the glycolytic pathway of bone cells appears to be responsive to the presence of parathyroid hormone. Third is the realization that bone is a target tissue for insulin and insulin-like growth factors — indeed, clinically, insulin deficiency has been linked with osteopenia and inhibition of normal bone growth and development.

While a great deal is known of the mechanism of insulin action on target tissues, information on the mode of action of this peptide hormone on bone is very limited. It is important to point out that insulin modulates the activity of a number of different pathways, many of which are tightly linked with carbohydrate metabolism. The hormone controls glycogen formation by regulating the phosphorylation status of glycogen synthase. In muscle, insulin activates a phosphoprotein phosphatase and dephosphorylates the synthase. This event results in stimulation of synthase activity and an increase in glycogenesis.

Using bone cells, Schmid et al. (1982) demonstrated that insulin stimulated the rate of incorporation of glucose into glycogen. It was also found that osteoblast-like cells exhibited a low level of basal glycogen synthase activity that was responsive to insulin. However, when compared to defined target tissues such as liver or muscle, the sensitivity and responsiveness were low (Ituarte et al. 1988).

As mentioned earlier, another agent that modulates glycogen metabolism is parathyroid hormone. In contrast to liver where the hormone stimulated glycogenolysis, in bone, parathyroid hormone promoted glycogenesis through a cAMP mechanism (Schmid et al., 1982). The stimulatory effect appeared to be specific for calvaria cells.

The mechanism that regulates glucose entry into bone and other tissues is poorly understood. In some tissues, glucose transport is related to cAMP synthesis. For example, in adipocytes, stimulation of cAMP formation inhibits glucose uptake. Van Valen and Keck (1988) used forskolin to probe glucose transport mechanism in bone cells. They observed that forskolin, a diterpine, served as a potent and reversible inhibitor of glucose transport that was independent of cAMP levels. To explain the response, they suggested that the diterpine modified the fluidity of the plasma membrane. Accordingly, the change in the rate of glucose transport was due to the forskolin interacting directly with the glucose carrier. Aside from this study there is little information available on the nature of the bone cell glucose carrier.

Lipids

A number of tissues of the body have high lipid requirements and can utilize fatty acids for energy. Before we develop the argument that bone cells may do so, the reader should realize that lipid metabolism is related to both the glycolytic and oxidative energy-generating systems in the cell. Fatty acids can undergo oxidative catabolism to form a two-carbon fragment acetyl CoA. In the presence of adequate quantities of oxaloacetate, this intermediate can then be completely oxidized in the TCA cycle. Oxaloacetate is regenerated in the TCA cycle from malate; it can also be formed from glutamine (see next section). For many tissues, when the rate of lipid oxidation is very high, oxaloacetate is formed by carboxylation of pyruvate.

The importance of lipids in osteoblast function, especially in relationship to the calcification process, has been stressed by a number of authorities (this topic is reviewed in Chapter 4). Few studies have been reported, however, to assess the lipid nutritional requirements of bone or isolated osteoblasts. Experiments conducted on the inhibitory action of diphosphonates on glycolysis, however, indicated that bone could utilize nonglycolytic pathways for energy metabolism. Work performed by Morgan et al. (1973) and Guenther et al. (1979) demonstrated that diphosphonates inhibited the production of lactate and increased the cellular glycogen content while increasing the production of CO_2 from acetate, leucine and citrate. Felix and Fleisch (1981) and Felix et al. (1986) blocked glucose utilization with diphosphonates and showed that both palmitate and octanoate could provide energy for calvarial cells. In a recent report, Adamek et al. (1987) examined the fatty acid requirements of cultured rat calvaria as well as a number of bone cell populations. They showed that palmitate was actively oxidized by all cells, although the osteoblast-like cells had slower rates of lipid oxidation than other populations. They reported that palmitate could undergo mitochondrial oxidative decarboxylation and be degraded to CO_2 and citrate. It was calculated that 40 to 80% of the energy needs of the cell could be obtained from lipid oxidation. As might be expected, lipid metabolism was found to be under hormonal control. Fatty acid oxidation was stimulated by 1,25- and 24,25-dihydroxyvitamin D_3 and it was inhibited by insulin.

Catherwood *et al.* (1988) investigated the requirements of ROS 17/2.8 cells for lipid, especially in their proliferative phase. Removal of lipoproteins from serum decreased the rate of cell proliferation; addition of lipoproteins restored proliferative activity. The addition of lipid to serum-free media permitted a parathyroid hormone-induced change in cAMP levels; this response was further attenuated by 1,25-dihydroxyvitamin D_3. The results of these studies suggested that aside from serving as a fuel for osteoblast energy needs, lipids are important in transduction of hormonal signals and for expression of the osteoblastic phenotype especially during the proliferative phase of the cell cycle.

Glutamine Metabolism by Cells in Culture

Within the past decade there has been an enormous interest in the use of culture techniques for the study of bone cell function. This paradigm has provided many new insights into cellular metabolism as well as providing a defined milieu for examining the effects of hormones, vitamins and nutritional factors on bone formation and resorption. For these reasons it is important to consider the mechanism by which cells generate energy in culture. As we mentioned above, there has been very little data published on bone cells, and much of what we know must be inferred from other cell types. The following comments are confined to considering the metabolism of the two major nutrients of all cultured cells: glucose and the amino acid glutamine. The pathways are outlined in Fig 4. and are described below. They are all common pathways of intermediary metabolism. However, it is of considerable interest to us that the metabolic fluxes in the different paths suggest that there may be a suppression of the activity of citrate-metabolizing enzymes of the TCA cycle. As we mentioned earlier, Dixon and Perkins (1952) came to a similar conclusion about the metabolism of bone cells, although direct measurement of enzyme activities did not support that claim.

Studies by numerous investigators have shown that in culture, cells utilize glucose as a major source of energy. Most of the glucose is degraded by glycolysis to pyruvate and a very high percentage of the pyruvate is reduced to lactate. Of the remainder, a small amount of pyruvate is converted to alanine. Alanine forms a very useful "sink" for amino groups formed by trans- and deamination reactions. The total level of oxidative metabolism of pyruvate via the TCA cycle is limited and cells generate low levels of CO_2. The rate of glucose utilization for lactate, alanine and pyruvate synthesis was 30-fold greater than oxidation to CO_2 (Lanks *et al.*, 1986; Zielke *et al.*, 1980; Reitzer *et al.*, 1979).

Aside from glucose, cultured cells require L-glutamine for energy generation (Eagle, 1959); partial degradation of glutamine results in the formation of intermediates for the synthesis of a number of cellular and extracellular compounds. The importance of this compound and a number of other amino

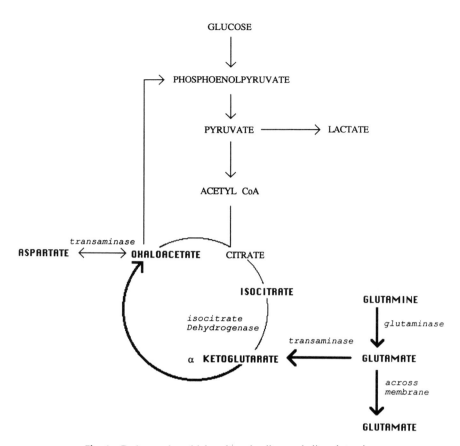

Fig. 4   Pathways by which cultured cells metabolize glutamine.

acids for the normal development of bone was first reported Biggers *et al.* (1961). A more recent study of chondrocyte metabolism by Handley *et al.* (1980) showed that amido groups derived from glutamine were utilized in glycosoaminoglycan synthesis. It is worthwhile noting that one reason for medium glutamine supplementation is that these cells have no measurable glutamine synthetase activity. As osteoblasts have a similar glutamine requirement as chondrocytes, it is likely that they are also deficient in the synthetase.

Experiments performed with a considerable number of cell types have gone a long way towards elucidating how glutamine is oxidized by cells in culture (Reitzer *et al.*, 1979; Zielke *et al.*, 1984; Lanks, 1987; Brand *et al.*, 1987; Lanks and Li, 1988). As with glucose metabolism, there is incomplete oxidation of glutamine and few of the carbon atoms are converted to CO_2. Hence, we need to consider the synthesis of compounds that accumulate within the cells or the medium. Fig. 4 shows that the first step in the metabolism of glutamine is its hydrolysis to glutamate by a phosphate-dependent glutaminase. Over 70% of the glutamate is transaminated to form α-ketoglutarate (although there is some glutamate dehydrogenase activity, this is limited in cells of fibroblast lineage).

Further metabolism of α-ketoglutarate results in the formation of a large number of compounds that include pyruvate, lactate, proline, oxaloacetate, citrate and aspartate. It is likely that α-ketoglutarate undergoes oxidation in mitochondria to form oxaloacetate. Most of the oxaloacetate is then transaminated to form aspartate; a small proportion is converted to citrate. The total amount of aspartate formed is dependent on the glucose concentration of the medium. Studies by Moreadith and Lehninger (1984) using mitochondrial preparations showed that the pyruvate concentration modulates aspartate and citrate formation. As most of the pyruvate is formed through glycolysis it is evident that the glucose concentration of the medium will influence the metabolism of glutamine. Using a number of different fibroblast cell lines, Lanks and Li (1988) noted that the rate of CO_2 production from glucose and glutamine was positively correlated, as was the formation of citrate and aspartate.

To a much lesser extent, oxaloacetate is converted into phosphoenolpyruvate and then pyruvate by phosphoenolpyruvate carboxykinase and pyruvate kinase. As each of these steps and the subsequent synthesis of lactate from pyruvate requires energy, it is not surprising that a limited amount of these compounds are formed. Studies performed by Ishikawa *et al.* (1985) using cultured chondrocytes suggest that a similar pathway may be functional in cartilage. However, whether these pathways are operative in bone cells has not been established.

Oxygen Tension and Bone Energy Metabolism

In bone, as with almost all other tissues, oxygen is required for the generation of metabolic energy (ATP). Oxygen diffuses into mitochondria from the vascular supply and is reduced to water by electrons generated by the cytochrome oxidase system. The rate of oxygen uptake by mitochondria is proportional to the rate at which ADP is phosphorylated to form ATP. It is convenient to consider the oxidative phosphorylation system of the mitochondrion in terms of a multi-substrate Michaelis-Menten enzyme. The rate of the enzyme, v, may then be expressed in terms of the concentrations of the substrates (ADP, Pi, O_2) and of the associated Michaelis-Menten constants (Ka, Kp, Ko, vmax). Thus

$$v = \frac{vmax}{(1 + [ADP]/Ka + [Pi]/Kp + [O_2]/Ko)}$$

The variety of studies on bone cells *in vivo* and *in vitro* which we describe here indicates that anaerobic pathways can play an important role in energy metabolism. This may occur even in experimental conditions which were not designed to be anoxic. It is not clear what factors regulate the choice of pathway, and much work still needs to be done in this area.

Aside from oxidative phosphorylation, oxygen has other functions in the cell. For example, oxygen serves as a substrate for a considerable number of enzyme systems, including those associated with oxygen radical formations. While the importance of oxygen radicals in bone metabolism has yet to be established, it is likely that osteoclasts may utilize these metabolites for the resorption process (Silverton *et al.*, 1989).

Because of the complex architecture of many tissues, the actual oxygen tension varies from site to site, and within a single tissue, considerable differences in oxygen concentration may exist. Measurements performed along sinusoids of the liver lobules indicate that intercellular oxygen values can differ by two orders of magnitude. Factors that regulate the local oxygen tension include: the number of cells per unit volume, the rate of cellular metabolism, the vascular supply and the rate of oxygen diffusion from the vascular supply to the cells. In bone, the mineral phase may serve to impede the rate at which the gas diffuses from the vascular supply. It is therefore probable that osteocytes (and some osteoblasts) exist in a milieu in which the oxygen supply is limiting. In the next few paragraphs we review briefly some of the salient responses of all cells to low oxygen tensions.

Investigations performed with whole cells and isolated mitochondria indicate that in soft tissues the vascular supply provides sufficient oxygen for normal rates of energy metabolism. A recent study by Wilson *et al.* (1988) showed that mitochondrial function depends on oxygen tension well into the physiological range. As a result of this dependence, mitochondria may function as "tissue oxygen sensors that convert information concerning the cytosolic oxygen concentration to a metabolic message".

As will be discussed later, there is information to suggest that the oxygen tension is low in the tissue fluid surrounding the bone cell. It should be noted that in other tissues, limited periods of hypoxia can be tolerated as the cell can adjust its energy needs to the available oxygen tension. During hypoxia, nucleotide turnover is lowered by decreased activity of $Na^+ K^+$ ATPase; as a result, there is maintenance of the mitochondrial pH gradient and membrane potential. Metabolically, the cell responds to the low oxygen challenge by increased reliance on anaerobic glycolysis. In this way, activities essential for cell survival are sustained although the functional state of the tissue is limited.

There is a recognizable stage induced by very low oxygen tensions which Hochachka called "metabolic arrest" (Hochachka, 1986). This state is seen as a mechanism directed at preserving cellular function by decreasing both oxidative and nonoxidative metabolism. If maintained for an extended time, it would result in "metabolic death" — indeed, the point of "no return" is seen in a number of ischemic states and has been attributed to ATP depletion (Vogt and Farber, 1968; Chance *et al.*, 1985).

Of direct relevance to the study of bone is the observation that when cells of soft tissues become de-energized by a lack of oxygen there is decreased synthesis of ATP and an accumulation of AMP. This latter compound can be further degraded to adenosine. Some AMP can be converted to inosine monophosphate by AMP deaminase or to inosine and hypoxanthine by a 5′nucleotidase (see below).

$$ATP \rightarrow ADP \rightarrow AMP \rightarrow adenosine \rightarrow inosine \rightarrow$$

$$hypoxanthine \rightarrow xanthine \rightarrow uric\ acid$$

Measurement of adenosine, inosine and hypoxanthine levels in cultured bone by Fredholm and Lerner (1984) indicated a slow continuous increase in purine metabolites in the culture medium as well as marked adenosine deaminase activity. A similar small increase in inosine and hypoxanthine was observed as the cells of the epiphyseal growth plate matured (Matsumoto *et al.*, 1988). These results would indicate that in these two bone-forming systems cells may become more hypoxic with time.

As indicated above, measurement of purine levels in bone provides some indirect evidence that the oxygen tension may be low. In the next section, the oxygen status of developing bone, mature bone and the endochondral growth plate will be discussed in terms of the local vascularity and tissue energy needs. From a practical viewpoint, it is easier to describe the vascular supply than trying to measure the actual oxygen tension at a specific site.

Oxygen Supply to Developing Bone

A common theme in developmental biology is that a determinant of cy-todifferentiation and tissue development is accessibility to nutrient supplies. In the embryo, nutrient accessibility is dependent on the temporal and spatial localization of the vascular system (Caplan and Koutropos, 1973). In a discussion of this topic, Caplan (1985) questioned whether the vascular sys-tem is the "driver of developmentally derived limb patterns in the embryo of specific phenotypes or is it an exquisitely sensitive responder to cellular and extracelluar changes which then reflect developmental events".

Reviewing the available evidence, Caplan concluded that the developing vascular system is both a driver and a responder.

In a detailed analysis of first bone formation in the developing avian embryo, Pechak *et al.* (1986 a,b) suggested that at stage 32, a tissue diffusion barrier is formed (made up of multi-cell layers, osteoid and eventually min-eral) which restricts nutrient flow from the vasculature into the core cartilage. The effects of the mineral diffusion barrier could affect the metabolism of osteoblasts and osteocytes. From an anatomical point of view, the oxygen tension of groups of bone cells would be dependent on their proximity to the vascular supply. Osteoblasts that are close to the vascular supply would be expected to be able to synthesize the proteins of the matrix and regulate osteoid mineralization. These cells would have normal rates of oxidative metabolism. Further away from the oxygen supply, as cells become surrounded by calcified matrix, they would experience a decrease in oxygen tension. As a result, the rate of many biosynthetic reactions, especially those that relate to the synthesis of the extracellular matrix proteins, would be decreased. Pechak et al. (1986) suggested that in the central cartilage core region of the developing long bone, the diffusion barrier may modify the cartilage phenotype. At the core, chondrocytes lose much of their biosynthetic activity and become hypertrophic. These workers speculated that the decrease in metabolic activity of the hypertrophic cells results in a lowered rate of synthesis of cellular and matrix proteins. If this occurred, the decreased synthesis of anti-angiogenesis factors would facilitate invasion of the cartilage space by blood vessels. This clever hypothesis, which brings together many facets of cartilage and bone development and which has obvious clinical value, is worthy of careful experimental validation.

The Oxygen Supply to Mature Bone

The cells of bone receive oxygen from a limited number of sources. In the long bone diaphysis, the nutrient artery is the major source of oxygen. Ascending and descending branches of this artery supply blood to Haversian bone. Periosteal arteries provide blood to cells located in the periosteum and the superficial regions of the bone. The metaphysis and cells of the epiphysis are supplied with blood from the nutrient artery and from metaphyseal-epiphyseal vessels (for detailed discussion of the vascular supply to bone, the reader should consult Rhinelander, 1980).

The blood flow to bone cells can be determined using radio-labeled microspheres. Using this technique, Li et al. (1989) showed that the rates of blood flow to periosteal cortical bone and endosteum were very similar. For example, in dogs, the blood flow to tibial cortical and endosteal bone was 4.46 and 4.55 ml/min/100 g bone, respectively. The rate of blood flow to cancellous bone was much higher (16.01 ml/min/100 g). Silverton et al. (1988) used a similar technique to measure the blood flow to metaphyseal bone, the growth plate and secondary ossification centers of newborn piglets. Table 3 clearly shows that compared with brain, the rate at which blood flows through bone is surprisingly rapid, i.e., the metaphyseal rate is almost 70% of the brain rate and two and a half times the rate of the growth plate and the secondary growth centers.

The blood flow values express differences in tissue architecture, cell number and metabolic activity. The blood flow to the metaphysis and cancellous

Table 3.
Rate of Blood Flow to Bone and Brain Tissue of the Pig

	Growth plate	Metaphysis	2° Growth center	Brain
Blood flow	20 ± 2	50 ± 7	19 ± 2	79 ± 7

Note: Blood flow was measured in ml/min/100 cm^3.

From Silverton *et al.* (1989).

bone reflects the high level of vascularity of these zones as well as the bio-synthetic activity of the resident bone cells. In contrast, the periosteum, the endosteum and the growth plate are less vascularized; they have a lower cell density and for the most part they are sites of limited oxidative activity.

It is important to make two comments about the functional architecture of the vascular supply to bone. First, in common with developing bone, in mature bone and in periosteal and Haversian bone formative events are organized in relationship to blood vessels. In the periosteum, bone is laid down circumferentially around a penetrating blood vessel. The vessel is separated from the osteoblast layer by a zone of fibroblastic cells that prob-ably contains pro-osteoblasts. Roberts *et al.* (1987) examined the recruitment of fibroblast-like cells to the osteoblast layer in relationship to the afferent blood vessel. It was shown that there was an osteogenic differentiation gra-dient radiating from the blood vessel and that pro-osteoblasts were predom-inant about 20 μm from the blood vessel. It is likely that the presence of the nondifferentiated cell layer would set up, and may even regulate, an oxygen and nutrient gradient between the vessel and the osteoblast layer. For os-teocytes buried in the calcified matrix, low oxygen concentration would be expected, as osteoid and mineralized matrix would form a diffusion barrier that would hinder the movement of ions and gases.

We can not yet describe the metabolic status of osteocytes. Few studies have been performed on these cells due to difficulties in extracting osteocytes from bone and maintaining their phenotype *in vitro*. Moreover, experiments that have been reported have not been performed in environments that mimic those that exist *in vivo*. Nevertheless, it is probable that osteocytes live in an atmosphere where oxygen is limiting, so we would expect that they would have a low level of metabolic activity.

Studies performed on healing bone defects such as those induced during fracture healing illustrate the importance of a good blood supply to bone formation. In this condition, there is a massive local hyperemia and, after a short time period, rapid deposition of woven bone. The importance of oxygen in controlling bone deposition and growth is supported by studies in which hyperoxia has been shown to stimulate osteogenesis, hydroxylation of proline and the synthesis of collagen (Lewis and Irving, 1970; Gray *et al.*, 1979). Studies of bone defects by McInnis *et al.* (1980) showed that bone formation was related directly to blood flow. Indeed, these workers believe that the increase in blood flow in new bone may be secondary to increased metabolic demands of cells of the forming bone.

Results of studies performed with other tissues suggest that the oxygen supply to a tissue can be self-regulatory. For example, when a muscle is at rest there is a decrease in oxygen requirements. As a result, vessels that supply the muscle become vasoconstricted. Subsequently, when the muscle performs mechanical work there is an active vasodilation caused by agents such as adenosine, histamine, H^+ and lactate (Nishiki et al., 1978). It is not known whether a mechanism for local regulation of blood flow and oxygen supply exists in bone. A careful evaluation of blood vessels of bone would help to determine whether this type of control exists and whether it is active at a specific stage of bone formation.

Oxygen Supply to Osteoblasts in Culture

The literature is replete with studies of osteogenesis using mineralizing cell culture systems. A common feature of these cultures is that mineral is first seen in the center of nodules formed by cells layering on top of each other. The formation of these nodules and the subsequent deposition of mineral has been linked to the formation of localized zones of low oxygen tension within the bone cell layer (Osdoby et al., 1981). It is possible that the local concentrations per se are less important than the juxtaposition of regions with differing concentrations. Indeed, within a nodule, or a multicell spheroid, gradients with respect to oxygen, lactate, protons and nutrients have been shown to exist (Sutherland, 1986). In terms of the mechanism of bone formation these same gradients may serve to produce local microenvironments which favor mineralization. Although details of these events in bone-forming systems are scanty, they are, nevertheless, worthy of more detailed investigation.

Oxygen Supply to the Epiphysis

The blood supply to the epiphysis is complex and varies from species to species. In mammalian long bones, tissue in the resting and proliferating regions of the cartilage is almost avascular; endochondral bone is highly vascularized (see Table 3). The exact relationship between the vascular supply to the plate and the deposition of mineral has been the subject of considerable scrutiny. Trueta and his colleagues (1953, 1960) drew attention to the position of metaphyseal vessels in relationship to the calcification of bone and cartilage; in terms of the site of the initial placement of mineral, these workers questioned whether the metaphyseal vessels ended as regular capillaries or irregular sinusoids. Arsenault (1987) examined the microvasculature of the epiphyseal-metaphyseal junction of the long bone of the rat and showed that the venous return occurred below the epiphysis. Since the vascular tree terminated as capillary sprouts, he concluded that an hypoxic region existed in newly mineralized cartilage.

Howlett and co-workers (1979, 1980, 1984) described the vasculature of the avian plate. In pre-mineralized cartilage, a small number of epiphyseal vessels provide oxygen and nutrients to chondrocytes in the resting and proliferating regions. A second group of vessels originating in the metaphysis supply blood to calcified cartilage and bone. These vessels also provide oxygen to cells in the hypertrophic region. Although there appears to be some limited communication between the two groups of vessels, Howlett *et al.* (1984) write that there are no patent blood vessels to form a functional anastomosis. At the periphery of the metaphyseal vessels, perivascular cells that are morphologically and functionally distinct from neighboring chondrocytes have been described by Cole and Wezeman (1985). In humans, cartilage canals contain a muscular arteriole, a venule and capillaries. As these structures are extremely thin and fenestrated, oxygen exchange between the capillary and the cartilage would be maximum (Rodriguez *et al.*, 1985). There is evidence of spaces or "fenestrae" in the matrix surrounding each chondrocyte. These gaps in the matrix would facilitate transport of oxygen from the blood vessels to each of the chondrocytes (Boyde and Shapiro, 1987).

In a series of important studies, Brighton and his colleagues (Brighton and Heppenstall, 1971 a,b; Brighton and Krebs, 1972; Heppenstall, *et al.*, 1975) determined the oxygen tension in the growth plate, in a healing bone defect and in a non-displaced fracture during fracture repair. A major finding was that an oxygen gradient existed in these tissues that was related to status of repair, cell maturation and degree of mineralization. The highest oxygen tension was seen in the proliferative region where the oxygen tension was 50 mm Hg. Cells in the resting and hypertrophic region could be considered to be hypoxic as the oxygen tension was reduced to 25 mm Hg. In the chondrogenic stage of fracture callus repair, the oxygen tension decreases to 20 to 30 mm Hg. If bone was present, the recorded oxygen tension increased to 40 to 50 mm Hg (Heppenstall *et al.*, 1975). The values for the oxygen levels in cartilage are in line with measurements of ATP and NADH in the different cartilage zones. Hence, it is likely that the metabolic state of these cells reflects the low oxygen tension and the limited vascular supply to the hypertrophic region.

Calcium, Mitochondrial Activity, and Oxidative Metabolism

Much of the work that links energy metabolism with mineral formation and bone growth has been performed using cells of the endochondral growth plate. Endochondral ossification is characterized by the formation of a zone of cartilage in which cells undergo sequential proliferation and hypertrophy; in most species, as the cartilage becomes calcified, it is invaded by vascular elements. Bone is subsequently deposited on and in the calcified cartilage matrix. Investigators have long recognized the inherent advantages of working with the endochondral system. The greatest advantage is that there is spatial and temporal separation of the individual zones so it is possible to isolate selected regions of the physis for biochemical and morphological evaluation. More recently, chondrocytes isolated from the plate have been shown to exhibit in culture similar developmental stages as those described *in situ*. Hence, adequate systems now exist to examine endochondral bone formation both *in vitro* and *in vivo*.

Endochondral ossification is not confined to long bones. Similar cellular events are seen in almost all the bones of the body (including most of the bones of the developing head). In addition, ossification associated with fracture repair and implantation of bone stimulating factors is endochondral in nature. However, the cartilage model is not seen during endosteal and periosteal bone formation, nor is it present during turnover and modeling. In the latter cases, bone is formed without the appearance of an intervening and transient cartilagenous phase.

The following critique will focus almost entirely on studies performed on cells of the endochondral growth plate. Hence, considerable emphasis is given to describing the energy status of growth plate chondrocytes and relating it to the initiation of mineralization. It has been proposed that the energy status of the cells regulates the deposition of mineral, i.e., a change in chondrocyte energy metabolism causes mineral to be formed in the extracellular matrix (Shapiro and Greenspan, 1969; Lehninger, 1970; Brighton and Hunt, 1978a).

Aspects of the theory that will be discussed are (a) high levels of calcium and phosphate ions exist in mitochondria (we will review studies that link the presence of these ions in chondrocyte and osteoblast mitochondria to mineral formation) and (b) and (c) specific mechanisms exist in hard tissues for the control of calcium and phosphate ion uptake and release by mitochondria, respectively. In (b) and (c) we will consider the hypothesis that chondrocytes and osteoblasts regulate the deposition of mineral by regulating the flow of calcium and phosphate ions to the extracellular matrix. We discuss the assumption that cells expend energy for the synthesis of specific macromolecules that are required for mineral deposition and formation.

Presence of Calcium and Phosphate Ions in Mitochondria

In direct support of the mitochondrial theory of mineralization was the observation by Matthews and his colleagues that electron-dense granules were present in mitochondria of the epiphyseal growth plate. Using pyroantimonate staining and microincineration techniques, they showed that the particles contained calcium and phosphorus atoms *in situ* (Matthews *et al.*,

1968). Also, mitochondrial granules were seen in osteoblasts (Martin and Matthews, 1970). Manston and Katchburian (1984) reported that large granules were present in early calcifying bone. In addition to these studies, there have been reports of granules in other forms of bone (Kjaer and Mathiessen, 1975; Maunsbach and Lucht, 1973). It is appropriate to mention that granules have also been detected in cells in which there is a high calcium flux (shell gland of the chicken, hepatopancreas of the molting crab, intestinal mucosa cells after calcium loading).

An important study by Brighton and Hunt (1974, 1978 a,b) indicated that mitochondrial inclusion granules existed in the hypertrophic chondrocyte. At the calcification front, loss of mitochondrial granule staining coincided with the appearance of mineral in matrix vesicles. The chemical nature of the granules observed in cells of the endochondral growth plate was characterized in a number of different ways. For example, Landis and Glimcher (1982) studied the granules *in situ* and showed that the calcium:phosphorus molar ratio varied from 1.0 in the nonmineralized regions of the growth plate to 1.2 to 1.5 in the hypertrophic region. Based on the ratio values and the electron diffraction pattern, they concluded that the mitochondrial mineral was brushite ($CaHPO_4,2H_2O$; $Ca/P = 1.0$). Using an *in vitro* system, Wuthier *et al.* (1985) modeled mitochondrial mineral formation. It was shown that the type of mineral formed is dependent on subtle variations in solution chemistry. The study also highlighted the observation that ATP regulates the solid phase transitions of the mineral. Thus, in the presence of this nucleotide a relatively stable form of calcium phosphate was formed with a low calcium:phosphate ratio. In the absence of ATP, this intermediate converted spontaneously into brushite. The findings from this study confirmed reports that adenine nucleotides, magnesium and bicarbonate ions regulate the type of mineral formed in calcifying systems (Blumenthal *et al.*, 1977). As the ATP-magnesium chelate plays such an important role in mineral development, it is likely that the energy status of the mitochondrion could influence the type of mineral that accumulates in the organelle.

At this stage, it is important to point out that none of the above observations prove that chondrocyte mitochondria regulate the mineralization process. Indeed, for more than 20 years it has been known that in the presence of phosphate ions and a respiratory substrate, mitochondria isolated from cells of soft tissues accumulate large quantities of calcium and form an insoluble subcrystalline precursor of a calcium-deficient apatite (Weinbach and von Brand, 1965, 1967; Thomas and Greenawalt, 1968; Brierley and Slautterback, 1964). Moreover, many observers have pointed out that the conditions that were used to fix, stain and section hard tissues can result in artifact formation. Any type of aqueous fixation may result in ion relocation, precipitation, and mineral phase change (Boyde and Shapiro, 1987). As far as section staining is concerned, Landis and Glimcher (1982) noted that pyroantimonate staining for calcium is non-specific; many monovalent and divalent cations react with this stain. Moreover, when a pyroantimonate calcium deposit is formed, detection by X-ray microanalysis is difficult due to overlap of calcium and antimony peaks. Freeze-drying techniques induce mineral deposition from physiological solution. Likewise, while aqueous fixation alone can cause the appearance of granules, nonaqueous fixation can induce mineral precipitation. Nevertheless, despite all of the caveats noted above, sufficient studies have been reported that would support the concept that cells participating in the mineralization process do have elevated intramitochondrial levels of calcium and phosphate ions.

Uptake of Calcium and Phosphate Ions by Mitochondria

To gain a more complete understanding of mitochondrial function in endochondral bone formation, experiments have been conducted using both isolated mitochondria and permeabilized whole cell preparations. Questions that were addressed included:

- Do mitochondria of cartilage and bone cells accumulate calcium? Is the mechanism of uptake or the extent of uptake different from that of organelles of nonmineralizing tissues?
- If mitochondria contain elevated calcium loads, how does calcium loading affect mitochondrial energy metabolism? What is the mechanism of calcium efflux? Is calcium exported from the cell in concert with a cell-derived particle (matrix vesicle) or as calcium phosphate granules?

Probably the most difficult problem facing investigators was to isolate respiring mitochondria from cells of the epiphyseal growth plate. Although mitochondria had been isolated from a wide variety of soft tissues, components of the cartilage extracellular matrix interfered with the isolation procedure and the mitochondria became uncoupled due to loading with calcium solubilized from the mineral phase. A review of the early literature reveals few studies of mitochondrial function in calcifying tissues. In 1972, Arsenis (1972) noted that calcium is actively accumulated by mitochondria isolated from costochondral cartilage. Meyer and Kunin (1969, 1973) also described the use of isolated mitochondrial preparations. However, in common with Arsenis, they failed to provide details of the metabolic state of the preparations that were used. Lee and Shapiro (1974, 1978) and Shapiro and Lee (1975) reported methods for isolating respiring mitochondria from the premineralized region of the chick growth cartilage. The respiratory characteristics of these organelles in terms of oxygen uptake values and P/O ratios in the presence of different substrates indicated that these organelles respire in a similar fashion to mitochondria isolated from other sources (see Table 4 and Fig. 5). Thus, ADP stimulated oxygen metabolism, while the clear "cut off", when ADP was limiting, showed that the phosphorylating activity of

Table 4.
Oxygen Uptake, P/O Ratio, Respiratory Control Index, and Dehydrogenase Activity of
Mitochondrial Fraction Derived from Chick Epiphyseal Cartilage

Substrate	Oxygen consumption	P/O ratio	Respiratory control index	Dehydrogenase activity
Succinate	0.053	1.7	3.9	1.57 ± 0.34
Malate	0.016	2.2	2.0	0.61 ± 0.15
Isocitrate (NAD linked)	0.017	2.3	2.7	0.61 ± 0.41
Isocitrate (NADP linked)	0.033	2.5	3.0	1.13 ± 0.58
Oxoglutarate	0.014	2.2	2.5	0.43 ± 0.07
Glycerol-3-phosphates	0.021	1.4	1.5	0.45 ± 0.04

From Lee, N. H. and Shapiro, I. M. (1974). *Calcif. Tissue Res.*, **16:** 277–282.

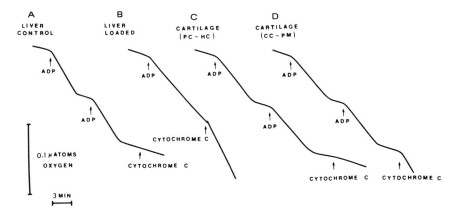

Fig. 5 Respiratory characteristics of mitochondria. The curves plot the oxygen tension as a
function of time in a cuvette with actively respiring mitochondria. The oxygen uptake rate is
the negative slope of the curve. ADP was added at the times indicated to stimulate oxidative
metabolism. (A) Liver mitochondria. (B) Liver mitochondria loaded with calcium to the level
found in cartilage mitochondria. Note that ADP has only a minor stimulatory effect on the
oxidative rate and there is no clear "cut off". (C) Precalcified cartilage mitochondria. ADP
stimulates oxidative phosphorylation and a clear "cut off" can be seen. (D) Cartilage mitochondria isolated from the calcifying region of the growth plate. Although ADP was seen to
stimulate respiration, the observation that cytochrome c further excited oxygen uptake suggested
that some of these mitochondria may be damaged.

the organelles was intact. The same extraction technique was used to isolate
mitochondria from the calcifying region of the plate; in this case, although
the mitochondria continued to respire, some damage was seen — when
treated with exogenous cytochrome oxidase there was an increase in the
respiratory rate.

Using the technique described above, it was possible to gain some quantitative data on mitochondrial calcium loading. Lee and Shapiro (1978)
showed that the calcium content of the mitochondria in cells of the epiphysis
was 10 to 30 times greater than organelles prepared from noncalcifying

tissues. Sucrose gradient centrifugation techniques permitted chondrocyte mitochondria to be separated on the basis of their buoyant density. In pre-mineralized cartilage, mitochondria formed a low density-low calcium (70 to 460 nmol/mg protein) band and high density-high calcium (280-700 nmol/mg protein) band. The presence of heterogeneous populations of mitochondria of differing density lent support to a concept put forward by Arsenis (1972) that mitochondria with differing functions may exist in cartilage cells (Shapiro et al., 1976; Meyer and Kunin, 1973; Yamamoto and Gay, 1988).

Aside from calcium content, hard tissue mitochondria appeared to be different from soft tissue mitochondria in terms of the control of oxidative phosphorylation. For example, when calcium was being accumulated by chondrocyte organelles there was minimum disturbance of mitochondrial respiratory function. At high calcium loads, cartilage mitochondria respired and exhibited coupled oxidative phosphorylation. In contrast, in soft tissues there was rapid loss of receptor control if the concentration of intramito-chondrial calcium was elevated by loading (see Fig. 5B, and Rossi and Lehninger, 1963). In damaged tissues, intramitochondrial calcium can accumulate. The presence of the cation caused a rapid decrease in receptor control and activation of phospholipases. As a result, there was membrane damage, and frequently cell death. One interpretation of these results is that mitochondria of a calcifying tissue are adapted to function in an environment in which there are large calcium fluxes of the kind expected to occur in the cytosol during bone formation.

An exciting approach to studying mitochondrial function in cells of a hard tissue was reported by Iannotti et al. (1985). The method described was superior to earlier techniques that relied on homogenization and differential centrifugation procedures. Instead, the cell membrane was permeabilized chemically to permit small molecules, such as a calcium fluorescent dye (Quin 2), to enter the cytosol. In addition, a dual-wavelength spectropho-tometer was utilized to measure mitochondrial cytochrome absorption spec-tra. With these techniques, these workers showed that chondrocytes con-tained nearly 1000 nmol calcium/mg mitochondrial protein (this calcium concentration was 50 times greater than values reported for hepatocytes). Over 75% of the total calcium in these cells was located in the mitochondria. In the same study, it was shown that the capacity for cation uptake by chondrocyte mitochondria was twofold greater than that of mitochondria of a nonmineralizing tissue. The results of these experiments as well as those performed on isolated mitochondria lend strong support for the view that chondrocyte mitochondria have unique features for both calcium storage and uptake.

Aside from examining the mechanism of calcium uptake by chondrocytes, experiments have been conducted to characterize the kinetics of calcium transport by chondrocyte mitochondria (Lee and Shapiro, 1978). In the presence of succinate, within a short time period, mitochondria accumulated

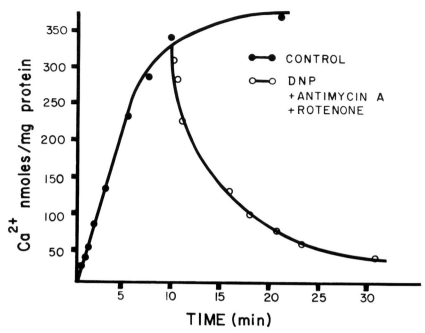

Fig. 6 Calcium uptake and efflux from growth plate mitochondria. The mitochondria were permitted to accumulate calcium in the presence of succinate for 10 min, after which time the uncoupler dinitrophenol (DNP) was added to the medium. The graph shows uptake and release of calcium. To monitor non-energy supported uptake of calcium, antimycin A and rotenone were added to the mitochondrial incubation medium.

over 300 nmol calcium/mg protein (see Fig. 6). This rate of uptake was similar to values reported for rat liver mitochondria during state 4 respiration.

In summary, although the total number of experiments performed with isolated mitochondria of growth cartilage cells are few, the data suggest that during proliferation and hypertrophy there is an elevation in the total quantity of cell calcium. Furthermore, as the total calcium load rises, there is a dramatic increase in the concentration of calcium in the extrudable pool. Still to be tested is the hypothesis that calcium in this latter pool is used to initiate the mineralization process.

Release of Calcium and Phosphate Ions by Mitochondria

If calcium ions contained within the extrudable pool are to be used for mineral formation, then mechanisms must exist that promote release of this cation from mitochondria. Moreover, the release mechanism must be under tight metabolic control. Studies performed with mitochondria containing low endogenous calcium loads (200 to 480 nmol/mg protein) showed that the presence of the uncoupler dinitrophenol (DNP) caused extrusion of more than 80% of the total mitochondrial calcium. Iannotti and his colleagues

(Iannotti et al., 1985) also studied the calcium extrusion phenomenon. Their investigations revealed that bovine growth plate mitochondria can release over 50% of the accumulated calcium. The results of these two experiments suggest that calcium is not simply binding to molecules of high calcium affinity, but is being maintained within the mitochondria by an energy-dependent process.

The mitochondrial extrudate has been subjected to analysis. Its calcium/phosphate ratio was found to be almost identical to the ratio found in the extracellular fluid of the longitudinal septa of the growth plate and very close to that of hydroxyapatite (Howell et al., 1968). It is worth noting that phosphoenolpyruvate, a product of glycolysis, caused calcium release from isolated chondrocyte mitochondria (see Fig. 2, and Shapiro and Lee, 1978). It is known that there is a switch from respiration to glycolysis as the cells in the growth cartilage mature with an accumulation of products of glycolysis. Thus, a mechanism can be discerned that could regulate mitochondrial calcium discharge.

In terms of a physiological role in endochondral bone formation, it is difficult to assess the importance of the glycolytic regulatory system. Phosphoenolpyruvate, along with a number of other agents such as phosphate ions, prostaglandins, palmityl CoA and oxaloacetate, release calcium by causing the collapse of the mitochondrial transmembrane potential. If this event occurred in vivo, it could cause irreversible damage to mitochondria. Therefore, other mechanisms which maintain the mitochondrial potential must be operative. There is now good evidence to indicate that a sodium-calcium exchange system also exists, while a calcium-hydrogen antiporter is present in a number of tissues. It remains to be determined whether these systems are functional in the cells of endochondral bone and to ascertain whether the systems become activated at a specific stage of cytodifferentiation.

Before leaving this discussion, it is important to point out that in 1978, Lehninger and colleagues examined the relationship between redox status of mitochondria and calcium transport. They claimed that oxidation of pyridine nucleotides promoted calcium efflux from isolated mitochondria. Later, these results were disputed. Palmer and Pfeiffer (1981) noted that NAD oxidation alone could not release all of the stored calcium ions. Nonetheless, both groups of investigators did ponder the importance of redox-related events as modulators of calcium transport in vivo. We examine this relationship in the next section.

Redox Measurements

As indicated earlier, there is little information available concerning the energy state of bone. For this discussion, therefore, it is necessary to draw heavily on work performed on the redox status of the growth plate in the authors' laboratories. We examined the relationship between cell redox state, chondrocyte maturation, and mineral deposition in the growth plate (Shapiro *et al.*, 1982, 1988; Kakuta *et al.*, 1986). Our approach was to freeze-trap the tissue to preserve its metabolic state and then to record the spatial distribution of pyridine (NAD, NADH) and adenine (ATP, ADP) nucleotide concentrations. As a delay in freezing, even by a few seconds, is known to result in a major redox change, great care was taken to preserve the metabolic status of the tissue. This was accomplished by rapidly freezing cartilage at $-155°C$ and storing the tissue in liquid nitrogen for subsequent optical (microfluorimetric) and biochemical investigations.

We used two complementary methods for determining pyridine nucleotide values. Measurements with high spatial resolution (tissue volumes of the order of $0.1 \times 0.1 \times 0.1$ mm) were made using a scanning microfluorimetric technique (Quistorff *et al.*, 1985). For this purpose, a computer-driven scanning-microflurometer was used to record optical fluorescence measurements of NADH at 455 nm (the NAD fluorescence yield at this wavelength is very low) in a raster of points across the tissue surface. Following the fluorescent scans of the growth plate, the tissue samples were examined by scanning electron microscopy to correlate fluorescence/NADH distribution with the morphology of the tissue. Although the method gives excellent information on the distribution of NADH across the tissue, it does not provide absolute values. For this information, the NAD and NADH levels of sections of growth cartilage were measured directly using a chemical technique which required volumes of tissue of about 1 mm³.

Our initial fluorescence measurements were made with a relatively low spatial resolution of 100×100 μm in the plane of the scan and about 50 μm normal to the plane. The fluorescence distributions across normal chick and rabbit epiphyseal growth plates was found to be very similar and are displayed in Fig. 7. The fluorescence may arise from high NADH levels or be nonspecific. The high fluorescence of articular cartilage has previously been shown to be due to intrinsic fluorescence of the cartilage and not related to the presence of NADH. Direct biochemical assays of pyridine nucleotides confirmed that the fluorescence of the growth plate was due to NADH and demonstrated that as the chondrocytes matured, the total NAD + NADH levels in each zone remained constant (Fig. 8). Therefore, the NADH values are indicative of changes in cell oxidative activity.

As far as adenine nucleotide concentrations were concerned, the values of ATP and GTP in selected zones of the growth plate are shown in Fig. 9. The ATP content of the tissue was highest in the precalcified zones (resting and proliferative cartilage); low levels of ATP were present in hypertrophic cartilage. In contrast to the pyridine nucleotide measurements, there were profound regional differences in the total cell ATP + ADP + AMP values. Together, the adenine and pyridine measurements provide ample proof that each of the distinct zones of the growth plate has a very distinct redox state.

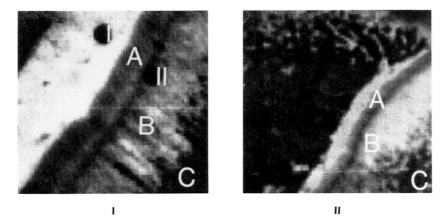

Fig. 7 Digital images showing the distribution of NADH across epiphyseal growth plate. (I) Chick and (II) rabbit. White indicates high fluorescence which is due to high levels of cellular NADH. The dark region in the proliferative cartilage indicates a high level of oxidative metabolism. The different zones are (A) proliferative cartilage, (B) hypertrophic cartilage, and (C) calcified cartilage-bone.

Energy Status of Resting and Proliferating Cartilage

The redox states of the resting and proliferating cartilage are very similar to that seen in a number of other tissues where oxygen is limiting. Compared with values obtained from highly oxygenated tissues such as liver, the ATP/ADP ratio (about 2), the energy charge ratio (greater than 0.7), and the NAD/NADH ratio (about 10) suggest that the tissue metabolism is neither entirely glycolytic nor entirely oxidative.

Energy Status of Hypertrophic Cartilage

From a functional viewpoint, the initial events associated with mineral deposition occur in the hypertrophic region. At the beginning of this zone there is minimum vascular supply, and therefore it is not surprising that the cells show biochemical changes consistent with reduced oxygen tension. It should be added that if cellular metabolic activity drives the mineralization process, then maximum changes in the redox state would be expected to be seen in this region. Indeed, the hypertrophic zone exhibits characteristics of hypoxia: the NADH levels were high, the energy charge was less than 0.7 and the ATP/ADP ratio was below 1. The ATP concentration was less than that of the resting/proliferating zones; on a DNA basis there was a sixfold decrease in the ATP concentration. However, there was very little change in the ADP levels, so that there is a decrease in the total ATP + ADP content of the tissue. This observation is unusual in that a change in energy charge ratio is usually accomplished by a reciprocal change in ATP and ADP levels. GTP metabolism was similar to that of ATP in that the GTP concentration in the hypertrophic zone is fivefold less than in the proliferative region.

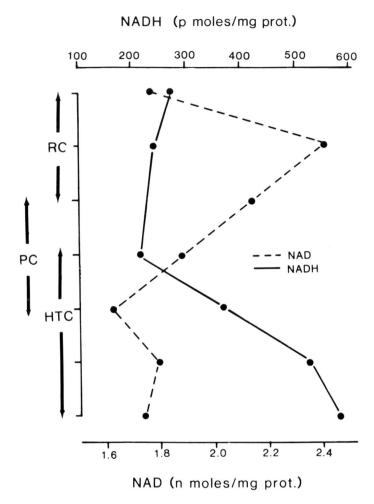

Fig. 8   Plot of the NADH and NAD levels across the avian epiphyseal growth plate. RC, resting cartilage; PC, proliferating cartilage; HTC, hypertrophic cartilage.

Redox Change and Mineralization

It is important to relate changes in energy metabolism to other mineralization-related events in a hard tissue. In terms of a mechanism to explain the observed changes in energy metabolism, as we have stated earlier, we favor a causative model in which the redox events cause, rather than follow, mineral deposition. An elevation in cellular NADH levels would impede mitochondrial calcium accumulation while the high NADH/NAD ratio would facilitate calcium and phosphate ion release from mitochondria. Both of these redox-related events could increase the extracellular calcium and phosphate ion product and thereby favor mineral formation.

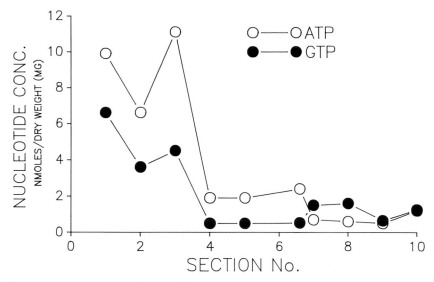

Fig. 9 Concentrations of ATP and GTP in sections of the chick growth cartilage. Sections 1–3, resting and proliferating cartilage; sections 4–7, hypertrophic cartilage.

In studies of elemental pools of hypertrophic cells, we pointed out that a limiting factor in the induction of tissue mineralization was the availability of phosphate ions (Boyde and Shapiro, 1980; Kakuta *et al.*, 1986). Thus, while the extracellular matrix contained some calcium ions, there was a deficiency in phosphorus; we also showed that chondrocytes contained high levels of total phosphorus. Subsequently, in a study of phosphate pools in the same tissue, we suggested that low molecular weight phosphorylated components may serve as a reservoir of phosphorus for the initiation of mineralization. The arguments presented here would support such a role for the adenine nucleotides. At the calcification front, increased degradation of ATP accompanied by a drop in ATP synthesis would provide a ready source of inorganic phosphate ions for the extracellular pool. Indeed, the drop in total ATP + ADP levels would be explained in terms of continued breakdown of adenine nucleotides to liberate phosphate ions. Since nucleotide synthesis and degradation is under strict metabolic control, regulation of this pathway would provide a mechanism for cellular regulation of mineral formation.

While the redox measurements may provide a clue to the mechanism that controls ion transport in mineralization, it is still not known what signal triggers these events. Brighton and his colleagues proposed that the signal for mineralization was the drop in the oxygen tension. However, if this were the case, then the first evidence of mineralization would be expected to be located at sites distant from the metaphyseal vessels. Morphologic studies of the mineralizing chick cartilage show that this assumption is not valid. Indeed, the first evidence of mineralization is associated with the chondro-

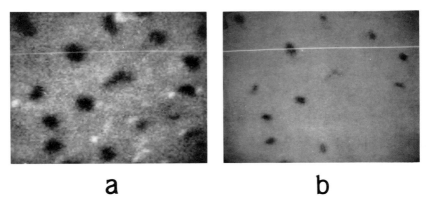

a   b

Fig. 10 Optical scans across a transverse plane through the mid hypertrophic region of the chick epiphyseal growth plate. (a) Fluorescent image: the white areas are regions with high NADH content. (b) Scattered, reflected light image: Because the tissue scatters light, the positions and size of the holes made by the channels are indicated by the dark regions. The dark fluorescence areas in "a" at the positions of the vessels are larger than the size of the channels indicated by "b". Therefore the channels are surrounded by an annulus of tissue with low fluorescence indicating that the perivascular cells have a lower NADH content than the rest of the tissue.

cytes which lie closest to the blood vessels (Boyde and Shapiro, 1987). Moreover, redox studies of cartilage performed with high spatial resolution indicated that the hypertrophic region was not uniformly reduced and that the redox levels depended on the proximity of the cells to the vascular channels.

High Resolution Redox Studies

We have reinvestigated the redox status of hypertrophic cartilage using a microfluorimetry system in which spatial resolution was about 20 μm (Shapiro *et al.*, 1988). With this system we were able to study the influence of the vascular canals on cartilage metabolism. Fig. 10b shows a microfluorimetric scan of cartilage in the early hypertrophic region. The most prominent feature of the scan is the presence of areas of low fluorescence scattered throughout the field. Each of these dark areas corresponds to the position of a penetrating blood vessel. Fig. 10a is a simultaneously recorded scan of light which is scattered and reflected directly from the tissue. The dark regions indicate the size as well as the position of the blood vessels. These areas are smaller than the dark regions shown in the fluorescence scan, indicating that there is a perivascular zone about 40 to 60 μm wide with a low fluorescence yield around each vessel. The low level of fluorescence would suggest that cells in this perivascular region have a higher level of oxidative metabolism than cells that are distant (greater than 150 μm) from the vascular channels. Morphologically, this zone of cells which exhibit a raised level of oxidative metabolism corresponds to cartilage perivascular cells (Cole and Wezeman,

1985). Mineralization is initiated by the chondrocytes which lie just outside of this zone in the cartilage matrix.

While we do not exclude the importance of nonoxidative metabolism and oxygen gradients on the functional development of cartilage and bone, the results of this study point to a specific role for perivascular cells in cartilage mineralization. For this reason, we now reject the view that mineralization of growth cartilage is simply a result of a change in chondrocyte energy metabolism due to an imposed hypoxic event.

If we are right in the assumption that the vascular channels direct mineralization in growth cartilage, questions must be asked concerning species specificity. Are the events described here, in terms of a perivascular calcification system, unique for avia, or do similar events occur in growth cartilages of other species? At first sight, the avian growth cartilage appears to be unique in that it is supplied with both epiphyseal vessels for the resting-proliferating zones and with metaphyseal vessels for the hypertrophic region (Howlett, 1980; Howlett *et al.*, 1984). In contrast, the mammalian growth plate appears to be almost avascular. However, more recent studies indicate that while the nonmineralizing region has a very poor blood supply, channels are seen in hypertrophic and calcifying cartilage. Interestingly, Cole and Wezeman (1985) reported that perivascular cells in the mouse epiphysis were morphologically distinct from chondrocytes; moreover, vascular channels appeared to be associated with both mineral formation and matrix resorption. We therefore suggest that despite the apparent paucity of channels in mammalian cartilage, the initiation of mineralization is still governed by the blood supply to the perivascular cells, as discussed above.

Conclusion

In this chapter, we have attempted to review those studies that have been directed at defining the metabolic state of cells of bone *in vivo* and *in vitro* and relate this information to the mineralization process. Despite somewhat embarrassing gaps in knowledge, especially those gaps that relate to the metabolism of cells in culture, the investigations highlighted a number of unique features of bone-forming cells. In the most well-studied system, the epiphysis, cells appear to undergo a complex series of development-related changes in metabolism. Other studies indicated that these cells are specialized with respect to energy-dependent transport of calcium and phosphate ions and apatite deposition.

Considerable space in the review was devoted to assessing the importance of the vascular system in terms of oxygen delivery, in the regulation of bone metabolism and in the initial formation of mineral. It was noted that in comparison with most soft tissues, both bone and cartilage may appear to be poorly vascularized. However, hard tissues contain blood vessels and the vessels are located at sites where there is a raised level of metabolic activity. Indeed, as was described earlier with respect to endochondral bone deposition, mineral formative units can be discerned that are in intimate association with the local blood supply. Similar types of structures are seen at other calcifying sites. In fetal long bones, a cylinder of "first bone" is synthesized in close proximity to the external blood supply (Pechak *et al.*, 1986 a,b). In Haversian bone, cells in the osteon form a tube of mineralizing matrix located around a central penetrating vascular channel — the most active cells in this unit are perivascular in location.

It is likely that the common anatomical theme that has been described above may have some functional significance. Perivascular cells in the metabolic unit, in both calcifying cartilage and bone, have immediate access to nutrients, oxygen and calcium ions. These cells would be expected to exhibit a high level of oxidative metabolism and to be active in those reactions that are required for biomineralization. In terms of control of mineralization, it is tempting to speculate that the perivascular cells may utilize much of their metabolic energy to regulate the rate of ion flow from the vascular supply to the preformed matrix.

Acknowledgments

This review was supported by NIH grants AR-34411, DE-06533, DE-09684, and DE-08239. The review was written while Irving M. Shapiro was on sabbatical leave at the Department of Orthopedic Surgery, Jefferson Medical College, Philadelphia.

References

Adamek, G., Felix, R., Guenther, H. L., and Fleisch, H. (1987). Fatty acid oxidation in bone tissue and bone cells in culture. Characterization and hormonal influences. *Biochem. J.*, **248**: 129–137.

Akisaka, T., Tamamoto, T., and Gay, C. V. (1988). Ultracytochemical investigation of calcium-activated adenosine triphosphate (Ca^{2+}-ATPase) in chick tibia. *J. Bone Min. Res.*, **3**: 19–25.

Aprille, J. R. (1988). Regulation of the mitochondrial adenine nucleotide pool size in liver: mechanism and metabolic role. *FASEB*, **2**: 2547–2556.

Arsenault, A. L. (1987). Microvascular organization of the epiphyseal-metaphyseal junction of growing rats. *J. Bone Min. Res.*, **2**: 143–149.

Arsenis, C. (1972). Role of mitochondria in calcification. Mitochondrial activity distribution in the epiphyseal plate and accumulation of calcium and phosphate ions by chondrocyte mitochondria. *Biochem. Biophys. Res. Commun.*, **46**: 1928–1974.

Berridge, M. J. and Galione, A. (1988). Cytosolic calcium oscillators. *FASEB J.*, **2**: 3074–3082.

Biggers, J. D., Gwatkin, R. B. L., and Heyner, S. (1961). Growth of embryonic avian and mammalian tibae on a relatively simple chemically defined medium. *Exp. Cell Res.*, **25**: 41–58.

Blaustein, M. P. (1977). Effects of internal and external cations and of ATP on sodium-calcium and calcium-calcium exchange in squid axons. *Biophys. J.*, **20**: 79–111.

Blumenthal, N. C., Betts, F. C., and Posner, A. S. (1977). Stabilization of amorphous calcium phosphate by Mg and ATP. *Calcif. Tissue Res.*, **23**: 245–250.

Boland, C. J., Fried, R. M., and Tashjian, A. H. (1986). Measurement of cytosolic free Ca concentrations in human and rat osteosarcoma cells: actions of bone resorption-stimulating hormones. *Endocrinology*, **118**: 980–989.

Borle, A. B., Nichols, N., and Nichols, G. (1960a). Metabolic studies of bone *in vitro*. I. Normal bone. *J. Biol. Chem.*, **235**: 1206–1210.

Borle, A. B., Nichols, N., and Nichols, G. (1960b). Metabolic studies of bone *in vitro*. II. The metabolic pattern of accretion and resorption. *J. Biol. Chem.*, **235**: 1211–1214.

Boyde, A. and Shapiro, I. M. (1980). Energy dispersive X-ray elemental analysis of isolated epiphyseal growth plate chondrocyte fragments. *Histochemistry*, **69**: 85–94.

Boyde, A. and Shapiro, I. M. (1987). Morphological observations concerning the pattern of mineralization of the normal and the rachitic chick growth cartilage. *Anat. Embryol.*, **175**: 457–466.

Brand, K., Hintzenstern, J. V., Langer, K., and Fekl, W. (1987). Pathways of glutamine and glutamate metabolism in resting and proliferating rat thymocytes: comparison between free and peptide-bound glutamine. *J. Cell. Physiol.*, **132**: 559–564.

Brierley, G. P. and Slautterback, D. B. (1964). Studies on ion transport. IV. An electron microscope study of the accumulation of Ca^{2+} and inorganic phosphate by heart mitochondria. *Biochim. Biophys. Acta*, **82**: 183–187.

Brighton, C. T. and Heppenstall, R. B. (1971a). Oxygen tension of the epiphyseal plate distal to an arteriovenous fistula. *Clin. Orthop.*, **80**: 167–171.

Brighton, C. T. and Heppenstall, R. B. (1971b). Oxygen tension in zones of the epiphyseal plate, the metaphysis and diaphysis. An *in vitro* and *in vivo* study in rats and rabbits. *J. Bone Jt. Surg.*, **53A**: 719–728.

Brighton, C. T. and Hunt, R. M. (1974). Mitochondrial calcium and its role in growth plate calcification. Histochemical localization of calcium in electron micrographs of the epiphyseal growth plate with K-pyroantimonate. *Clin. Orthop. Rel. Res.*, **100**: 406–416.

Brighton, C. T. and Hunt, R. M. (1978a). The role of mitochondria in growth plate calcification as demonstrated in a rachitic model. *J. Bone Jt. Surg.*, **60**: 630–639.

Brighton, C. T. and Hunt, R. M. (1978b). Electron microscopic pyroantimonate studies of matrix vesicles and mitochondria in the rachitic growth plate. *Metab. Bone Dis. Rel. Res.*, **1**: 199–204.

Brighton, C. T. and Krebs, A. G. (1972). Oxygen tension of healing fractures in the rabbit. *J. Bone Jt. Surg.*, **54A**: 323–329.

Caplan, A. I. (1985). The vasculature and bone development. *Cell Diff.*, **16**: 1–11.

Caplan, A. I. and Koutroupas, S. (1973). The control of cartilage and muscle development in the chick limb: the role of differential vascularization. *J. Embryol. Exp. Morphol.*, **29**: 571–583.

Carafoli, E. (1987). Intracellular calcium homeostasis. In: *Annual Review of Biochemistry*, Richardson, C. C., Ed., Annual Reviews, Palo Alto, CA, 395–434.

Catherwood, B. D., Addison, J., Chapman, G., Contreras, S., and Lorang, M. (1988). Growth of rat osteoblast-like cells in a lipid-enriched culture medium and regulation of function by parathyroid hormone and 1,25-dihydroxyvitamin D. *J. Bone Min. Res.*, **3**: 431–438.

Chance, B., Leigh, J. S., Clark, B. J., Maris, J., Kent, J., Nioka, S., and Smith, D. (1985). Control of oxidative metabolism and oxygen delivery in human skeletal muscle: a steady state analysis of the work/energy cost transfer function. *Proc. Natl. Acad. Sci. U.S.A.*, **82**: 8384–8388.

Chesnoy-Marchais, D. and Fritsch, J. (1988). Voltage-gated sodium and calcium currents in rat osteoblasts. *J. Physiol.*, **398**: 291–311.

Chu, L. L., Macgregor, R. R., and Hamilton, J. W. (1971). A bioassay for parathyroid hormone-based hormonal inhibition of CO_2 production from citrate in mouse calvarium. *Endocrinology*, **89**: 1425–1431.

Cohn, D. V. and Forscher, B. K. (1962). Effect of parathyroid extract on the oxidation in vitro of glucose and the production of $^{14}CO_2$ by bone and kidney. *Biochim. Biophys. Acta*, **65**: 20–26.

Cole, A. A. and Wezeman, F. H. (1985). Perivascular cells in cartilage canals of the developing mouse epiphysis. *Am. J. Anat.*, **174**: 119–129.

Dixon, T. F. and Perkins, H. R. (1952). Citric acid and bone metabolism. *Biochem. J.*, **52**: 260–265.

Eagle, H. (1959). Amino acid metabolism in mammalian cell cultures. *Science*, **130**: 432–437.

Felix, R. and Fleisch, H. (1981). Increase in fatty acid oxidation in calvarial cells cultured with diphosphonates. *Biochem. J.*, **196**: 237–245.

Felix, R., Fleisch, H., and Schenk, R. (1986). Effects of halogen methylenebisphonates on bone cells in culture and on bone resorption *in vivo*. *Experientia*, **42**: 302–304.

Ferrier, J., Illeman, A., and Zashek, E. (1985). Transient and sustained effects of hormones and calcium on membrane potential in a bone cell clone. *J. Cell. Physiol.*, **122**: 53–58.

Ferrier, J. and Ward, A. (1986). Electrophysiological differences between bone cell clones: membrane potential responses to parathyroid hormone and correlation activity with the cAMP response. *J. Cell. Physiol.*, **126**: 273–242.

Ferrier, J., Ward-Kesthley, A., Heersche, J. N. M., and Aubin, J. E. (1988). Membrane potential changes, cAMP stimulation and contraction in osteoblast-like UMR 106 cells in response to calcitonin and parathyroid hormone. *Bone Mineral*, **4**: 133–145.

Ferrier, J., Ward-Kesthley, A., Homble, F., and Ross, S. (1987). Further analysis of spontaneous membrane potential activity and the hyperpolarizing response to parathyroid hormone in osteoblast-like cells. *J. Cell Physiol.*, **130**: 344–351.

Flanagan, B. and Nichols, G. (1964). Metabolic studies of bone *in vitro*. Glucose metabolism and collagen biosynthesis. *J. Biol. Chem.*, **239**: 1261–1265.

Fredholm, B. B. and Lerner, U. (1984). Adenine nucleotide levels and adenosine metabolism in cultured calvarial bone. *Acta Physiol. Scand.*, **120**: 551–555.

Gray, D. H., Katz, J. M., and Speak, K. S. (1979). The effect of varying oxygen tensions on hydroxyproline synthesis in mouse calvaria *in vitro*. *Clin. Orthop. Rel. Res.*, **146**: 275–281.

Guenther, H.L., Guenther, H.E., and Fleisch, H. (1979). Effects of hydroxyethane-1,1-diphosphonate and dichloromethanediphosphonate on rabbit articular chondrocytes in culture. *Biochem. J.*, **184**: 203–214.

Handley, C. J., Speight, G., Leyden, K. M., and Lowther, D. A. (1980). Extracellular matrix metabolism by chondrocytes. 7. Evidence that L-glutamine is an essential amino acid for chondrocytes and other connective tissue cells. *Biochim. Biophys. Acta*, **627**: 324–331.

Hekkelman, J. W. (1961). The effect of parathyroid extract on the isocitric dehydrogenase activity of bone tissue. *Biochim. Biophys. Acta*, **47**: 426–427.

Heppenstall, R. B., Grislis, G., and Hunt, T. K. (1975). Tissue gas tensions and oxygen consumption in healing bone defects. *Clin. Orthop. Rel. Res.*, **106**: 357–365.

Hochachka, P. W. (1986). Defense strategies against hypoxia and hypothermia. *Science*, **231**: 234–241.

Howell, D. S., Pita, J. C., Marquez, J. F., and Madruga, J. E. (1968). Partition of calcium, phosphate and protein in the fluid phase aspirated at calcifying sites in epiphyseal cartilage. *J. Clin. Invest.*, **47**: 1121–1132.

Howlett, C. R. (1979). The fine structure of the proximal growth plate of the avian tibia. *J. Anat.*, **128**: 377–399.

Howlett, C. R. (1980). The fine structure of the proximal growth plate and metaphysis of the avian tibia: endochondral osteogenesis. *J. Anat.*, **130**: 745–768.

Howlett, C. R., Dickson, M., and Sheridan, A. K. (1984). The fine structure of the proximal growth plate of the avian tibia: vascular supply. *J. Anat.*, **139**: 115–132.

Iannotti, J. P., Brighton, C. T., Stambough, J. L., and Storey, B. T. (1985). Calcium flux and endogenous calcium content in isolated mammalian growth plate chondrocytes, hyaline cartilage chondrocytes and hepatocytes. *J. Bone Jt. Surg.*, **67A**: 113–120.

Ishikawa, Y., Chin, J. E., Hubbard, H. L., and Wuthier, R. E. (1985). Utilization and formation of amino acids by chicken epiphyseal chondrocytes: comparative studies with cultured cells and native cartilage tissue. *J. Cell. Physiol.*, **123**: 79–85.

Ituarte, E. A., Ituarte, H. G., and Hahn, T. J. (1988). Insulin and glucose regulation of glycogen synthase in rat calvarial osteoblast-like cells. *Calcif. Tissue Int.*, **42**: 351–357.

Kakuta, S., Golub, E. E., Haselgrove, J. C., Chance, B., Frasca, P., and Shapiro, I. M. (1986). Redox studies of the epiphyseal cartilage: pyridine nucleotide metabolism and the development of mineralization. *J. Bone Min. Res.*, **1**: 433–440.

Kjaer, I. and Matthiessen, E. (1975). Mitochondrial granules in human osteoblasts with a reference to one case of osteogenesis imperfecta. *Calcif. Tissue Res.*, **17**: 173–176.

Klingenberg, M. (1989). Molecular aspects of the adenine nucleotide carrier from mitochondria. *Arch. Biochem. Biophys.*, **270**: 1–14.

Landis, W. J. and Glimcher, M. J. (1982). Electron optical and analytical observations of rat growth plate cartilage prepared by ultracryomicrotomy. *J. Ultrastruct. Res.*, **78**: 227–268.

Lanks, K. W. (1987). End products of glucose and glutamine metabolism by L929 cells. *J. Biol. Chem.*, **262**: 10093–10097.

Lanks, K. W., Hitti, I. F., and Chin, N. W. (1986). Substrate utilization for lactate and energy production by heat shocked L929 cells. *J. Cell. Physiol.*, **127**: 451–456.

Lanks, K. W. and Li, P.-.W. (1988). End products of glucose and glutamine metabolism by cultured cell lines. *J. Cell. Physiol.*, **135**: 151–155.

Laskin, D. M. and Engel, M. B. (1956). Bone metabolism and bone resorption after parathyroid extract. *Arch. Pathol.*, **62**: 296–302.

Lee, N. H. and Shapiro, I. M. (1974). Oxidative phosphorylation by chondrocyte mitochondria. *Calcif. Tissue Res.*, **16**: 277–282.

Lee, N. H. and Shapiro, I. M. (1978). Ca^{2+} transport by chondrocyte mitochondria of the epiphyseal growth plate. *J. Membrane Biol.*, **41**: 349–360.

Lehninger, A. L. (1970). Mitochondria and calcium ion transport. *Biochem. J.*, **119**: 129–138.

Lehninger, A. L., Vercesi, A., and Bababunmi, E. A. (1978). Regulation of Ca^{2+} release from mitochondria by the oxidation-reduction state of pyridine nucleotides. *Proc. Natl. Acad. Sci. U.S.A.*, **75**: 1690–1694.

Lewis, E. A. and Irving, J. T. (1970). An autoradiographic investigation of bone remodelling in the rat calvarium grown in organ culture. *Arch. Oral Biol.*, **15**: 769–773.

Li, G., Bronk, J. T., and Kelly, P. J. (1989). Canine bone blood flow estimated with microspheres. *J. Orthop. Res.*, **7**: 61–67.

Lieberherr, M. (1987). Effects of vitamin D3 metabolites on cytosolic free calcium in confluent mouse osteoblasts. *J. Biol. Chem.*, **262**: 13168–13173.

Lowik, C. W., Van Leeuwen, J. P., Van Der Meer, J. M., Van Zeeland, J. K., Scheven, B. A., and Hermann-Erlee, M. P. (1985). A two receptor model for the action of parathyroid hormone on osteoblasts: a role for intracellular free calcium and cAMP. *Cell Calcium*, **6**: 311–326.

Luben, R. A. and Cohn, D. V. (1976). Effects of parathormone and calcitonin on citrate and hyaluronate metabolism in cultured bone. *Endocrinology*, **98**: 413–419.

Manston, J. and Katchburian, E. (1984). Demonstration of mitochondrial mineral deposits in osteoblasts after anhydrous fixation and processing. *J. Microsc.*, **134**: 177–182.

Martin, J. H. and Matthews, J. L. (1970). Mitochondrial granules in chondrocytes, osteoblasts and osteocytes. An ultrastructural and microincineration study. *Clin. Orthop. Rel. Res.*, **68**: 273–278.

Matsumoto, H., DeBolt, K., and Shapiro, I. M. (1988). Adenine, guanine and inosine nucleosides of chick growth cartilage: relationship between energy status and the mineralization process. *J. Bone Min. Res.*, **3**: 347–352.

Matthews, J. L., Martin, J. H., Lynn, J. A., and Collins, E. J. (1968). Calcium incorporation in the developing cartilaginous epiphysis. *Calcif. Tissue Res.*, **1**: 330–336.

Maunsbach, A. B. and Lucht, U. (1973). Elemental composition of lysosomal and mitochondrial inclusions studied in the electron microscope by X-ray analysis. *J. Ultrastruct. Res.*, **44**: 435–439.

McInnis, J. C., Robb, R. A., and Kelly, P. J. (1980). The relationship of bone blood flow, bone tracer deposition and endosteal new bone formation. *J. Lab. Clin. Med.*, **96**: 511–522.

Meyer, W. L. and Kunin, A. S. (1969). The inductive effect of rickets on glycolytic enzymes of rat epiphyseal cartilage and its reversal by vitamin D and phosphate. *Arch. Biochem. Biophys.*, **129**: 438–446.

Meyer, W. L. and Kunin, A. S. (1973). Effects of cortisone, starvation and rickets on oxidative enzyme activities of epiphyseal cartilage from rats. *Arch, Biochem. Biophys.*, **156**: 122.

Moreadith, R. W. and Lehninger, A. L. (1984). The pathway of glutamate and glutamine oxidation by tumor cell mitochondria. *J. Biol. Chem.*, **259**: 6215–6221.

Morgan, D. B., Monod, A., Russell, R. G. G., and Fleisch, H. (1973). Influence of dichloro-methylene diphosphonate (Cl2MDP)and calcitonin on bone resorption, lactate production and phosphatase and pyrophosphatase content of mouse calvaria treated with parathyroid hormone. *Calcif. Tissue Res.*, **13**: 287–294.

Neuman, W. F., Neuman, M. W., and Brommage, R. (1978). Aerobic glycolysis in bone: lactate production and gradients in calvaria. *Am. J. Physiol.*, **234(1)**: C41–C50.

Nijweide, P. J. and Van der Plas, A. (1979). Regulation of calcium transport in isolated periosteal cells, effects of hormones and metabolic inhibitors. *Calcif. Tissue Res.*, **29**: 155–161.

Nishiki, K., Erecinska, M., and Wilson, D. F. (1978). Evaluation of oxidative phosphorylation in hearts from euthyroid, hypothyroid and hyperthyroid rats. *Am. J. Physiol.*, **235**: C212–C219.

Osdoby, P. and Caplan, A. I. (1981). First bone formation in the developing chick limb. *Dev. Biol.*, **86**: 147–156.

Palmer, J. K. and Pfeiffer, D. R. (1981). The control of Ca^{2+} release from heart mitochondria. *J. Biol. Chem.*, **256**: 6742–6750.

Pechak, D. G., Kujawa, M. J., and Caplan, A. I. (1986a). Morphological and histochemical events during first bone formation in embryonic chick limbs. *Bone*, **7**: 441–458.

Pechak, D. G., Kujawa, M. J., and Caplan, A. I. (1986b). Morphology of bone development and bone remodeling in embryonic chick limbs. *Bone*, **7**: 459–472.

Pershadsingh, H. A. and McDonald, J. M. (1980). A high affinity calcium-stimulated mag-nesium-dependent adenosine triphosphatase in rat adipocyte plasma membranes. *J. Biol. Chem.*, **255**: 4087–4093.

Prentki, M., Glennon, M. C., Thomas, A. P., Morris, R.L., Matschinsky, F. M., and Corkey, B. E. (1988). Cell-specific patterns of oscillating free Ca^{2+} in carbomylcholine-stimulated insulinoma cells. *J. Biol. Chem.*, **263**: 11044–11047.

Quistorff, B., Haselgrove, J. C., and Chance, B. (1985). High spatial resolution readout of metabolic organ structures; an automated low temperature redox scanning instrument. *Anal. Biochem.*, **148**: 389–400.

Reitzer, L. J., Wice, B. M., and Kennel, D. (1979). Evidence that glutamine not sugar is the major energy source for cultured HeLa cells. *J. Biol. Chem.*, **254**: 2669–2676.

Rhinelander, F. W. (1980). The blood supply of the limb bones. In: *Scientific Foundations of Orthopaedics and Traumatology*, Owen, R., Ed., WB Saunders, Philadelphia, 126–151.

Roberts, W. E., Chambers, D. W., and Burk, D. T. (1987). Vascularly oriented differentiation gradient of osteoblast precusor cells in rat periodontal ligament: implications for osteoblast histogenesis and periodontal bone loss. *J. Perio. Res.*, **22**: 461–467.

Rodriguez, J. I., Delgado, E., and Paniagua, R. (1985). Multivacuolated cells in human cartilage canals. *Acta Anat.*, **124**: 54–57.

Rossi, C. S. and Lehninger, A. L. (1963). Stoichiometric relationships between mitochondrial ion accumulation and oxidative phosphorylation. *Biochem. Biophys. Res. Commun.*, **11**: 441–446.

Rouleau, M. F., Mitchell, J., and Goltzman, D. (1988). *In vivo* distribution of parathyroid hormone receptors in bone: evidence that a predominant osseous target cell is not the mature osteoblast. *Endocrinology,* **123**: 187–191.

Schatzmann, H. J. and Vincenzi, F. F. (1969). Calcium movements across the membrane of human red cells. *J. Physiol.,* **201**: 369–395.

Schmid, C. H., Steiner, T. H., and Froesch, E. R. (1982). Parathormone promotes glycogen formation from [14C]glucose in cultured osteoblast-like cells. *FEBS Lett.,* **148**: 31–34.

Scott, B. L. and Glimcher, M. J. (1971). Distribution of glycogen in osteoblasts of the fetal rat. *J. Ultrastruct. Res.,* **36**: 565–586.

Shapiro, I. M., Burke, A., and Lee, N. H. (1976). Heterogeneity of chondrocyte mitochondria. A study of the Ca^{2+} concentration and density banding characteristics of normal and rachitic cartilage. *Biochim. Biophys. Acta,* **451**: 583–591.

Shapiro, I. M., Golub, E. E., Chance, B., Piddington, C., Oshima, O., Tuncay, O., Frasca, P., and Haselgrove, J. C. (1989). Linkage between energy status of perivascular cells and mineralization of the chick growth cartilage. *Dev. Biol.,* **128**: 372–379.

Shapiro, I. M., Golub, E. E., Kakuta, S., Haselgrove, J. C., Havery, J., Chance, B., and Frasca, P. (1982). Initiation of endochondral calcification is related to changes in the redox state of hypertrophic chondrocytes. *Science,* **217**: 950–952.

Shapiro, I. M. and Greenspan, J. S. (1969). Are mitochondria directly involved in biological mineralization?. *Calcif. Tissue Res.,* **3**: 100–102.

Shapiro, I. M. and Lee, N. H. (1975). Effects of Ca^{2+} on the respiratory activity of chondrocyte mitochondria. *Arch. Biochem. Biophys.,* **170**: 627–633.

Shapiro, I. M. and Lee, N. H. (1978). The effects of oxygen, phosphoenolpyruvate, and pH on the release of calcium from chondrocyte mitochondria. *Metabol. Bone Dis. Rel. Res.,* **1**: 173–177.

Shen, V., Hruska, K., and Avioli, L. V. (1988). Characterization of a $(Ca^{2+} + Mg^{2+})$-ATPase system in the osteoblast plasma membrane. *Bone,* **9**: 325–329.

Shen, V., Kohler, G., and Peck, W. A. (1983). A high affinity, calmodulin-responsive $(Ca^{2+} + Mg^{2+})$-ATPase in isolated bone cells. *Biochim. Biophys. Acta,* **727**: 230–238.

Silverton, S. F., Wagerle, L. C., Robiolo, M. E., Haselgrove, J. C., and Forster, R. E. (1989). Oxygen gradients in two regions of the epiphyseal growth plate. *Adv. Exp. Med. Biol.,* **248**: 809–815.

Somjen, D., Kaye, A. M., and Binderman, I. (1984). Stimulation of creatine kinase BB activity by parathyroid hormone and by prostaglandin E_2 in cultured bone cells. *Biochem. J.,* **225**: 591–596.

Somjen, D., Kaye, A. M., Rodan, G. A., and Binderman, I. (1985). Regulation of creatine kinase activity in rat osteogenic sarcoma cell clones by parathyroid hormone, prostaglandin E_2 and vitamin D metabolites. *Calcif. Tissue Int.,* **37**: 635–638.

Somjen, D., Zor, U., Kaye, A. M., and Binderman, I. (1987). Parathyroid hormone induction of creatine kinase activity and DNA synthesis is mimicked by phospholipase C, diacylglycerol and phorbol ester. *Biochim. Biophys. Acta,* **931**: 215–223.

Star, A. M., Iannotti, J. P., Brighton, C. T., and Armstrong, P. F. (1987). Cytosolic calcium concentration in bovine growth plate chondrocytes. *J. Orthop. Res.,* **5**: 122–127.

Stewart, P. J., Hefley, T. J., Charlesworth, J., Minick, O. T., and Stern, P. H. (1986). Electron microscopic analysis of enzymatically isolated neonatal mouse bone cells: effects of PTH on glycogen storage pools. *J. Bone Min. Res.,* **1**: 132(A).

Streeten, E. A., Ornberg, R., Curcio, F., Sakaguchi, K., Marx, S., Aurbach, G. D., and Brandi, M. L. (1989). Cloned endothelial cells from fetal bovine bone. *Proc. Natl. Acad. Sci. U.S.A.,* **86**: 916–920.

Sutherland, R. M. (1986). Importance of critical metabolites and cellular interactions in the biology of microregions of tumors. *Cancer,* **58**: 1668–1680.

Thomas, R. S. and Greenawalt, J. W. (1968). Microincineration, electron microscopy and electron diffraction of calcium phosphate-loaded mitochondria. *J. Cell Biol.,* **39**: 55–76.

Trueta, J. and Amato, V. P. (1960). The vascular contribution to osteogenesis III changes in growth cartilage. *J. Bone Jt. Surg.*, **42B**: 571–587.

Trueta, J. and Harrison, M. H. M. (1953). The normal vascular anatomy of the femoral head in adult man. *J. Bone Jt. Surg.*, **35B**: 442–461.

Tsien, R. Y. (1981). A non-disruptive technique for loading calcium buffers and indicators into cells. *Nature*, **290**: 527–28.

Vaes, G. and Nichols, G. J. R. (1961). Metabolic studies of bone *in vitro*. III. Citric acid metabolism and bone mineral solubility. Effects of parathyroid hormone and estradiol. *J. Biol. Chem.*, **236**: 3323–3329.

Van Valen, F. and Keck, E. (1988). Forskolin inhibition of glucose transport in bone cell cultures through a cAMP independent mechanism. *Bone*, **9**: 89–92.

Van Reen, R. (1959). Metabolic activity in calcified tissues: aconitase and isocitric dehydrogenase activities in rabbit and dog femurs. *J. Biol. Chem.*, **234**: 1951–1954.

Vogt, M. T. and Farber, E. (1968). On the molecular pathology of ischemic renal cell death. Reversible and irreversible cellular and mitochondrial metabolic alterations. *Am. J. Pathol.*, **53**: 1–26.

Weinbach, E. C. and von Brand, T. (1965). The isolation and composition of dense granules from Ca^{++} loaded mitochondria. *Biochem. Biophys, Res. Commun.*, **19**: 133–137.

Weinbach, E. C. and von Brand, T. (1967). Formation, isolation and composition of dense granules from mitochondria. *Biochim. Biophys. Acta*, **148**: 256–266.

Wilson, D. F., Rumsey, W. L., Green, T. J., and Vanderkooi, J. M. (1988). The oxygen dependence of mitochondrial oxidative phosphorylation measured by a new optical method for measuring oxygen concentration. *J. Biol. Chem.*, **263**: 2712–2718.

Wolinsky, I. and Cohn, D. V. (1969). Oxygen uptake and $^{14}CO_2$ production from citrate and isocitrate by control and parathyroid hormone treated bone maintained in tissue culture. *Endocrinology*, **84**: 28–35.

Wong, G. L., Luben, R. A., and Cohn, D. V. (1977). 1,25-Dihydroxycholecalciferol and parathormone: effects on isolated osteoclast-like and osteoblast-like cells. *Science*, **197**: 663–665.

Wuthier, R. E., Rice, G. S., Wallace, J. E. B., Weaver, R. L., LeGeros, R. Z., and Eanes, E. D. (1985). *In vitro* precipitation of calcium phosphate under intracellular conditions: formation of brushite from an amorphous precursor in the absence of ATP. *Calcif. Tissue Int.*, **347**: 401–410.

Yamamoto, T. and Gay, C. V. (1988). Ultrastructural analysis of cytochrome oxidase in chick epiphyseal growth plate cartilage. *J. Histochem. Cytochem.*, **36**: 1161–1166.

Ypey, D. L., Ravesloot, J. H., Buisman, H. P., and Nijweide, P. J. (1988). Voltage activated ionic channels and conductance in embryonic chick osteoblast cultures. *J. Memb. Biol.*, **101**: 141–150.

Zielke, H. R., Sumbilla, C. M., Sevdalian, D. A., Hawkins, R. L., and Ozand, P. T. (1980). Lactate: a major product of glutamine metabolism by human diploid fibroblasts. *J. Cell. Physiol.*, **104**: 433–441.

Zielke, H. R., Zielke, C. L., and Ozand, P. T. (1984). Glutamine: a major energy source for cultured mammalian cells. *Fed. Proc.*, **43**: 121–125.

6

Effects of Vitamins A, C, D, and K on Bone Growth, Mineralization, and Resorption

ROBERTO NARBAITZ
Department of Anatomy
Faculty of Health Sciences
University of Ottawa
Ottawa, Canada

Introduction

Vitamins A, C, and D have been known for many years to be of special importance for bone growth, differentiation and function. The recent isolation of vitamin K-dependent proteins from bone matrix has added this vitamin to the classical trio. In this chapter I shall cover the literature on the actions of these four vitamins, but special emphasis will be given to the analysis of effects of vitamins A and D because knowledge on these fields is progressing very rapidly. Although clinical aspects of ongoing research will be covered when supporting experimental data, I purposely have emphasized pertinent basic research on animal models.

Vitamin A

Chemical Nature and Metabolism

A brief summary on the chemical structure and metabolism of the vitamin will suffice. The reader wishing a more detailed examination of this aspect is referred to J. A. Olson's (1988) review.

Vitamin A is now considered chemically as a member of the subgroup of retinoids, compounds which consist of four isoprenoid units joined in a head-to-tail manner (see Fig. 1). The typical form of vitamin A is retinol (all-trans retinol), a highly unsaturated primary alcohol soluble in most organic solvents but not in water. While retinol is the typical form, the term vitamin A usually encompasses all retinoids having a biological action similar to retinol. These include, among others, the free alcohol, its esters, the aldehyde (retinene) and the acid (retinoic acid).

The primary unit of biological activity for all forms of vitamin A is equivalent to the activity of 1 μg trans-retinol.

Food contains both retinol esters and pro-vitamins known as carotenes. Both esters and carotenes are hydrolyzed in the intestine to yield retinol. Fig. 1 illustrates the hydrolysis of β-carotene into two molecules of retinol. Retinoic acid is produced by several cell types from retinol or retinene.

All forms of vitamin A must be emulsified in the intestine before they can be absorbed and transported to the liver as chylomicra. Hepatocytes will esterify most forms of vitamin A, which will then be stored by specialized cells known as "stellate" cells or "lipocytes". In normal conditions these cells contain 90% of the vitamin A of the body. Retinoic acid differs from other forms in that it is not stored by the liver.

Hepatocytes produce a plasmatic protein (retinol-binding protein) which transports all of the circulating forms of the vitamin with the exception of retinoic acid. This binding protein adheres to receptors in the target cells so that retinol can penetrate their cytoplasm.

The best known physiological role of vitamin A is the formation of visual pigment. Retinol is transformed in the retinal rods into retinal (retinene).

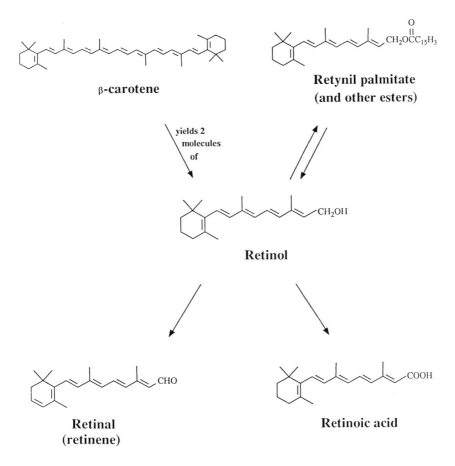

Fig. 1 Chemical structures of β-carotene and of some of the most important forms of vitamin A.

Retinoic acid, however, cannot be transformed into retinal and does not play any role in the visual cells. In all other tissues, including bone, both retinol and retinoic acid are active and appear to act on cells in a manner different from that observed in rods and cones. Thus, rather than becoming incorporated as a cytoplasmic component, they bind to a cytoplasmic receptor protein, together with which they become incorporated into the nucleus where they influence the genome. Thus, the way they act on cells appears to be similar to the way in which steroid hormones, thyroid hormones and 1,25-(OH)$_2$D$_3$ act.

The fact that cells contain different binding proteins for retinol and retinoic acid would appear to indicate that these two compounds have a different function. However, no differences have been found between the effects of retinoic acid and retinol in most differentiated cells. Differences in the degree of activity of these two compounds have been attributed to the fact that retinoic acid has a much shorter life, so that repeated or continuous administration is required in order to obtain effects comparable in magnitude to those produced by retinol. The fact that retinoic acid is produced in the organism (from retinol or retinal), has a very short life, and is transported by the blood to the target cells suggests that it should be considered to be a hormone rather than a vitamin. It has been recently been shown that retinoic acid is produced very early in the limb buds of chick embryos where it acts as a morphogen (Thaller and Eichele, 1987).

Effects of Hypovitaminosis A

Although hypovitaminosis A is known to produce skeletal alterations in man, the importance of these alterations is obscured by the severity of retinal, corneal and skin lesions; these demand treatment before the deficiency has become severe enough to induce significant bone lesions. The nature of the bone alterations produced by the deficiency is better known from experimentally induced deficiencies in several laboratory animals (see review by Barnicot and Datta, 1972).

It was first found that rats fed a diet deficient in vitamin A presented a disproportion between the size of the brain and the size of the cranial cavity: the brain was distorted and dislocated towards the foramen magnum. Similarly, a disproportion between the size of the spinal cord and the cavity of the vertebral canal produced distortion of the spinal cord and herniation of nerve roots into the intervertebral foramina.

The causal relationship between the bone changes and the resulting neural alterations was best demonstrated by Mellanby (1944) in dogs reared on a diet deficient in vitamin A. This author found degenerative changes of the 2nd, 5th and 8th cranial nerves. It was in studying the lesions of the 8th nerve that he concluded that the changes in the nerves were due to their compression by overgrown bone. More importantly, overgrowth of facial bones, unaccompanied by nervous lesions, was also found. The term "overgrowth" is perhaps inappropiate since, with the exception of the case of the auditory meatus in which narrowing of the canal results from the formation of bone which normally is not formed at this place, in most other sites the lesions consist of a failure of osteoclasts to destroy bone which normally should disappear during the process of remodeling (Barnicot and Datta, 1972). These works suggested that hypovitaminosis A affects the function of both osteoblasts and osteoclasts. By showing that bone resorption decreases and bone formation increases when vitamin A is lacking, these classical studies suggested that the main action of the vitamin is to stimulate bone resorption and inhibit bone formation. This idea was further supported by the results of contemporary studies on experimental hypervitaminosis A.

Effects of Hypervitaminosis A

Early studies found an increase in bone fractures in young rats receiving large doses of fish liver oil concentrate; the conclusion that the bone lesions were due to hypervitaminosis A was put into question because the concentrates administered to the animals also contained vitamin D (see review by Barnicot and Datta, 1972). However, similar bone lesions were later observed in experiments using crystalline vitamin A (Barnicot and Datta, 1972).

It was shown that bones break because of thinning of the cortex in many regions due to excessive resorption. Fractures appear so consistently that Cashin and Lewis (1984) have proposed that this property can be used for a test ("tibial bone-breaking strain") to detect the degree of hypervitaminosis A. Calcification, on the other hand, appears to proceed normally in the animals with hypervitaminosis A.

In addition to their propensity to fracture, changes in the shape of long bones were observed which were interpreted as resulting from a combination of excessive bone resorption at some sites and failure to grow new bone at others (Wolbach, 1947; Barnicot and Datta, 1972). Histological studies showed an increase in the number of osteoclasts in the regions with excessive resorption. Thinning of the cortex due to excessive osteoclastic resorption was sometimes accompanied by the formation of osteoid at the endosteal surface (Wolbach, 1947; Barnicot and Datta, 1972). Bone changes produced by hypervitaminosis A have also been quantitated through morphometric procedures (Lopez *et al.*, 1982).

When young, rather than mature, animals were treated, an inhibition of growth in length was observed in the long bones (Wolbach, 1947); these bones show thinning of their epiphyseal plates. It appears as if an excessive resorption of the hypertrophic zone fails to be compensated for by growth of the proliferative zone (Barnicot and Datta, 1972).

While the above-described studies have been conducted mainly on laboratory rodents, similar results have been obtained in dogs and chicken (see review by Barnicot and Datta, 1972).

Vitamin A and Bone and Cartilage Resorption

Classical studies, summarized previously, demonstrated a decrease in bone and cartilage resorption in animals deficient in vitamin A and an increase in resorption in the case of hypervitaminosis A. It is tempting to conclude from these experiments that one of the main functions of vitamin A is to stimulate bone and cartilage resorption.

Numerous experiments have been carried out to try to establish whether this effect of vitamin A is a direct one or if it is mediated by hormonal factors. That resorption results from a direct action of the vitamin on the bone was first suggested by Barnicot's experiments (reviewed in Barnicot and Datta, 1972). This investigator placed small fragments of crystalline vitamin A acetate into direct contact with small pieces of parietal bone and grafted both together into the skulls of young mice: the vitamin crystals produced resorption of the contacting bone. The idea that vitamin A acts directly on bone was later supported by *in vitro* experiments showing that the vitamin can promote resorption of mineral from cultured bones pre-labeled with ^{45}Ca (Raisz, 1965); Reynolds (1968) confirmed these results and showed, in addition, that vitamin A-induced resorption can be blocked by calcitonin. The idea that vitamin A acts directly on osteoclasts is supported by the fact that these cells possess a cytoplasmic retinol-binding protein (Teti *et al.*, 1986).

More recently, Hough *et al.* (1988) observed that rats injected with the vitamin showed an increase in urinary hydroxyproline excretion (which is indicative of bone resorption) but had normal serum levels of parathyroid homone, 25-hydroxyvitamin D_3 and 1,25-dihydroxyvitamin D_3 (calcitriol). These experiments appear to suggest that the bone-resorbing activity of vitamin A is not mediated by any of the aforementioned powerful bone resorbers. The fact that vitamin A acts directly on bone cells does not exclude the possibility that it might interact at a cellular level with other hormonal factors. Thus, Petkovich *et al.* (1984) found that retinoic acid can stimulate binding of calcitriol to cultured osteosarcoma cells and it has been suggested that vitamin A might act by increasing the receptors for calcitriol in osteoclasts or their predecessors. Osteoclasts are now believed to originate through fusion of macrophages originated from monocytes, and calcitriol appears to be capable of stimulating this cellular fusion (Miyaura *et al.*, 1986).

On the other hand, the idea that vitamin A can increase the responsivity of osteoclasts to calcitriol does not agree well with the results of previous experiments showing that vitamin A is capable of preventing or improving the symptoms of hypervitaminosis D (Clark and Smith, 1964; Metz *et al.*, 1985). Additional clarification of this aspect of the problem is required.

That vitamin A can also induce cartilage resorption was suggested by the previously discussed classical experiments on hypervitaminosis A. These experiments had shown that the growth of long bones was greatly affected and that epiphyseal cartilages became very narrow due to increased resorption at the hypertrophic zone not compensated for by an increase in cell proliferation at the growth zone. That this is a direct effect of the vitamin on cartilage cells is suggested by numerous *in vitro* experiments from the group of Fell at Cambridge.

Fell and Mellanby (1950) showed that when the cartilaginous primordia of long bones from mouse embryos were grown on media containing vitamin A, the cartilaginous matrix lost its capacity to stain metachromatically. It was later shown by the same group that the incorporation of radioactive sulfate by the cultured primordia was greatly decreased. Subsequently, it was demonstrated (Fell and Thomas, 1960) that a proteolytic enzyme, papain, when added to the culture medium could mimic the effects of vitamin A on the cartilage matrix. Lucy *et al.* (1961) demonstrated that the changes induced by vitamin A were due to the liberation by the cells of cathepsin C. It was finally concluded (Weston *et al.*, 1969) that the vitamin's effects were due to increased permeability of the lysosomes in the chondrocytes and that this increased permeability allowed the exit of cathepsin, which then produced the matrix changes.

Vitamin A and Bone and Cartilage Formation

Classical experiments with hypervitaminosis A suggested that the vitamin not only can increase the resorption of bone, but that it can also inhibit its formation. This has been supported by studies by Tyler and Dewitt-Stott (1986) who showed that the vitamin inhibits membrane bone formation in an *in vitro* system; this would suggest that this growth inhibition results from a direct effect of the vitamin on bone cells. In addition, it would appear that vitamin A can affect the synthesis of several components of the bone matrix including collagen (Dickson and Walls, 1985).

The idea that some of these actions of vitamin A result from its interaction with calcitriol in osteoblasts is suggested by the experiments of Chen and Feldman (1985) showing that retinoic acid can modulate the receptors for calcitriol in these cells. The meaning of this interaction is not clear since Grigoriadis *et al.* (1986), working with osteoblast-like cells from an osteosarcoma cell line, found that although retinoic acid modulates receptors for calcitriol it does not increase the biological response of these cells to the hormone. It must be cautioned that the results of experiments with cultured cells, and especially of those that involve tumor cell lines, might not reflect the behavior of normal tissues *in vivo*.

Vitamin A appears also to affect the synthesis of cartilage matrix, producing inhibition of the synthesis of glycosaminoglycans and proteoglycans (Solursch and Meier, 1973; Vasan and Lash, 1975).

Vitamin C

Vitamin C, chemically L-ascorbic acid, has the formula shown in Fig. 2. Vitamin C is synthesized in the liver in most animals; either glucose and glucuronic acid or galactonic acid can serve as precursors. Certain animals such as guinea pigs and primates, including man, cannot synthesize the vitamin and depend on its ingestion for survival. It is present in large amounts in fruits and fresh vegetables. It is highly thermolabile and is destroyed at temperatures over 60°C. In animals which cannot synthesize the vitamin, a deficit in the consumption of vitamin C-rich food produces the typical symptomatology of scurvy. The manifestations of scurvy in man have been known since the era of long sea voyages, during which the intake of fruits and fresh vegetables was greatly reduced. Of the various manifestations of scurvy, we shall describe only those found in bones.

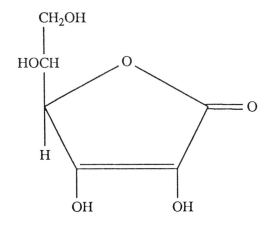

L-ascorbic acid

Fig. 2 Chemical structure of vitamin C (L-ascorbic acid).

The first observation in classical studies was that bone fractures in scorbutic patients were difficult to heal. It was also claimed that long-time healed fractures could again break through resorption or softening of the calluses, but these claims were never confirmed experimentally. The delay in the healing of fractures is probably related to the fact that vitamin C is required for the synthesis of bone matrix, as discussed below.

The main bone histological lesions observed in scurvy in both guinea pigs and in the human (see review by Bourne, 1972) consist of subperiosteal hemorrhages, thinning of the diaphysis of the long bones and alterations in shape and size of their metaphyses.

The main mechanism by which changes in the shape of the bones take place is related to the inability of the osteoblasts to produce normal bone matrix. In the diaphysis, bone trabeculae are thin and without osteoid seams. In the case of the metaphysis, the zone in which the degenerating cartilage is replaced by bone trabeculae, the weak calcified remnants of cartilaginous matrix fracture repeatedly and intermingle with irregularly arranged bone trabeculae. This zone of abnormal bone trabeculae is not only clearly distinguishable in histological sections but also in X-ray pictures where it is seen as a "scorbutic band" or "Trummerfeld". The well-known scorbutic metaphyseal deformities are apparently due to mechanical stress; the weak "scorbutic band" cannot support weight and becomes compressed and deformed by the overlying epiphyseal cartilage. This mechanism has been demonstrated experimentally: when weight-bearing stress is prevented by placing a cast around a leg, the deformity is prevented (Follis, 1948).

All of the above-described bone abnormalities are probably related to the fact that ascorbic acid is required for the synthesis of collagen and, possibly, glycosaminoglycans. That vitamin C has a direct effect on collagen synthesis was suggested by experiments with embryonic bone rudiments maintained *in vitro*. The addition of ascorbic acid to the medium significantly increased collagen synthesis (Jeffrey and Martin, 1966a,b; Reynolds, 1967). The differentiation *in vitro* of chondrocytes from undifferentiated cells also requires ascorbic acid (Hall, 1981).

It is now known that vitamin C is required for the hydroxylations of proline into hydroxyproline and lysine into hydroxylysine (see review by Hornig *et al.*, 1988). Hydroxylation of proline is required for the formation and stabilization of the triple helical structure of collagen and hydroxylation of lysine is essential for glycosylation and formation of hydroxylysine-derived cross-links. The enzymes required for both hydroxylations are inactivated in the absence of ascorbic acid (Hornig *et al.*, 1988). It is also believed that, in addition to acting on proline and lysine hydroxylation, ascorbic acid can directly stimulate collagen peptide synthesis (Murad *et al.*, 1981).

Ascorbic acid appears to also be important for glycosaminoglycan synthesis in cartilage (Bird *et al.*, 1986). It is possible that this is also true for the bone, but sufficient supporting evidence is still lacking.

Vitamin D

Structure and Metabolism

Excellent reviews describing the structure and metabolism of vitamin D are available in the literature (Lawson and Davie, 1979; Norman, 1980; De Luca, 1988). Here, we shall only summarize established knowledge in the field. The vitamin normally synthesized by animals is known as cholecalciferol or vitamin D_3 (see Fig. 3). Mammals and birds carry on this synthesis in the skin and feathers, respectively. A pre-vitamin (7-dehydrocholesterol) is transformed there into cholecalciferol through the action of sunlight; this is a photolytic conversion and does not involve enzymatic activity. In addition, animals obtain pre-formed vitamin from food.

A similar compound, ergocalciferol or vitamin D_2, can be produced by irradiating ergosterol (a secosterol of plant origin). It is this synthetic vitamin D_2 that is added to milk in North America; it is also the form used in medical prescriptions. This vitamin D_2 is metabolized by the organism in the same way as described below for vitamin D_3.

Whether synthesized in the skin or absorbed through the intestine, vitamin D_3 is inactive on target tissues; it must be hydroxylated in position 25 by liver cells before becoming active. The resulting compound, 25-hydroxycholecalciferol (25-D_3), is the main circulating form of the vitamin. Although 25-D_3 is active on target tissues, the vitamin is further activated by hydrox-

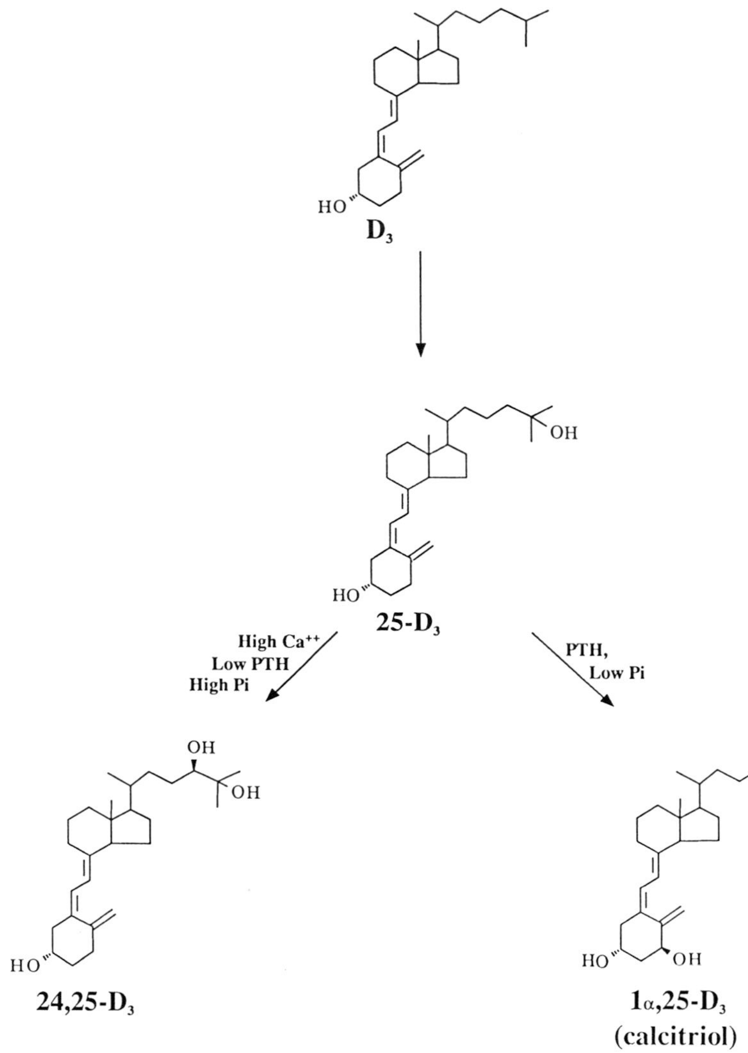

Fig. 3 Chemical structures of vitamin D and its most important metabolites.

ylation in position 1; the resulting metabolite, 1α,25-dihydroxycholecalciferol
(calcitriol), is many times more active than 25-D₃. Although various tissues
are able to produce calcitriol in *in vitro* experiments, in the living organism
the synthesis takes place mainly in proximal convoluted tubules of the kidney.
While hydroxylation in position 25 by liver cells is not regulated to a great
extent, hydroxylation in position 1α by kidney cells is a very closely regulated
process. Thus, calcitriol is synthesized in accordance with the momentary
requirements of calcium and phosphate. Hypocalcemia stimulates the synthesis of calcitriol directly and by increasing the circulating levels of para-

thyroid hormone. In the case of hypophosphatemia, the synthesis of the metabolite is stimulated directly by low tissue levels of phosphate (see review by DeLuca, 1988).

While high levels of parathyroid hormone and low levels of phosphate are recognized as the main stimulators of the synthesis of calcitriol, this process can also be modulated by other hormones such as estrogens, growth hormone and prolactin. This modulation appears to be important in periods of life with high demands of calcium and phosphate such as pregnancy, lactation and growth spurts during childhood. The fact that calcitriol (a) is very active, (b) is synthesized by one organ in accordance with the changing needs of the organism, and (c) is transported through the blood in order to act on target tissues has prompted various authors to consider it a real steroid hormone (Norman, 1980).

During hypercalcemia and/or hyperphosphatemia, the synthesis of calcitriol decreases greatly, but another metabolite, 24R,25-dihydroxycholecalciferol (24R,25-D_3), is produced instead by the same kidney cells. This compound is much less active than calcitriol and 25-D_3. It has, however, a longer life than calcitriol and can be re-activated by hydroxylation into 1,24,25-trihydroxycholecalciferol (1,24,25-D_3).

The vitamin D absorbed through the intestine is transported in chylomicrons. Metabolites of vitamin D, however, are transported in the serum bound to a specific vitamin D-binding protein which is synthesized by hepatocytes. This binding protein binds preferentially to 25-D_3 and 24,25-D_3 and, with less affinity, to calcitriol and vitamin D_3 itself.

In common with other steroid hormones, calcitriol acts on target cells by binding to a specific cytoplasmic D-binding protein, together with which it translocates into the nucleus, where it acts on the genome regulating the synthesis of one or more proteins. The cytoplasmic protein preferentially binds calcitriol and, with less intensity, other active metabolites. The utilization of autoradiographic methods to search for target cells for calcitriol has permitted the confirmation of previously proposed target cells (intestinal epithelium, osteoblasts, kidney's distal tubule epithelium), but also allowed the recognition of other previously unsuspected targets such as skin, pituitary, parathyroid glands, mammary glands, numerous neurons, etc. (Stumpf et al., 1979; Narbaitz et al., 1980, 1981b, 1983).

As with other steroid hormones, calcitriol appears to affect the synthesis of different proteins by its target cells. A vitamin D-dependent calcium-binding protein (calbindin) was isolated from the intestine of chicken and has been later identified in numerous target cells for calcitriol. Jande and Schreiner (1982) localized this protein in bones. It has been shown that calcitriol also regulates the production of other proteins such as carbonic anhydrase in the chick embryo's chorioallantoic membrane (Narbaitz et al., 1981a) and osteocalcin in bone cells (Price, 1985).

One of the main targets for calcitriol is the intestinal epithelium. In response to the hormone, there is an increase in the absorption of Ca and P. Calcitriol also stimulates bone resorption. By acting both on the intestine and on the bone, calcitriol is capable of increasing the serum levels of Ca and inorganic phosphorus (Pi). In analyzing the effects of vitamin D metabolites on bone, it is sometimes difficult to discriminate the effects which result from their direct action on bone cells from those which are secondary to alterations in Ca and Pi homeostasis induced by the same or by derived metabolites.

Vitamin D Deficiency

A large proportion of what we now know on the action of vitamin D on bone and cartilage derives from the study of bone changes in rickets and osteomalacia, two forms of vitamin D deficiency. Both deficiency states occur spontaneously in man and domestic animals and can be reproduced with ease in the laboratory.

Rickets, which reached epidemic proportions at the end of the last century and the beginning of the present one, coincided with the industrial revolution which created over-crowding in cities and in which children were submitted to deficient exposure to sunlight and diets which were inadequate both in amount and in quality. In addition to lack of growth, asthenia and muscular weakness, the expression of this condition includes characteristic skeletal deformities such as enlarged epiphysis, "knock knees" or "bow legs" and "pigeon chest". The most serious forms of the disease became infrequent after their relation to a deficiency in vitamin D was understood. The histological changes characteristic of the condition have been described long ago (see review by Harris, 1956) and will be summarized here briefly.

The characteristic skeletal lesions result mainly from inadequate calcification of bone structures. In the case of epiphyseal cartilage, calcium fails to be deposited in the matrix at the zone of provisional calcification; as a result, this zone fails to be resorbed. Since the cartilage continues proliferating but is not resorbed at the same rate, it increases in breadth; at the same time, in the zone directly underlying the cartilage there is an irregular proliferation of undermineralized bone trabeculae and atypical distribution of blood vessels.

On the other hand, mineralization is also deficient in bone trabeculae in the diaphysis. The characteristic bending of leg bones in rickets (bow legs) results precisely from the undermineralization of cortical bone in the diaphysis of the tibiae. This mineralization defect is visualized histologically as an increase in the width of osteoid seams, i.e., the zone of bone matrix located between the layer of osteoblasts and the fully mineralized matrix. The unmineralized bone matrix stains differently, probably due to a different carbohydrate content; the molecular structure of collagen in osteoid is perhaps also altered (Mechanic et al., 1975; Baylink et al., 1980). These changes are generally defined as "matrix immaturity"; osteoid must "mature" before it can be mineralized (Baylink *et al.*, 1980).

Osteomalacia is the form of vitamin D deficiency which occurs when the deficiency starts after completion of growth and disappearance of epiphyseal plates. In this case, the lesions affect only the bones, which are undermineralized and have a tendency to bend. Again, the histological expression of this condition is an increase in the width of osteoid seams.

Both in rickets and in osteomalacia, histological lesions heal rapidly after treatment with vitamin D. Less frequent cases of rickets are found which do not respond to treatment with vitamin D (vitamin D-resistant rickets). Genetic defects consisting of either the inability to produce calcitriol because of the lack of 25-hydroxycholecalciferol 1-hydroxylase (Type I) or the inability of target tissues to respond (Type II) have been described in man (see review by DeLuca, 1988). Animal models for both of these varieties have been studied (Eicher *et al.*, 1976; Yamaguchi *et al.*, 1986).

The condition of rickets can be reproduced with ease in dogs and chickens by submitting the animals to diets deficient in vitamin D (see review by Harris, 1956). In rats, rickets can only be induced by administering diets which are deficient in vitamin D but which are also poor in P or contain a high Ca/P ratio (Harrison *et al.*, 1958).

After the discovery of the active metabolites of vitamin D, numerous experiments were carried out to establish the relative capacity of the various metabolites to heal rickets. It was found that 25-D cures the lesions to the same extent as vitamin D_3, but conflicting reports were made initially on the capacity of calcitriol to heal experimental rickets. It has been found, however, that since this metabolite has a very short half-life, successful treatment requires repeated administration (Dickson *et al.*, 1984). In the case of rats, both a diet with adequate amounts of Ca and P and low doses of calcitriol are required in order to heal or prevent rickets. Large doses or inadequate Ca/P ratio in the diet induce hypercalcemia with normal or lower than normal levels of P and produce signs of hypervitaminosis as described below (Gunness-Hey *et al.*, 1988).

Hypervitaminosis D

Our knowledge on the mechanisms of action of vitamin D on bone has also been enriched by the analysis of spontaneous and experimentally induced hypervitaminosis D (Harris, 1956).

Chronic hypervitaminosis D results in an increase in absorption of Ca and P from the gut and resorption of the same elements from the bone. As a result of these effects there is usually hypercalcemia and hyperphosphatemia and, consequently, calciuria and phosphaturia. Finally, deposition of calcium salts in extraskeletal tissues occurs principally in kidney and large blood vessels.

The first experiments on hypervitaminosis D detected two types of skeletal changes: a proliferation of osteoid trabeculae at the endosteal side of long bones and an increase in osteoclastic bone resorption (see review by Harris, 1956). Based on the fact that an increase in osteoid was considered to be pathognomic of rickets, the term "hypervitaminosis D rickets" was coined to designate the bone changes observed in hypervitaminosis D. However, unlike in rickets, in hypervitaminosis D, endosteal bone proliferates extensively to the point that, in the most severe cases, it completely fills the marrow cavity (Harris, 1956). In late stages of the chronic experiments vitamin D-induced osteoclastic bone resorption becomes more prominent and supersedes osteoid formation. All of the above-described findings were repeatedly confirmed using different animals and diets (Harris, 1956).

As in vitamin D deficiency, the type of skeletal effects of hypervitaminosis D in rats varies with the content of Ca and P in the diet. In general, when large doses of vitamin D_3 are administered chronically to animals fed a diet with a well-balanced content of Ca and P, the excess of vitamin produces an increase in the proliferation of bone trabeculae and a moderate amount of osteoclastic bone resorption. On the other hand, if the animals are fed a diet which is poor in P or contains a large Ca/P ratio, osteoclastic resorption becomes predominant (Harris, 1956).

While all classical studies were conducted by administering large doses of vitamin D, identical results can be obtained using 25-D_3 or calcitriol. Due to the short half-life of calcitriol, repeated doses at daily intervals are required in order to obtain similar results (Boyce and Weistrode, 1983; Hock et al., 1986; Wronski et al., 1986). In the chick embryo, calcitriol-induced osteoid proliferation can be elicited with a single injection (Narbaitz and Tolnai, 1978; Narbaitz and Fragiskos, 1984).

Mechanisms for Vitamin D Effects on Bone and Cartilage Mineralization

That vitamin D is required for normal bone and cartilage mineralization was first suggested by the fact that both the epiphyseal cartilage and bone trabeculae fail to mineralize adequately in rickets.

It was recognized early that rickets is usually associated with hypocalcemia and/or hypophosphatemia which result from decreased efficiency of the absorption of Ca and P from the gut; it was concluded that the defects observed in cartilage and bone mineralization were secondary to the humoral changes.

The concentration of Ca and P in the blood from vitamin D-deficient animals varies according to the diet. As indicated earlier, in the case of rats, bone and cartilage undermineralization do not occur unless the D-deficient animals are fed a diet which is poor in phosphate or has a high Ca/P ratio (Harrison et al., 1958). The resulting hypophosphatemia is probably responsible for bone and cartilage undermineralization.

It has been customary to indicate that mineralization of bone and cartilage requires a "normal CaXP product" in the blood. It probably would be more accurate to define the relationship between Ca and P levels and mineralization by expressing that "mineralization requires normal serum levels of both Ca and P". This is so, because in some cases Ca and P levels vary in opposite directions and a mineralization defect occurs despite a normal CaXP product; thus, in vitamin D deficiency in the chick embryo, low serum levels of Ca coexist with high P levels (Narbaitz and Tsang, 1989). High levels of Ca with normal or lower than normal levels of phosphate will also inhibit mineralization in rats (Gunness-Hey et al., 1988).

The idea that the low serum levels of P usually found in rickets are responsible for the lack of bone and cartilage mineralization is supported by the fact that lesions very similar to those found in this condition also appear in clinical conditions in which hypophosphatemia occurs, but is unrelated to D deficiency.

Bone and cartilage lesions typical of rickets heal very rapidly after the administration of vitamin D and the healing of the lesions is preceded by normalization of blood concentrations of Ca and P. Moreover, epiphyseal plates isolated from rachitic animals mineralize when placed in normal serum or in solutions containing normal amounts of Ca and P (Anderson et al., 1975). In addition, normal mineralization of both cartilage and bone has been observed in D-deficient rats in which the concentrations of Ca and P in blood were normalized after intravenous infusion of a solution containing those elements in adequate proportion (Underwood and DeLuca, 1984).

All the above-described findings lead to the generally accepted conclusion that the main mechanism by which vitamin D prevents or heals rickets is the normalization of Ca and P levels in the blood. It is also agreed that the most active metabolite involved in this action is calcitriol.

As indicated earlier, a deficit in mineralization also occurs in hypervitaminosis D. The fact that undermineralization occurs both as a result of a deficit and as a result of an excess of the vitamin is not surprising because alterations in the levels of Ca and P in blood are present in both cases.

Hypervitaminosis D stimulates the growth of bone trabeculae and undermineralization occurs mainly in the newly formed trabeculae which are growing much faster than in normal animals; there is probably not an inhibition of mineralization but a failure of mineralization to keep pace with the increased rate of matrix deposition. The combination of hypercalcemia with normal or lower than normal levels of phosphate is associated most frequently with these lesions.

Thus, both in D deficiency and in hypervitaminosis D, the deficit in cartilage and bone mineralization can be explained without assuming that vitamin D metabolites exert a direct control on the process of mineralization. One should, however, keep an open mind on this subject since the complex mechanisms leading to mineralization are still incompletely known. There is some, still inconclusive and/or circumstantial, evidence supporting the idea of a direct effect of D metabolites on bone mineralization.

In the first place, a direct action of vitamin D on bone cells is suggested by the fact that cytoplasmic and nuclear receptors for calcitriol have been demonstrated in pre-osteoblasts, osteoblasts and osteocytes (Narbaitz et al., 1983). There is debate on the possible existence of specific receptors for 24,25-D_3 (Manolagas and Deftos, 1981; Fine et al., 1985).

A second line of evidence suggesting a direct effect of D metabolites on bone mineralization emerged from the demonstration that, in cultured bones from chick embryos, mineralization occurs when a combination of calcitriol and 24,25-D_3 is added to the culture medium and does not occur if calcitriol or 24,25-D_3 is added independently (Endo et al., 1980). In addition, it has been shown that calcitriol and 24,25-D_3 can affect in opposite directions alkaline phosphatase activity and the phospholipidic composition of plasma membranes and matrix vesicles from chondrocytes of the epiphyseal plates (Boyan et al., 1988; Hale et al., 1986).

The third line of evidence, suggesting a direct action of the metabolites on bone mineralization, comes from clinical (Bordier et al., 1978; Rasmussen et al., 1980) and experimental (Tam et al., 1986) studies in which mineralization was evaluated morphometrically with or without tetracycline labeling; these studies conclude that vitamin D metabolites other than calcitriol, and most probably 24,25-D_3, appear to stimulate mineralization through a direct action on bone cells. However, in clinical studies and in experiments with intact animals it is difficult to discriminate between the actions of both metabolites since both calcitriol and 24,25-D_3 can be converted by the organism into 1,24,25-D_3, a metabolite which acts like calcitriol although it is less active. Partial clarification of this problem came from experiments using an analog of calcitriol in which the two positions 24 are blocked by fluorine and cannot be hydroxylated. Rachitic animals treated with this compound have no detectable 24,25-D_3 in their blood and despite this show normal mineralization of epiphyseal cartilage and bone (Miller et al., 1981). These experiments appear to indicate that hydroxylation in position 24 is not indispensable for mineralization to occur.

Vitamin D and Bone Formation

The classical studies on hypervitaminosis D were the first to suggest that vitamin D might directly affect bone growth. As discussed previously (section on Hypervitaminosis D), the administration of large doses of the vitamin induces the proliferation of many trabeculae, most of them at the endosteal side of long bones; in extreme cases these trabeculae completely fill the marrow cavity.

In most experiments in which excessive formation of bone trabeculae was detected, there was also hypercalcemia; it is not clear if growth stimulation results from a direct action of the vitamin on bone cells or from the concomitant hypercalcemia. The fact that osteoprogenitor cells are known to be targets for calcitriol (Narbaitz et al., 1983) makes the first alternative attractive. However, Gunness-Hey et al. (1988), working on rats, found that when calcitriol is administered in low doses, which do not induce hypercalcemia, there is no increase in bone mass. They concluded that the hypercalcemia is the main reason for the increase in bone mass which occurs with high doses of the vitamin or its metabolites. A similar conclusion has been reached in the case of hypervitaminosis D in chick embryos (see section "Vitamin D in the Chick Embryo").

The increase in new bone formation induced by calcitriol results mainly from an increase in proliferation and differentiation of pre-osteoblastic cells. It has been suggested that in addition to the increased rate of proliferation of these cells, the rate of matrix production by osteoblasts and osteocytes might also be increased. This suggestion would agree with the results of in vivo experiments showing that vitamin D_3 increases the synthesis of bone collagen in rachitic rats (Canas et al., 1969). However, calcitriol itself appears to inhibit, and not to stimulate, the synthesis of collagen (Raisz et al., 1978; Hock et al., 1982).

Osteocalcin, another important component of bone matrix, is a vitamin K-dependent protein; the effects of calcitriol on its synthesis will be discussed in the section dedicated to vitamin K.

Vitamin D and Bone Resorption

The fact that vitamin D might play a role in regulating osteoclastic bone resorption was first suggested by the classical experiments on hypervitaminosis D discussed in a previous section. It was later observed that parathyroid hormone fails to induce resorption in the absence of vitamin D (Harrison et al., 1958; Rasmussen et al., 1963) and it was concluded that, rather than producing bone resorption by itself, vitamin D acted by making bone more sensitive to the action of parathyroid hormone. An impaired response to parathyroid hormone has been confirmed in bone cells isolated from calvariae of vitamin D-deficient rats (Crowell et al., 1981). This does not exclude the possibility that vitamin D metabolites might also act on their own, inducing bone resorption (Holtrop et al., 1981).

That vitamin D might influence resorption through a direct action on bone cells was first suggested by the experiments of Barnicott (1948). Following previous experiments in which he had successfully demonstrated direct action of vitamin A on bone grafts, he conducted similar experiments using vitamin D. He implanted a combination of pieces of bone with pellets of crystallized vitamin D into the head cavity of mice and showed that bone resorption only occurred in the region of the bone which was in direct contact with the pellet of vitamin (Barnicott, 1948). The concept of a direct action on bone cells is today generally accepted as true but only with regard to vitamin D active metabolites and not to vitamin D itself.

Further clarification of this aspect of the problem came from the results of experiments in which the amount of bone resorption was evaluated by measuring the release of ^{45}Ca from prelabeled bones cultured on media to which the vitamin D metabolites were added. Thus, Trummel et al. (1969) showed that the release of ^{45}Ca from long bones of fetal rats could be stimulated by low doses of 25-D_3 but only inconsistently by very large doses of vitamin D_3 itself. Likewise, Reynolds et al. (1973) compared the effects of 25-D_3 and calcitriol on prelabeled mouse calvaria and concluded that calcitriol was 100 times more potent than 25-D_3.

Resorption induced in vivo by calcitriol has also been confirmed using morphometric evaluation of osteclasts and hydroxyproline excretion (Holtrop et al., 1981; Marie and Travers, 1983). Contradictory results in previous works have been interpreted on the basis of differences in dose or, most importantly, in the Ca/P ratio in the diet.

Calcitriol-induced bone resorption is more evident when animals are fed diets poor in calcium. When the diet contains sufficient calcium, the resorptive response to calcitriol is less notable; this is probably because in this situation calcitriol preferentially stimulates calcium absorption from the gut, and the resulting hypercalcemia triggers calcitonin secretion, which in turn blunts the response of osteoclasts. A similar mechanism is probably at play in the chick embryos, as will be discussed in the following section.

The mechanisms by which active vitamin D metabolites influence bone resorption have been debated. On the one hand, in cultured bones, calcitriol-induced bone resorption appears to depend mainly on an increase in the activity of existing osteoclasts (Holtrop and Raisz, 1979). The idea of a direct action of calcitriol on osteoclasts has been contradicted by experiments in which osteoclasts isolated from neonatal rabbit bones failed to respond to calcitriol (Chambers et al., 1985) and also by the fact that osteoclasts have not been shown to possess receptors for calcitriol. These receptors have been detected only in osteoblasts, osteocytes and osteoprogenitor cells (Narbaitz et al., 1983). It is possible that calcitriol might act by stimulating the release from osteoblasts or osteocytes of agents which, in turn, would activate osteoclasts, but the responsible agent(s) has (have) not been identified.

In long-term experiments, calcitriol not only stimulates the activity of existing osteoclasts, but also produces an increase in the number of osteoclasts. These cells are believed to originate by fusion of precursor mononuclear macrophagic cells. Calcitriol might act by stimulating the differentiation and/or fusion of precursor cells. In support of this idea, Shinna et al. (1986) succeeded in demonstrating that calcitriol activates in vitro the fusion of macrophages to form multinucleated osteoclasts and Teti et al. (1988) showed that the hormone increases the rate of fusion of monocytes with pre-existent osteoclasts.

The fact that calcitriol is capable of stimulating bone resorption at the same time that it increases the absorption of Ca and P from the gut allows the hormone to play an important role in the maintenance of Ca and P homeostasis. However, the regulation of osteoclastic function by calcitriol is not only related to Ca and P homeostasis. Resorption by osteoclasts is an important part of the continuous remodeling process undergone by bones to adapt to the requirements of growth and mechanical function, and calcitriol and/or other vitamin D metabolites are required for this remodelling process to take place. This is illustrated clearly by experiments in chick embryos described below.

Vitamin D in the Chick Embryo

During the last decade we have acquired a great amount of information on the mechanisms by which vitamin D regulates Ca and P metabolism in the chick embryo (Narbaitz, 1987). It is known that the embryo obtains the vitamin from the yolk and that it is capable of producing all metabolites including $25\text{-}D_3$, $24,25\text{-}D_3$ and calcitriol. Target cells for calcitriol have been identified in several embryonic tissues such as choriallantoic membranes, kidneys, gut, parathyroid glands and bones (Narbaitz *et al.*, 1980; Narbaitz, 1987).

A large part of what we know about the role of vitamin D in the regulation of Ca and P in the embryo has been learned from the analysis of the effects of D deficiency and hypervitaminosis D.

It has been known for many years that the eggs from vitamin D-deficient hens have very low hatchability, but the exact mechanisms by which the deficiency affects embryonic development have only recently been clarified. An effective method of inducing vitamin D deficiency in the embryos was suggested by works from two laboratories (Sunde *et al.*, 1978; Henry and Norman, 1978). This consists of substituting calcitriol for the normal vitamin D content in the diet of the laying hens. The eggs from these hens have very low hatchability and have been confirmed to be deficient in all vitamin D metabolites. These D-deficient embryos are hypocalcemic and hyperphosphatemic and have bones with a low ash content (Narbaitz *et al.*, 1987). These changes can be corrected by the injection of calcitriol. The hypocalcemia observed in D deficiency is probably due to reduced intake of calcium from the shell since it is known that vitamin D regulates shell solubilization (see review by Narbaitz, 1987). On the other hand, the hyperphosphatemia is probably due to reduced utilization of P for bone mineralization and/or increased resorption from the filtrate in the kidney tubules.

Histological studies of the bones from deficient embryos (Narbaitz and Tsang, 1989) have shown that bone trabeculae have the wide osteoid seams typical of rickets and osteomalacia. Treatment with a single injection of calcitriol, $25\text{-}D_3$ or $24,25\text{-}D_3$ reverts this histological change.

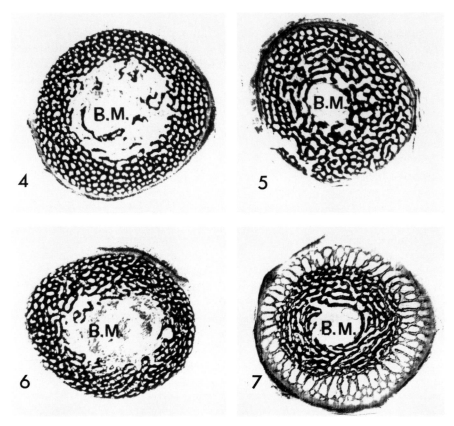

Figs. 4–7 Cross sections of tibiae from 17-day-old embryos.
Fig. 4 Control; note the large bone marrow cavity (B.M.) containing portions of old, partially resorbed trabeculae.
Fig. 5 D-deficient embryo; note the small marrow cavity with preservation of nearly intact inner bone trabeculae.
Fig. 6 D-deficient embryo treated with 10 ng calcitriol.
Fig. 7 D-deficient embryo treated with 100 ng calcitriol; note small marrow cavity and a subperiosteal rim of elongated undermineralized bone trabeculae. Toluidine blue-alizarin. (Magnification ×27.)

In normal embryos a continuous remodeling process occurs. Growth in diameter of the diaphysis takes place because new bone trabeculae are continuously being formed at the subperiosteal side while the older trabeculae at the endosteal side are being resorbed so that the marrow cavity also increases in width. As shown by Narbaitz and Tsang (1989), the resorption process at the endosteal side either does not occur or is greatly inhibited in D-deficent embryos; as a result, the marrow cavity remains small and has a smooth contour (see Fig. 5 and compare with Fig. 4). Treatment of deficient embryos with a single dose of calcitriol restores the normal remodeling process (Fig. 6).

Hypervitaminosis can be produced in chick embryos with a single dose of calcitriol, 25-D_3, or 1,24,25-D_3 (Narbaitz and Tolnai, 1978; Narbaitz and Fragiskos, 1984). The injected embryos are hypercalcemic, apparently due to a stimulation of absorption of calcium from the shell (Narbaitz, 1987). The concomitant hypophosphatemia appears to be due to phosphaturia (Rad and Narbaitz, 1989).

The injection of a high dose of calcitriol produces in long bones a response comparable to that induced in adult animals: stimulation of the rapid growth of numerous undermineralized trabeculae. (Narbaitz and Tolnai, 1978; Narbaitz and Fragiskos, 1984). These osteoid trabeculae, however, are subperiosteal rather than endosteal and form a rim or "halo" around the bone (Fig. 7). The deficit of bone mineral in these new trabeculae is probably due to the concomitant hypophosphatemia; as soon as the levels of phosphate return to normal, the osteoid trabeculae mineralize rapidly (Narbaitz and Fragiskos, 1984).

The above-mentioned stimulation of bone growth appears to be due to the concomitant hypercalcemia and not to a direct effect of calcitriol on bone cells. Recent experiments (Narbaitz et al., 1988) appear to confirm this idea. When portions of tibia were grafted on the chorioallantoic membrane of normal embryos, they responded to calcitriol stimulation with significant subperiosteal bone growth (Fig. 8). However, when similar portions of tibia were grafted on the chorioallantoic membranes of "shell-less" cultured embryos, they failed to respond to calcitriol in a similar way (Fig. 9; compare with Fig. 8). This lack of response was most probably due to "shell-less" cultured embryos having very low levels of blood calcium. That these levels increase after calcitriol injection but do not reach normal levels supports the conclusions of Gunness-Hey et al. (1988) who found that the increase in bone mass observed in rats after the injection of calcitriol occurs only when the doses used produce significant hypercalcemia.

The injection of large doses of calcitriol to chick embryos tends to reduce bone resorption at the endosteal side of the diaphysis of long bones (Narbaitz and Tolnai, 1978). This appears to be at odds with the fact that calcitriol is considered to be a powerful bone resorber. However, since the administration of calcitriol also produces a very significant hypercalcemia and hypercalcemia is known to stimulate calcitonin secretion (Baimbridge and Taylor, 1980), it is possible that it is the rise in the levels of this hormone that blunts the effects of calcitriol on bone resorption.

In summary, the effects of vitamin D on the embryonic bone are comparable to those in adult birds and mammals. Most experiments in the embryo suggest that vitamin D is required for bone resorption but that changes in bone mineralization and bone growth are secondary to concomitant alterations in the concentrations of Ca and/or P in the blood. Differences in the humoral responses to both D deficiency and hypervitaminosis D depend on the fact that some of the target organs on which the vitamin acts

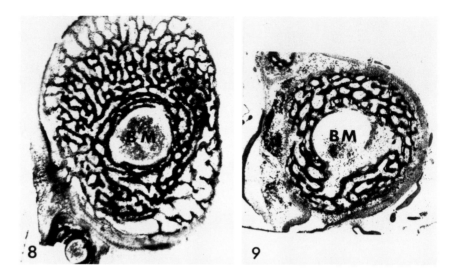

Fig. 8 Cross section of tibia grafted on a normal embryo injected with 100 ng calcitriol on the 14th day of incubation and sacrificed on day 17. Note the growth of a subperiosteal rim of elongated, partially mineralized trabeculae. (Toluidine blue-alizarin. Magnification ×45.)
Fig. 9 Cross section of tibia grafted on a shell-less cultured embryo, injected on day 14 with 100 ng calcitriol and sacrificed on day 17. The subperiosteal rim has not formed. (Toluidine blue-alizarin. Magnification ×45.)

in the embryo are different from those on which it acts in the adult (in the embryo the shell and the yolk are the source for Ca and P rather than the gut). The fact that bones grow and differentiate very rapidly in the embryo allows the use of short-term treatments for the analysis of responses to the different vitamin D metabolites.

Vitamin K

Chemical Structure and Metabolism

An excellent review on the structure and metabolism of vitamin K was published by R. E. Olson (1988). We shall summarize here only the most important information on the subject.

Vitamin K_1, known as phylloquinone, is an homologue of vitamin K found in plants (see Fig. 10). Vitamin K_2, known as menaquinone and found in animal tissues, constitutes, in reality, a family of homologues differing only in the number of isoprenyl units in the molecule (menaquinone-1 to menaquinone-7). Some of the homologues are products of bacterial biosynthesis in the gut. Menadione is a provitamin which can be converted by liver cells into menaquinone-4, but only a small fraction of the provitamin absorbed is actually transformed into the vitamin. Absorption of all forms of the vitamin requires solubilization by bile and pancreatic juices.

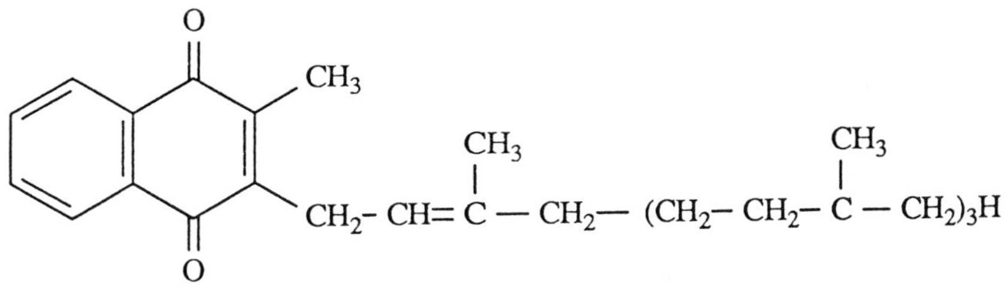

Vitamin K$_1$

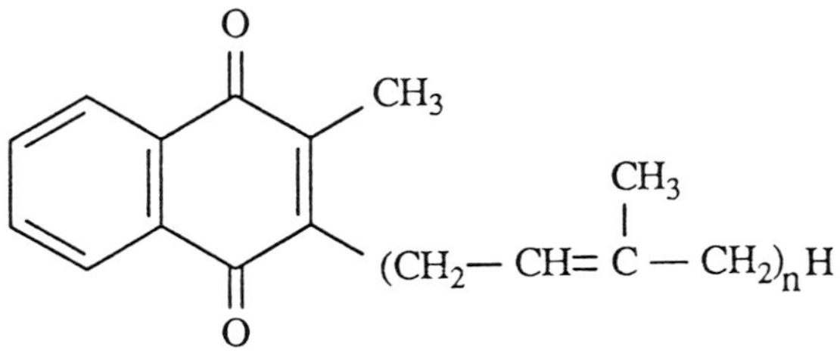

Vitamin K$_2$

Fig. 10 Chemical structures of vitamin K$_1$ (phylloquinone) and K$_2$ (menaquinone).

The absorbed vitamin is transported by chylomicrons; specific carriers for the vitamin have not been identified in the blood. The turnover of the vitamin in the body is rapid and the total body pool is relatively small. Part of the vitamin is recycled in the liver; thus, the vitamin is converted into an epoxide which can be reconverted into active vitamin.

Since there is enough vitamin K in regular mixed diets and since a large proportion of the daily requirements can also be satisfied by the vitamin synthesized by the intestinal flora, deficiency only occurs as a result of disease or of the ingestion of chemicals capable of inhibiting vitamin K synthesis. Among these, the best known are dicumarol, a substance isolated from spoiled clover, and warfarin, a synthetic derivative of dicumarol with higher solubility. Dicumarol and warfarin appear to act by inhibiting the recycling of the vitamin: they act on the enzyme required to change the epoxide into the vitamin.

Vitamin K is required for the synthesis of a series of proteins containing γ-carboxyglutamate. It acts by facilitating the posttranslational carboxylation of glutamate. These proteins include prothrombin and other plasmatic proteins required for coagulation and, in the case of bone, osteocalcin and matrix Gla protein. The possible role of these bone proteins is the subject of intensive experimentation by several laboratories.

Osteocalcin and Bone Mineralization

Osteocalcin (bone Gla protein or BGP) is a relatively abundant protein isolated from chicken (Hauschka et al., 1975) and calf (Price et al., 1976) bones. Osteocalcin is secreted by osteoblasts (Bronkers et al., 1985); part of the protein produced by the osteoblasts leaks into the blood. It has been proposed that the concentration of osteocalcin in the blood could serve as a parameter to measure the amount of bone matrix being laid at a given period (see review by Price, 1985).

Hauschka and Reid (1978) showed that the amount of osteocalcin in the bones from chick embryos increases as mineralization progresses and suggested that the protein might play a role in bone mineralization.

Osteocalcins, both of bovine and chicken origin, bind in vitro to apatite and prevent the growth of initial crystalls of apatite (Price et al., 1976; Hauschka and Reid, 1978). On the basis of these data it has been proposed that the osteocalcin might also act in vivo by inhibiting mineralization. This idea has yet to receive adequate support from experiments in vivo. Thus, no alteration in the mineralization process of bone has been observed in rats made deficient in vitamin K by the administration of warfarin despite the fact that the content in osteocalcin of these bones was reduced to 2% of the normal (Price et al., 1982). The only histological change observed in the skeleton of the rats treated with warfarin was an obturation of epiphyseal plates and their replacement by bone trabeculae; it was detected several months after the initiation of the treatment and was attributed to excessive mineralization (Price, 1985). It is not clear if the obturation of the epiphyseal plates is a direct effect of a reduction in the concentration of osteocalcin in the epiphyseal plates since determinations in separated epiphyseal plates were not made. Since epiphyseal cartilages, as well as cartilages from other regions, contain other vitamin K-dependent protein, i.e., matrix Gla protein, it is possible that the cartilage alterations produced by warfarin are related to the deficit of this component rather than osteocalcin.

Additional interest in the possible roles of osteocalcin was stimulated by the demonstration that the in vitro synthesis of this protein by osteoblasts can be increased significantly by calcitriol (Price and Baukol, 1980). In addition, rats treated with warfarin respond to large doses of calcitriol with a decrease in mineralization (Price and Sloper, 1983). It has been proposed that the presence of calcitriol-stimulated osteocalcin in the bones would be related to calcitriol's role in maintaining Ca homeostasis (Price, 1985). Thus, osteocalcin would bind calcium and prevent it from being deposited as apatite; it would increase its availability to the extracellular compartment. This attractive hypothesis requires the support of additional verification.

Matrix Gla Proteins

A second vitamin K-dependent protein was isolated from bone matrix by the group of Price (see review by Price, 1987). This protein has similarities with osteocalcin and might have arisen in evolution by gene duplication. It has a wider distribution than osteocalcin; in addition to bone, it is present in epiphyseal, nasal, tracheal, intracostal and sternal cartilages (Price, 1987). Its role in bone formation and mineralization has yet to be adequately explored.

References

Anderson, H. C., Cecil, R., and Sajdera, S. W. (1975). Calcification of rachitic rat cartilage *in vitro* by extracellular matrix vesicles. *Am. J. Pathol.*, **79**: 237–245.

Baimbridge, K. G. and Taylor, T. G. (1980). Role of calcitonin in calcium homeostasis in the chick embryo. *J. Endocrinol.*, **85**: 171–185.

Barnicot, N. A. (1948). The local action of calciferol and oestradiol on bone. *J. Anat. (London)*, **85**: 120–134.

Barnicot, N.A. and Datta, S. P. (1972). Vitamin A and bone. In: *The Biochemistry and Physiology of Bone*, 2nd ed., Volume 2: Physiology and Pathology. Bourne, G. H., Ed., Academic Press, New York, 197–229.

Baylink, D. J., Morey, E. R., Ivey, J. L., and Stauffer, M. E. (1980). Vitamin D and bone. In: *Vitamin D. Molecular Biology and Clinical Nutrition*, Norman, A. W., Ed., Marcel Dekker, New York, 387–453.

Bird, T. A., Spanheimer, R. G., and Peterkofsky, B. (1986). Coordinate regulation of collagen and proteoglycan synthesis in costal cartilage of scorbutic and acutely fasted, vitamin C-supplemented guinea pigs. *Arch. Biochem. Biophys.*, **246**: 42–51.

Bordier, P., Rasmussen, H., Marie, P., Miravet, L., Gueris, J., and Ryckwaert, A. (1978). Vitamin D metabolites and bone mineralization in man. *J. Clin. Endocrinol. Metab.*, **46**: 284–294.

Bourne, G. H. (1972). Vitamin C and bone. In: *The Biochemistry and Physiology of Bone*, 2nd ed., Volume 2: Physiology and Pathology. Bourne, G. H., Ed., Academic Press, New York, 231–279.

Boyce, R. W. and Weistrode, S. E. (1983). Effect of dietary calcium on the response of bone to 1,25(OH)$_2$D$_3$. *Lab. Invest.*, **48**: 683–689.

Boyan, B. D., Schwartz, Z., Carnes, D. L., and Ramirez, V. (1988). The effects of vitamin D metabolites on the plama and matrix vesicle membranes of growth cartilage cells *in vitro*. *Endocrinology*, **122**: 2851–2860.

Bronkers, A. L. J. J., Gay, S., DiMuzio, M. T., and Butler, W. T. (1985). Immuno-localization of -carboxyglutamic acid-containing protein in developing rat bones. *Collagen Rel. Res.*, **5**: 17–22.

Canas, F., Brand, J. S., Neuman, W. F., and Terepka, A. (1969). Bone effects of vitamin D$_3$ in collagen synthesis in rachitic chick cortical bone. *Am. J. Physiol.*, **216**: 117–120.

Cashin, C. H. and Lewis, E. J. (1984). Evaluation of hypervitaminosis A in the rat by measurement of tibial bone breaking strain. *J. Pharmacol. Methods*, **11**: 91–95.

Chambers, T. J., McSheehy, P. M. J., Thomson, B. M., and Fuller, K. (1985). The effect of calcium-regulating hormones and prostaglandins oon bone resorption by osteoclasts disaggregated from neonatal rabit bones. *Endocrinology*, **60**:234–239.

Chen, T. L. and Feldman, D. (1985). Retinoic acid modulation of 1,25(OH)$_2$D$_3$ receptors and bioresponse in bone cells, species differences between rat and mouse. *Biochem. Biophys. Res. Commun.*, **132**: 74–80.

Clark, I. and Smith, M. R. (1964). Effects of hypervitaminosis A and D on skeletal metabolism. *J. Biol. Chem.*, **239**: 1266–1271.

Crowell, J. A., Jr., Cooper, C. W., Toverud, S. U., and Boass, A. (1981). Influence of vitamin D on parathyroid hormones-induced adenosine 3'5'-monophosphate production by bone cells isolated from rat calvariae. *Endocrinology*, **109**: 1715–1722.

DeLuca, H. F. (1988). The vitamin D story: a collaborative effort of basic science and clinical medicine. *FASEB J.*, **2**: 224–236.

Dickson, I. R., Hall, A. K., and Jande, S. S. (1984). The influence of dihydroxylated vitamin D metabolites on bone formation in the chick. *Calcif. Tissue Int.*, **36**: 114–122.

Dickson, I. and Walls, J. (1985). Vitamin A and bone formation. *Biochem. J.*, **226**: 789–795.

Eicher, E. M., Southard, J. L., Scriver, C. R., and Glorieux, F. H. (1976). Hypophosphatemia: mouse model for human familial hypophosphatemia (vitamin D-resistant) rickets. *Proc. Natl. Acad. Sci. U.S.A.*, **73**: 4667–4671.

Endo, H., Kiyoki, M., Kawashima, K., Naruchi, T., and Hashimoto, Y. (1980). Vitamin D_3 metabolites and PTH synergistically stimulate bone formation of chick embryonic femur *in vitro*. *Nature (London)*, **286**: 262–264.

Fell, H. B. Mellanby. E. (1950). Effects of hypervitaminosis A on foetal mouse bones cultivated *in vitro*. *Br. Med. J.*, **2**: 535–539.

Fell H. B. and Thomas, L. (1960). Comparison of the effects of papain and vitamin A on cartilage. II. The effects on organ culture of embryonic skeletal muscle. *J. Exp. Med.*, **111**: 719–743.

Fine, N., Binerman, D., Somjen, D., Earon, Y., Edelstein, S., and Wiesman, Y. (1985). Autoradiographic lcoalization of 24R,25-dihydroxyvitamin D_3 in epiphyseal cartilage. *Bone*, **6**: 99–104.

Follis, R. H. (1948). *The Pathology of Nutritional Diseases*. Blackwell, Oxford.

Grigoriadis, A. E., Petkovich, P. M., Rosenthal, E. E., and Heersche, J. N. M. (1986). Modulation by retinoic acid of 1,25-dihydroxyvitamin D_3 effects on alkaline phosphatase activity and parathyroid hormone responsiveness in an osteoblast-like osteosarcoma cell culture. *Endocrinology*, **119**: 932–939.

Gunness-Hey, M., Gera, I., Fonseca, J., Raisz, L. G., and Hock, J. M. (1988). 1,25 dihydroxyvitamin D_3 alone or in combination with parathyroid hormone does not increase bone mass in young rats. *Calcif. Tissue Int.*, **43**: 284–288.

Hale, L. N., Kemick, M. L. S., and Wuthier, R. E. (1986). Effect of vitamin D metabolites on the expression of alkaline phosphatase activity by epiphyseal hypertropic chondrocytes in primary cell culture. *J. Bone Min. Res.*, **1**: 489–495.

Hall, B. K. (1981). Modulaciton of chondrocyte activity *in vitro* in response to ascorbic acid. *Acta Anat. (Basel)*, **109**: 51–63.

Harris, L. J. (1956). Vitamin D and bone. In: *The Biochemistry and Physiology of Bone*, Bourne, G. H., Ed., Academic Press, New York, 581–622.

Harrison, H. C., Harrison, H. E., and Park, E. A. (1958). Vitamin D and citrate metabolism. Effect of vitamin D in rats fed diets adequate in both calcium and phosphorus. *Am. J. Physiol.*, **182**: 432–436.

Hauschka, P. V., Lian, J. B., and Gallop, P. M. (1975). Direct identification of the calicum binding amino acid, γ-carboxyglutamate, in mineralized tissue. *Proc. Natl. Acad. Sci. U.S.A.*, **72**: 3925–3929.

Hauschka, P. V. and Reid, M. L. (1978). Timed appearance of a calcium-binding protein containing γ-carboxyglutamic acid in developing chick bone. *Dev. Biol.*, **65**: 426–434.

Henry H. L. and Norman, A. W. (1978). Vitamin D: two dihydroxylated metabolites required for normal chick egg hatchability. *Science*, **201**: 835–837.

Hock, J. M., Kream, B. E. and Raisz, L. G. (1982). Autoradiographic study on the effects of 1,25-dihydroxyvitamin D_3 on bone collagen matrix synthesis in vitamin D replete rats. *Calcif. Tissue Int.*, **34**: 347–351.

Hock, J. M., Gunness-Hey, M., Poser, J., Olson, H., Bell, N. H., and Raisz, L. G. (1986). Stimulation of undermineralized matrix formation by 1,25 dihydroxyvitamin D_3 in long bones of rats. *Calcif. Tissue Int.*, **38**: 79–86.

Holtrop, M. E., Cox, K. A., Clark, M. B., Holick, M. F., and Anast, C. S. (1981). 1,25-dihydroxycholecalciferol stimulates osteoclasts in rat bones in the absence of parathyroid hormone. *Endocrinology*, **108**: 2293–2301.

Holtrop, M. E. and Raisz, L. G. (1979). Comparison of the effects of 1,25-dihydroxycholecal-ciferol, prostaglandin E_2, and osteoclast-activating factor with parathyroid hormone on the ultrastructure of osteoclasts in cultured long bones of fetal rats. *Calcif. Tissue Int.*, **29**: 201–205.

Hornig, D. H., Moser, U., and Glatthaar, B. E. (1988). Ascorbic acid. In: *Nutrition in Health and Disease*, Shils, M. E. and Young, V. R., Eds., Lea and Febiger, Philadelphia, 417–435.

Hough, S., Avioli, L. V., Muir, H., Gelderblom, D., Jenkins, G., Kurasi, H., Slatopolsky, E., Bergfeld, M. A., and Teitelbaum, S. L. (1988). Effects of hypervitaminosis A on the bone and mineral metabolism of the rat. *Endocrinology*, **122**: 2933–2939.

Jande, S. S. and Schreiner, D. S. (1982). Cellular localization of vitamin D dependent calcium binding protein by immunoperoxidase methods. In: *Vitamin D, Chemical, Biochemical and Clinical Endocrinology of Calcium Metabolism*, Norman, A. W., Schaefer, K., Herrath, D. V., and Grigoleit, H. G., Eds., Walter de Gruyter, New York, 203–208.

Jeffrey, J. J. and Martin, G. R. (1966a). The role of ascorbic acid in the biosynthesis of collagen. I. Ascorbic acid requirements by embryonic chick tibia in tissue culture. *Biochim. Biophys. Acta*, **121**: 269–280.

Jeffrey, J. J. and Martin, G. R. (1966b). The role of ascorbic acid in the biosynthesis of collagen. II. Site and nature of ascorbic acid participation. *Biochim. Biophys. Acta*, **121**: 281–291.

Lawson, D. E. M. and Davie, M. (1979). Aspects of the metabolism and function of vitamin D. *Vitam. and Horm.*, **37**:1–67.

Lopes, R. A., Souza, M. L., and Azoubel, R. (1982). Morphometric study of malformations induced by hypervitaminosis A on rat fetus Meckel cartilage, maxillary bone and mandible. *Anat. Anz.*, **152**: 329–336.

Lucy, J. A., Dingle, J. T., and Fell, H. B. (1961). Studies on the mode of action of excess of Vitamin A. 2. A possible role of intracellular proteases in the degradation of cartilage matrix. *Biochem. J.*, **79**: 500–508.

Manolagas, S. C. and Deftos, L. F. (1981). Comparison of 1,25-, 25, and 24,25-hydroxylated vitamin D_3 binding in fetal rat calvariae and osteogenic sarcoma cells. *Calcif. Tissue Int.*, **33**: 655–661.

Marie, P. J. and Travers, R. (1983). Continuous infusion of 1,25-dihydroxyvitamin D_3 stimulates bone turnover in the normal young mouse. *Calcif. Tissue Int.*, **35**: 418–425.

Mechanic, G. L., Toverud, S. U., Ramp, W. K., and Gonnerman, W. A. (1975). The effect of vitamin D on the structural crosslinks and maturation of chick bone collagen. *Biochim. Biophys. Acta*, **393**: 419–425.

Mellanby, E. (1944). Nutrition in relation to bone growth and the nervous system. *Proc. R. Soc.*, **B132**: 28–46.

Metz, A. L., Walser, M. M., and Olson, W. G. (1985). The interaction of dietary vitamin A and vitamin D related to skeletal development in the turkey poult. *J. Nutr.*, 115–929.

Miller, S. C., Halloran, B. P., DeLuca, H. F., Yamada, S., Takayama, H., and Jee, W. S. S. (1981). Studies on the role of 24-hydroxylation of vitamin D in the mineralization of cartilage and bone of vitamin D-deficient rats. *Calcif. Tissue Int.*, **33**: 489–497.

Miyaura, C., Segawa, A., Nagasawa, H., Abe, E., and Suda, T. (1986). Effects of retinoic acid on the activation and fusion of mouse alveolar macrophages induced by $1\alpha,25$-dihydroxy-vitamin D_3. *J. Bone Min. Res.*, **1**: 359–368.

Murad, S. Grove, D., Lindberg, K. A., Reynolds, G., Sivarajah, A., and Reynolds, G. (1981). Regulation of collagen synthesis by acorbic acid. *Proc. Natl. Acad. Sci. U.S.A.*, **78**: 2879–2882.

Narbaitz, R. (1987). Role of vitamin D in the development of the chick embryo. *J. Exp. Zool.*, **Suppl. 1**: 15–23.

Narbaitz, R., Duncan, M. A., and Kinson, G. (1988). Response to calcitriol of chick embryonic bones grown as chorioallantoic grafts. *Proc. Can. Fed. Biol. Soc.*, **31**: 91.

Narbaitz, R. and Fragiskos, B. (1984). Hypervitaminosis D in the chick embryo: comparative study of various vitamin D_3 metabolites. *Calcif. Tissue Int.*, **36**: 392–400.

Narbaitz, R., Kacew, S., and Sitwell, L. (1981a). Carbonic anhydrase activity in the chick embryo choriallantois: regional distribution. *J. Embryol. Exp. Morphol.*, **65**: 127–137.

Narbaitz, R., Stumpf, W. E., and Sar, M. (1981b). The role of autoradiographic and immunocytochemical techniques in the clarification of sites of metabolism and action of vitamin D. *J. Histochem. Cytochem.*, **29**: 91–100.

Narbaitz, R., Stumpf, W. E., Sar, M., DeLuca, H. F., and Tanaka, Y. (1980). Autoradiographic demonstration of target cells for 1,25-dihydroxycholecalciferol in the chick embryo chorioallantoic membrane, duodenum, and parathyroid glands. *G. Comp. Endrocrinol.*, **42**: 283–289.

Narbaitz, R., Stumpf, W. E., Sar, M., Huang, S., and DeLuca, H. F. (1983). Autoradiographic localization of target cells for 1α,25-dihydroxyvitamin D_3 in bones from fetal rats. *Calcif. Tissue Int.*, **35**: 177–182.

Narbaitz, R. and Tolnai, S. (1978). Effects produced by the administration of high does of 1,25-dihydroxycholecalciferol to the chick embryo. *Calcif. Tissue Res.*, **26**: 221–226.

Narbaitz, R. and Tsang, C. P. W. (1989). Vitamin D deficiency in the chick embryo. Effects on pre-hatching motility and on the growth and differentiation of bone, muscles and parathyroid glands. *Calcif. Tissue Int.*, **44**: 348–355.

Narbaitz, R., Tsang, C. P. W., and Grunder, A. A. (1987). Effects of vitamin D deficiency in the chick embryo. *Calcif. Tissue Int.*, **40**: 109–113.

Norman, A. W. (1980). 1,25-$(OH)_2$-D_3 as a steroid hormone. In: *Vitamin D, Molecular Biology and Clinical Nutrition*, Norman, A. W., Ed., Marcel Dekker, New York, 197–250.

Olson, J. A. (1988). Vitamin A, retinoids, and carotenoids. In: *Modern Nutrition in Health and Disease*, Shils, M. E. and Young, V. R., Eds., Lea and Febiger, Philadelphia, 292–312.

Olson, R. E. (1988). Vitamin K. In: *Modern Nutrition in Health and Disease*, Shils, M. E. and Young, V. R., Eds., Lea and Febiger, Philadelphia, 329–336.

Petkovich, P. M., Heersche, J. N. M., Tinker, D. O., and Jones, G. (1984). Retinoic acid stimulates 1,25-dihydrovitamin D_3 binding in rat osteosarcoma cells. *J. Biol. Chem.*, **259**: 8274–8280.

Price, P. A. (1985). Vitamin K-dependent formation of bone Gla protein (Osteocalcin) and its function. *Vitam. and Horm.*, **42**: 65–108.

Price, P. A. (1987). Vitamin K-dependent bone proteins. In: *Calcium Regulation and Bone Metabolism, Basic and Clinical Aspects*, Cohn, D. V. , Martin, T. J., and Meunier, P. J., Eds., Excerpta Medica, Amsterdam, 419–425.

Price, P. A. and Baukol, S. A. (1980). 1,25-Dihydroxyvitamin D_3 increases synthesis of the vitamin K-dependent bone protein by osteosarcoma cells. *J. Biol. Chem.*, **255**: 11660–11663.

Price, P. A., Otsuka, A. S., Poser, J. W., Kristaponis, J., and Raman, N. (1976). Characterization of a γ-carboxyglutamic acid containing protein from bone. *Proc. Natl. Acad. Sci. U.S.A.*, **73**: 1447–1451.

Price, P. A. and Sloper, S. A. (1983). Concurrent warfarin treatment further reduces bone mineral levels in 1,25-dihydroxyvitamin D_3-treated rats. *J. Biol. Chem.*, **258**: 6004–6007.

Price, P. A., Williamson, M. K., Haba, T., Dell, R. B., and Jee, W. S. S. (1982). Excessive mineralization with growth plate closure in rats on chronic warfarin treatment. *Proc. Natl. Acad. Sci. U.S.A.*, **79**: 7734–7738.

Rad, J. S. and Narbaitz, R. (1989). Role of calcitriol in phosphate regulation by the chick embryo. *Calcif. Tissue Int.*, **44**: 278–285.

Raisz, L. C. (1965). Inhibition by actinomycin D in bone resorption induced by parathyroid hormone or vitamin A. *Proc. Soc. Exp. Biol. Med.*, **119**: 614–617.

Raisz, L. G., Maina, D. M., Gworek, S., Dietrich, J. W., and Canalis, E. M. (1978). Hormonal control of bone collagen synthesis *in vitro:* inhibitory effect of 1-hydroxylated vitamin D metabolites. *Endocrinology*, **102**: 731–735.

Rasmussen, H., DeLuca, H., Amaud, C., Hauker, C., and von Stedingk, M. (1963). The relationship between vitamin D and parathyroid hormone. *J. Clin. Invest.*, **42**: 1940–1946.

Rasmussen, H., Baron, R., Broadus, A., Defronzo, R., Lang, R., and Horst, R. (1980). 1,25(OH)$_2$D$_3$ is not the only D metabolite involved in the pathogenesis of osteomalacia. *Am. J. Med.*, **69**: 360–368.

Reynolds, J. J. (1967). The effect of ascorbic acid on the growth of chick bone rudiments *in vitro*. *Exp. Cell. Res.*, **47**: 42–48.

Reynolds, J. J. (1968). Inhibition by calcitonin of bone resorption induced *in vitro* by vitamin A. *Proc. R. Soc. London (Biol. Sci.)*, **170**: 61–69.

Reynolds, J. J., Holick, M. F., and DeLuca, H. F. (1973). The role of vitamin D metabolites in bone resorption. *Calcif. Tissue Res.*, **12**: 295–301.

Shiina, Y., Yamaguchi, A., Yamana, H., Abe, R., Yoshiki, S., and Suda, T. (1986). Comparison of the mechanisms of bone resorption induced by 1,25-dihydroxyvitamin D$_3$ and lipolysaccharides. *Calcif. Tissue Int.*, **39**: 28–34.

Solursch, M. and Meier, S. (1973). The selective inhibition of mucopolysaccharide synthesis by vitamin A treatment of cultured chick embryo chondrocytes. *Calcif. Tissue Res.*, **13**: 131–142.

Stumpf, W. E., Sar, M., Reid, F. A., Tanaka, Y., and DeLuca, H. F. (1979). Target cells for 1,25-dihydroxyvitamin D$_3$ in intestinal tract, stomach, kidney, skin, pituitary and parathyroid. *Science*, **206**: 1188–1190.

Sunde, M. L., Turk, C. M., and DeLuca, H. F. (1978). The essentiality of vitamin D metabolites for chick development. *Science*, **200**: 1067–1069.

Tam, C. S., Heersche, J. N. M., Jones, G., Murray, T. M., and Rasmussen, H. (1986). The effect of vitamin D on bone *in vivo*. *Endocrinology*, **118**: 2217–2224.

Teti, A., Oreffo, R. O., Zambonin Zallone, A., Triffit, J. T., and Francis, M. J. (1986). The effect of retinol on osteoclasts is mediated by a specific cytosolic binding protein. *Boll. Soc. Ital. Biol. Sper.*, **62**: 1315–1309.

Teti, A., Volleth, G., Carano, A., and Zambonin Zallone, A. (1988). The effects of parathyroid hormone or 1,25-dihydroxyvitamin D$_3$ on monocyte-osteoclast fusion. *Calcif. Tissue Int.*, **42**: 302–308.

Thaller, C. and Eichele, G. (1987). Identification and spatial distribution of retinoids in the developing chick limb bud. *Nature*, **327**: 625–628.

Trummel, C. L., Raisz, L. G., Blunt, J. W., and DeLuca, H. F. (1969). 25-hydroxycholecalciferol: stimulation of bone resorption in tissue culture. *Science*, **163**: 1450–1451.

Tyler, M. S. and Dewitt-Stott, R. A. (1986). Inhibition of membrane bone formation by vitamin A in the embryonic chick mandible. *Anat. Rec.*, **214**: 193–197.

Underwood, J. S. and DeLuca, H. F. (1984). Vitamin D is not directly necessary for bone growth and mineralization. *Am. J. Physiol.*, **246**: E493–E498.

Vasan, N. S. and Lash, J. W. (1975). Chondrocyte metabolism as affected by vitamin A. *Calcif. Tissue Res.*, **19**: 00–107.

Weston, P. D., Barrett, A. J., and Dingle, J. T. (1969). Specific inhibition of cartilage. *Nature (London)*, **222**: 285–286.

Wolbach, S. B. (1947). Vitamin-A deficiency and excess in relation to skeletal growth. *J. Bone Jt. Surg.*, **29**: 171–192.

Wronsky, T. J., Halloran, B. P., Bikle, D. D., Globus, R. K., and Morey-Holton, E. R. (1986). Chronic administration of 1,25-dihydroxyvitamin D$_3$: increased bone but impaired mineralization. *Endocrinology*, **119**: 2580–2585.

Yamaguchi, A., Kohno, Y., Yamazaki, T., Takahashi, N., Shinki, T., Horiuchi, N., Suda, T., Koizumi, H., Tanioka, Y., and Yoshiki, S. (1986). Bone in the marmoset: a resemblance to vitamin D-dependent rickets Type II. *Calcif. Tissue Int.*, **39**: 22–27.

7

Biomineralization in the Integumental Skeleton of the Living Lower Vertebrates

LOUISE ZYLBERBERG, JACQUELINE GÉRAUDIE, FRANÇOIS MEUNIER, and JEAN-YVES SIRE
Equipe "Formations Squelettiques"
URA CNRS 1137
Laboratoire d'Anatomie comparée
Université Paris
Paris, France

Introduction and Terminology

The potentiality of the vertebrate skin to produce mineralized structures can be related to the function of the integument which acts as a barrier protecting the underlying soft tissues (reviewed in Spearman, 1973; Krejsa, 1979; Matoltsy and Bereiter-Hahn, 1986). In vertebrates, the concept of an integumental skeleton (= dermal skeleton or dermoskeleton) is thus linked to the presence of reinforcing mineralized structures such as scales, scutes, fin rays, osteoderms, etc. These derive, at least in part, from the embryonic dermatomal mesenchyme and they differentiate directly without an intermediate, transitory, cartilaginous stage (Romer, 1964) and are mostly considered as dermal bones *sensu lato* (reviewed in Francillon-Vieillot *et al.*, 1990). In these skeletal elements a wide spectrum of tissues is found, from true bony tissue to mineralized noncollagenous matrices; the latter tissues are peculiar to the dermal skeleton. These elements also demonstrate various processes of mineralization.

The polymorphism of the integumental skeleton in living lower vertebrates is the result of long evolutionary processes. Various primitive jawless fishes, the oldest known vertebrate fossils, had an extensive, heavily mineralized dermal "armor" and they had already differentiated a wide variety of dermal mincralizations (Hall, 1975; Smith and Hall, 1990). Bone tissue was restricted to this dermal skeleton and it is considered phylogenetically older than the endoskeleton (Romer, 1964). So the dermal skeleton is a convenient model to study the history of mineralization processes in the vertebrates.

Among primitive vertebrates, the integumental skeletal elements were very often associated with superficial dental tissues (Ørvig, 1951, 1967; Schaeffer, 1977). The dental components are organized as superficial isolated units, the "odontodes", or fused together, according to different patterns in various lineages, to form "odontocomplexes" (Ørvig, 1977). In evolved fishes, amphibians and reptiles, the dermal skeleton has lost the dental components.

From paleontological and comparative anatomical data, it is obvious that the general trend in integumental skeleton history is of reduction (Romer, 1964) even if extensive dermal skeletons have reappeared or been retained among unrelated lineages in each class of vertebrates, except the aves. Therefore, the presence of mineralized elements in the dermis is considered a primitive character for vertebrates (Schaeffer, 1977). A consequence of this reduction in fish is their improved swimming performance (Burdak, 1979). For most terrestrial tetrapods, the integumental skeleton is no longer of the heavy armor kind impeding locomotory performances (Moss, 1964, 1968b, 1972).

The loss or reduction of the various components forming the ancestral vertebrate integumental skeleton did not occur at similar rates within the different lineages. New combinations arose from either new reciprocal arrangements of the remaining components, their transformation and/or the appearance of new components (i.e., different from bone and tooth tissues) leading to a great variety of mineralized structures. These evolutionary processes give rise to convergences and/or parallelism occurring while the various structures differentiate. These structures are not necessarily homologous, even if they are the expression of a common developmental process which results in sheathing the body surface.

The terminology found in the literature is somewhat complex and confusing because the same term has often been used to define different structures or different terms have been used for the same structure. For instance, scales in fishes are mineralized dermal plates whereas scales in reptiles and birds are keratinous epidermal differentiations. In the same way, according to its peripheral location, the term exoskeleton has been used to collectively name various mineralized integumental elements as the antonym of endoskeleton which is restricted to the deepest elements of the skeleton. The vertebrate skeleton has usually been divided into endo- and exoskeleton not only when referring to its location but also to its embryological origin (reviewed in Patterson, 1977; Francillon-Vieillot *et al.*, 1990; Smith and Hall, 1990). However, from an overall zoological point of view, this is formally incorrect according to broad comparative perspectives, and we will restrict the concept of exoskeleton to the keratinous-rich hard tissues which differentiate peripherally from the external side of the skin, as invertebrate cuticles do. Conversely, among vertebrates, even if the integumental skeleton integrates enamel or enamel-like tissues irrespective of their epidermal origin, it differentiates within the dermis. These epidermal components are produced at the inner surface of the epidermis facing the dermis with which they establish close structural and functional relationships (Ørvig, 1977; Sire *et al.*, 1987). Thus, the current use of the term exoskeleton to refer to the superficial elements of the integumental mineralized elements of vertebrates as the antonym of endoskeleton is not appropriate, is best avoided and replaced by dermal skeleton.

We will only give here the definitions helpful for the present chapter. A recent terminology of bony tissues can be found elsewhere (Francillon-Vieillot *et al.*, 1990).

The dermal bones of the integumental skeleton can become secondarily associated with endoskeletal elements, especially in the head, fusing sometimes with them to form composite cranial bones. In this case, the mineralization processes in the dermal bones are ultimately undistinguishable from those occurring in the endoskeletal bones and both can be considered together and compared to the great diversity of mineralization processes encountered in the postcranial integumental skeleton. On the other hand, birds and mammals (with some exceptions such as armadillos) do not usually possess any integumental mineralized plates. However, the presence of dermal plates in armadillos demonstrates that the mammalian dermis has retained the ability to mineralize and to form bone (Moss, 1964, 1968a, 1972) which is also expressed in experimental and pathological circumstances (Boivin, 1975; Boivin *et al.*, 1987). For the above reasons, this review will be limited to the postcranial integumental skeleton and to lower vertebrates: osteichthyan fish, amphibians and reptiles.

We have also excluded from this review the placoid scales of the chondrichthyan fish because they are odontodes and thus are relevant to dental tissues. However, dental tissues as well as other mineralized tissues which are not bone will be mentioned when they constitute a structural entity with the dermal bone with which they are associated, as for instance in ganoid scales (dental tissues) or in reptilian osteoderms (other tissues).

The diversity and complexity of the dermal elements of the integumental skeleton of the lower vertebrates have lead us to describe their organization and structure before analyzing the mineralization processes. It is obvious that mineralization occurs within the tissues owing to the presence of specialized cells (scleroblasts [Klaatsch, 1890], osteoblasts, osteocytes) and their extracellular produces such as collagen, but also noncollagenous substances. These aspects will not be entertained here, but in other chapters of the treatise, especially Volume 3.

Structural Data

The Integumental Skeleton of the Osteichthyes

Scales and Related Structures

The scales of the living osteichthyan fish are considered to be derived from the ancestral rhomboid type known from the lower Devonian genus *Lophosteus*, possibly the oldest fossil representative of the Osteichthyes (Schultze, 1977).

A great polymorphism is observed among the osteichthyan scales according to their location, their local arrangement and their structural organization particularly when the earliest extinct fossil forms are considered. Osteichthyan scales can be morphologically subdivided into two types: the ancestral or primitive rhomboid scales and the derived elasmoid scales (Goodrich,

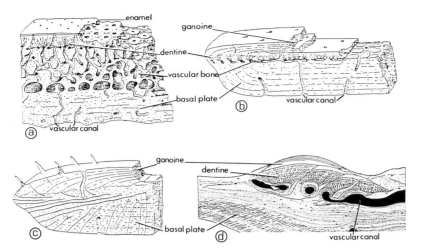

Fig. 1   Rhomboid scales. Three-dimensional reconstruction. (a) Cosmoid scale of *Megalichthys*. (b) Palaeoniscoid scale of *Eurynotus*. (c) Lepisosteoid scale of *Lepisosteus*. (a, b, c adapted from Goodrich, 1907.) (d) Odontocomplex topping a scale of *Plegmolepis*. (Adapted from Orvig, 1978b.)

1907; Bertin, 1958). These types of scales are found in the two main lineages or clades of Osteichthyes: Sarcopterygii and Actinopterygii. In the latter, dermal structures known as spines and scutes are also present in some un-related taxa and show structural characteristics which differ from both rhomboid and elasmoid scales.

Rhomboid scales.   The rhomboid scales are thick, adjacent plates often articulated to each other and are composed of two superimposed layers (Fig. 1): (1) a thick basal plate of parallel-fibered and vascularized bone, and (2) a superficial layer of tooth-derived material, the odontodes (Fig. 1d) or odontocomplexes (dentine and hypermineralized substance: either enameloid or enamel) (reviewed in Ørvig, 1967, 1968; Schaeffer, 1977; Meunier, 1984b).

The rhomboid scales are divided into two groups: the cosmoid scales of the early Sarcopterygii and the ganoid scales of the early Actinopterygii.

Cosmoid scales (Fig. 1a) are known only in fossils. They are thick osseous plates covered by a spongy bony layer comprising large vascular cavities. This layer is topped by odontodes associated with small chambers which open on the outer scale surface. Because of its characteristic organization this layer of odontodes is called cosmine (Ørvig, 1969; Thomson, 1975). The odontodes are deposited either in several superimposed layers surrounding a network of vascular canals (as in primitive cosmoid scales) or as a single layer on which enamel (or enameloid) is well developed. In the living Sarcopterygii dentine and enamel have disappeared in Dipnoi (Ørvig, 1968; Smith, 1977; Bemis, 1984), but in *Latimeria* (Fig. 6) odontodes are still present on the posterior field of the scales (Smith *et al.*, 1972; Castanet *et al.*, 1975). The spatial arrangement of the superficial dental tissues differs from the vascular system characterizing a cosmoid scale. Moreover, their thin, lamellar and imbricated scales should be better considered as scales of an elasmoid type of organization rather than as a rhomboid one (Meunier, 1983).

Ganoid scales are found in early primitive Actinopterygii and are still extant as the scales of some living Osteichthyes, Polypteridae and Lepisosteidae, in which they have retained several characters of the ancestral rhomboid scales. There are two types of ganoid scales: the paleoniscoid and lepidosteoid types (Goodrich, 1907). The paleoniscoid scales (Fig. 1b) are composed of a thick basal layer made of compact parallel-fibered and vascularized bone, a central vascularized layer of dentine and a superficial layer of ganoine (Aldinger, 1937; Gross, 1935, 1966; Schultze, 1966). The scales of the living Polypteridae have retained this typical structure of the paleoniscoid type (Sewertzoff, 1932; Kerr, 1952; Meunier, 1980). A small plywood-like structure made of several thick layers of regularly deposited collagenous fibrils has been recently discovered to be located between the dentine layer and the osseous basal plate (Sire, 1989, 1990).

In the lepidosteoid type the dentine layer is lacking (Fig. 1c); the ganoine lies directly on the surface of the osseous basal plate (Nickerson, 1893; Goodrich, 1907; Kerr, 1952; Meunier *et al.*, 1978; Thomson and McCune, 1984). In the extant Lepisosteidae, the parallel-fibered bone generally contains scarce vascular canals and numerous fine tubules: the non-vascular canals of Williamson (Williamson, 1849; Ørvig, 1951; Kerr, 1952; Meunier *et al.*, 1978). This peculiarity is found in the bones and scales of most Holostei.

At the ultrastructural level the collagenous stroma of the basal plate of the ganoid scales shows the same feature as bone (Figs. 31, 32).

Elasmoid scales. The elasmoid scales of Teleostei were subdivided by Goodrich (1907) into ctenoid and cycloid types according to the presence or absence of ctenii, namely superficial comb-like ornamentations of the posterior margin of the scales. However, even if the morphological aspects of these two types of scales differs, their structural organization does not show basic differences (Meunier, 1983). All cycloid and ctenoid scales are thin, flexible, lamellar and imbricated collagenous plates and both belong to the elasmoid type as defined by Bertin (1944). According to this definition, as already mentioned above, the scales of the modern Dipnoi, of *Latimeria* (Coelacanthidae) and of *Amia* (Holostei) are also of the elasmoid type (Kerr, 1952, 1955; Giraud *et al.*, 1978; Meunier and François, 1980; Meunier, 1983).

The surface of the elasmoid scale presents numerous ornamentations that vary in shape, size and organization from one species to another (Fig. 2a–e). They are generally characterized by concentrically disposed ridges, the *circuli* (Fig. 2a–c), that are interrupted by uncalcified grooves, the *radii* (Baudelot, 1873) (Fig. 2a, b, d, e), which allow flexibility. Indeed, these grooves are radially oriented but in Osteoglossiformes (Meunier, 1984a) and also in Dipnoi (Kerr, 1955; Brien, 1962; Meunier and François, 1980; Zylberberg,

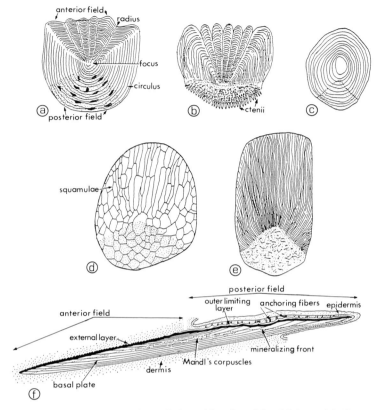

Fig. 2 a–e Superficial ornamentations of elasmoid scales of Osteichthyes. (a) *Cyprinus carpio* (Cyprinidae): Typical elasmoid scale. (b) *Perca fluviatilis* (Percidae): Ctenoid scale. (c) *Salmo fario* (Salmonidae): Cycloid scale without radii. (d) *Gnathonemus petersii* (Mormyridae): Scale with squamulae. (e) *Amia calva* (Amiidae): Scale with radial ridges. The uncovered posterior field of the scales is represented by the dotted areas. (a to e adapted from Meunier, 1983). (f) *Hemichromis bimaculatus* (Cichlidae): Diagram of a longitudinal section of an elasmoid scale. (Adapted from Sire, 1985.)

1988) they form a typical network defining mineralized small and numerous polygonal units, the *squamulae* (Fig. 2d). The superficial ornamentations probably participate in anchoring the scale in the skin (Lanzing and Wright, 1976; Sire, 1986, 1987), and anchoring fibrils (Figs. 69, 71, 72) arising from the superficial layer on the posterior field of the scale connect the epidermis and the dermis to the scale (Zylberberg and Meunier, 1981; Sire, 1985, 1986).

An elasmoid scale is typically composed of two layers (Goodrich, 1907; Bertin, 1958): a lamellar basal plate organized in a plywood-like structure (Meunier, 1983, 1984b) called isopedine (Meunier, 1987), covered by a thin ornamented superficial layer (= osseous layer or bony layer) (Fig. 2f). Isopedine has the histological and histochemical characteristics of a lamellar bone whereas the superficial layer shows different staining properties (Neave,

1936) which are those of a woven bone (Table 1). This latter layer contains acid mucopolysaccharides (Wallin, 1956; Maekawa and Yamada, 1970; Zylberberg and Nicolas, 1982). In the dipnoan *Protopterus annectens* it is noteworthy that a dense material rich in mucosubstances stained with ruthenium red forms a definite boundary between the external layer and the basal plate (Fig. 62). So far a similar structure is unknown in the typical elasmoid scales in the Teleostei.

The isopedine (Figs. 3, 5a) consists of several superimposed plies of thick collagen fibrils (Table 2). In each ply, the fibrils are parallel one to another but their direction changes from one ply to the next. This organization in a plywood pattern (Weiss and Ferris, 1954; Bouligand, 1972; Meunier and Géraudie, 1980) is a characteristic of all elasmoid scales (Giraud *et al.*, 1978; Meunier and François, 1980; Meunier, 1981; Meunier and Castanet, 1982; Meunier, 1987–88). Different types of plywood-like arrangements (twisted, orthogonal, etc.) have been described and their precise organization may be related to phylogeny (Meunier and Castanet, 1982; Meunier, 1984b, 1987–88).

In the scales of some Teleostei such as the Cyprinidae, "sheet-like structures" (Onozato and Watabe, 1979) composed of thin collagen fibrils (30 nm in diameter [Table 2]), the TC fibers (Figs. 3, 5a), are oriented vertically, perpendicular to the thick collagen fibrils of the isopedine. The TC fibers appear to be involved in the first stages of mineralization (Figs. 40, 43) (Schönbörner *et al.*, 1979; Zylberberg and Nicolas, 1982).

In the teleost scales, the isopedine is incompletely mineralized (Fig. 4). In Dipnoi it is either partially calcified *(Lepidosiren, Protopterus annectens)* or uncalcified *(Neoceratodus)* (Meunier and François, 1980). In *Latimeria* (Fig. 6), it is thick and uncalcified (Smith *et al.*, 1972; Castanet *et al.*, 1975; Meunier, 1982). It is noteworthy that even if it is not mineralized isopedine shows the histochemical characteristics of lamellar bone (Table 1). The plywood-like arrangement of the elasmoid scales occurring concomitantly with a regression of the mineralization increases the flexibility without much reducing their mechanical properties. Thus, compared to the organization of the rhomboid scales, that of the elasmoid ones allows better swimming performances.

In Teleostei, the superficial layer can be composed of two superimposed layers (Fig. 3): the "external layer" topped by the "outer limiting layer" (Schönbörner *et al.*, 1979) at least in the part of the scale covered by epidermis (Sire, 1985, 1987). The external layer (Fig. 5b) is always present and is the first part of the scale deposited during ontogeny (Waterman, 1970; Fouda, 1979a; Sire and Géraudie, 1983) and regeneration (Fouda, 1979b; Frietsche and Bailey, 1980; Sire and Géraudie, 1984). It consists of a woven-fibered bony tissue composed of thin collagen fibrils (about 30 nm in diameter [Table 2]) forming a loose meshwork (Zylberberg and Nicolas, 1982). The external layer is thin and once deposited does not thicken during subsequent growth of the fish (Sire and Meunier, 1981; Sire, 1985).

Table 1.
Staining and Histochemical Characteristics of Scales and Osteoderms Compared to the Dermis

	OSTEICHTHYES								AMPHIBIA		REPTILIA		
	Polypterus scales		Latimeria scales		Protopterus scales		Teleostei scales*		Gymnophiona scales**		Osteoderms		
	Ganoine	BP	SL	BP	SL	BP	SL	BP	Squamulae	BP	SL	BP	Dermis
Azan	blue	red	blue	red	blue	red	blue	red	blue	red	blue	red	blue
Delafield's hematoxylin-eosin							blue	red					
Mallory's trichrome	blue	red	blue	red	blue	red	blue	red	blue	red	blue	red	blue
Masson-Goldner's trichrome	green	red	green	red	green	red	green	red	green	red	green	red	green
One-step trichrome	green	red	green	red	green	red	green	red	green	red	green	red	green
PAS	+	+	+++	+	++	+	++	+	++	+	+++	++	+
Metachromasia	++	−	++	−	+	−	+	−	+	−	+	−	−
Alcian blue pH 3.2	++	−	++	−	+	−	+	−	+	−	+	−	−
Danielli's coupled tetrazonium reaction	−	+	+	++	+	++	+	++	+	++	+	++	++
Reaction for bone salts	+++	++	++	−	+	+	++	+	++	−	+	+	+

Row group labels (left margin): *Histological stainings* (Azan through One-step trichrome), *Mucosubstances* (PAS through Alcian blue pH 3.2), *Proteins* (Danielli's coupled tetrazonium reaction).

+++ very strongly positive
++   strongly positive
+   moderately positive
−   weakly positive
BP   Basal plate
SL   Superficial layers
*   Data from Neave (1936, 1940), Wallin (1956), Maekawa and Yamada (1970) and personal results.
**   Data from Gabe (1971a) and Zylberberg and Wake (1990).

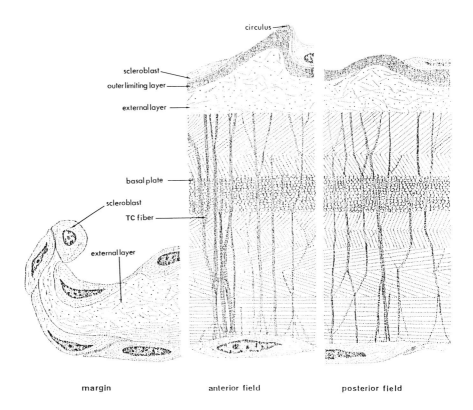

Fig. 3 *Carassius auratus* (Cyprinidae). Diagram of a section perpendicular to the surface of an elasmoid scale showing the organization of the isopedine and the TC fibers forming the characteristics "sheet-like structures" crossing the plies of the isopedine. (Adapted from Zylberberg and Nicholas, 1982.)

The outer limiting layer (Fig. 5b) is cyclically deposited throughout the life of the fish (Sire, 1985). This is the part of the scale richest in muco-substances (Zylberberg and Nicolas, 1982). It is entirely or nearly devoid of collagen fibrils depending on species, except in the region where it is crossed by anchoring fibers. The outer limiting layer develops preferentially at the level of these anchoring fibers forming the tubercules visible on the scale surface (Zylberberg and Meunier, 1981; Sire, 1986, 1987).

Scutes and spines. In various unrelated taxa of osteichthyan fishes, bony scutes and spines instead of typical elasmoid scales develop in the dermis (Bertin, 1958). They are similar in structure and formation to the osseous basal plate of the rhomboid scales from which they are considered to be derived after loss of the superficial dental components (Ørvig, 1968; Meunier, 1984b).

The sturgeons (Chondrostei) have small or large, but always thick, bony scutes (Goodrich, 1907; Weisel, 1975; Meunier *et al.*, 1978). In teleosts, scutes

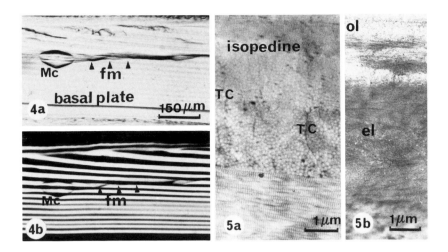

Fig. 4 *Etelis carbunculus* (Lutjanidae). Ground-section of an elasmoid scale. (a) Normal transmitted light. The basal plate is not entirely mineralized as shown by the location of the front of mineralization (fm) where a Mandl's corpuscle (Mc) is observed. (b) Polarized light. The black and white superimposed collagenous plies are characteristic of an orthogonal plywood-like structure.

Fig. 5 *Carassius auratus* (Cyprinidae). TEM. Demineralized elasmoid scale. (a) The twisted plywood-like structure of the isopedine is crossed by the TC fibers. (b) The external layer (el) contains a loose meshwork of thin collagen fibrils immersed in a granular ground substance. Collagen fibrils are not observed in the outer limiting layer (ol) containing only a fibrillar material.

are found in taxonomically distant families (Loricariidae, Callichthyidae, Syngnathidae, Gasterosteidae, for instance). They show a great diversity of shapes and organizations on the fish body. In armored catfishes, the scutes are large, imbricated plates, vascularized and mainly made of cellular bone; their outer surface is ornamented with numerous odontodes (Bhatti, 1938; Ørvig, 1977). In Gasterosteidae, Ostraciontidae, Agonidae and Syngnathidae, the scutes are composed of acellular bone (Williamson, 1851; Roth, 1920; Whitear and Mittal, 1986). Spine-like formations are found in Tetraodontidae, Diodontidae, etc. (Rosen, 1913). In some Thunnidae (Williamson, 1851; Meunier and Sire, 1981), and in *Makaira* (Istiophoridae) and *Ruvetus* (Gempylidae) (LaMonte, 1958; Bone, 1972), the scutes vary from round to elongated plates with a characteristic well-developed network of cavities. In *Thunnus alalunga,* cellular bony plates are found on the anterior part of the body and typical elasmoid scales on its posterior part (Meunier and Sire, 1981). Series of intermediate scales showing together characteristics of scutes (bone) and of elasmoid scales (isopedine) are present from the anterior to the posterior part of the body. In the part containing bony tissue, mineralization proceeds as in bone while in the part showing the characteristics of an elasmoid scale, mineralization processes are those observed in a typical elasmoid scale (Meunier and Sire, 1981). However, precise homol-

Table 2.
Diameter of Collagenous Fibrils in the Scales, Fin Rays, and Osteoderms

Species	Tissues	Diameter (nm)	Authors
OSTEICHTHYES	Scales		
Coelacanthidae			
Latimeria chalumnae	I	130	Giraud *et al.*, 1978
Protopteridae			
Neoceratodus forsteri	I	80–120	Meunier and François, 1980
Protopterus aethiopicus	I	100–140	Meunier and François, 1980
Amiidae			
Amia calva	I	60–120	Meunier, 1981
Salmonidae			
Onchorhynchus keta	I	30–60	Yamada, 1971
Salmo gairdneri	E.L.	30	Maekawa and Yamada, 1970
Salmo gairdneri	I	60	Maekawa and Yamada, 1970
Cyprinidae			
Carassius auratus	E.L.	20–30	Schönbörner *et al.*, 1979
Carassius auratus	I	65–100	Onozato and Watabe, 1979
Cyprinus carpio	I	100–120	Zylberberg, unpublished
Carassius auratus	T.C.	35–45	Zylberberg and Nicolas, 1982
Carassius auratus	A.F.	20	Zylberberg and Meunier, 1981
Cyprinus carpio	A.F.	30	Zylberberg and Meunier, 1981
Brachydanio rerio	I	20–25	Waterman, 1970
Poeciliidae			
Poecilia reticulata	E.L.	20–30	Schönbörner *et al.*, 1979
Poecilia reticulata	I	100	Zylberberg, unpublished
Gobiidae			
Pomatoschistus microps	E.L.	30	Fouda, 1979
Pomatoschistus microps	I	60–90	Fouda, 1979
Cichlidae			
Hemichromis bimaculatus	I	50–80	Sire and Géraudie, 1982
Hemichromis bimaculatus	E.L.	30–40	Sire, unpublished
Tilapia rendalli	E.L.	20–30	Schönbörner *et al.*, 1979
Tilapia mossambica	I	60–90	Lanzing and Wright, 1976
Pleuronectidae			
Hippoglossoides ellassodon	I	30–110	Brown and Wellings, 1969
	Fin rays		
Latimeria chalumnae	Act.	60–110	Géraudie and Meunier, 1981
Salmo gairdneri	Act.	40–80	Géraudie and Meunier, 1981
AMPHIBIANS	Scales		
Ichthyophiidae			
Ichthyophis kohtaoensis	B.P.	≈100	Zylberberg *et al.*, 1980
Caeciliidae			
Hypogeophis rostratus	B.P.	≈100	Zylberberg *et al.*, 1980
Microcaecilia unicolor	B.P.	≈100	Zylberberg and Wake, 1990
Dermophis mexicanus	B.P.	≈100	Zylberberg and Wake, 1990

Table 2. (continued)
Diameter of Collagenous Fibrils in the Scales, Fin Rays, and Osteoderms

Species	Tissues	Diameter (nm)	Authors
REPTILES	Osteoderms		
Anguiidae			
Anguis fragilis	S.L.	100	Zylberberg and Castanet, 1985
Anguis fragilis	B.P.	80	Zylberberg and Castanet, 1985
Gekkonidae			
Tarentola mauritanica		45–250	Levrat-Calviac and Zylberberg, 1986

Act. = Actinotrichia
A.F. = Anchoring fibres
B.P. = Basal plate
E.L. = External layer
I = Isopedine
S.L. = Superficial layer
T.C. = T.C. fibers

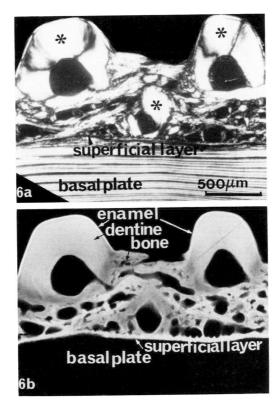

Fig. 6 *Latimeria chalumnae* (Crossopterygii). Ground-section of the posterior field of a scale. (a) Polarized light. Three odontodes (*) and vascular bone lie on the superficial layer which covers the whole surface of the basal plate where isopedine is organized in a double-twisted plywood-like structure. (b) X-ray microradiography. The mineralization is heterogeneous in the odontodes and in the superficial layer; the basal plate is not mineralized.

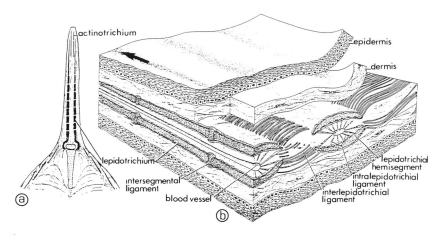

Fig. 7 Diagrams of the dermoskeleton is teleost fins. (a) Drawing of a longitudinal section of an unpair fin. The unmineralized actinotrichia are located in the tip of the fin and the most proximal lepidotrichial segment is connected by ligaments to the cartilagenous endoskeleton. (Adapted from Goodrich, 1904.) (b) Three-dimensional reconstruction of a fin showing the topographical location of the segmented lepidotrichium. The arrow indicates the direction of the apex where actinotrichia would be found. (Adapted from Beccera *et al.*, 1983.)

ogies between scutes and typical elasmoid scales are generally unknown in most families of Teleostei (Bertin, 1958; Whitear, 1986; Whitear and Mittal, 1986).

Ultrastructural studies in the developing scutes in the callichthyid *Corydoras arcuatus*, show that the body scute form in the dermis (Sire, unpub. res.). Initial and deep regions of the scute are built in part by metaplasis of the preexistent dermis whereas the superficial parts are formed by a layer of osteoblasts lining the scute surface. The study of several growing stages reveals that typical bony tissue is deposited first in all the regions of the scute, but when the growth slows down in older specimens, an atypical tissue, rich in microfilaments and devoid of collagen fibrils, is deposited, probably by the osteoblasts, on the external surface of the scute. This layer is well developed in adult scutes and shows, after decalcification, numerous electron-dense alignments of thin granules suggesting that this layer is deposited cyclically.

Fin Rays

The term "fin rays" covers three basic types of fish fin skeletal scaffolding, namely: 1) the bony lepidotrichia, 2) the bony spiny rays, both in Osteichthyes (except the Dipnoi) and 3) the camptotrichia in Dipnoi only (Goodrich, 1904). The unique presence of ceratotrichia in Selachians fins will not be discussed here since ceratotrichia that overlap a large cartilaginous skeletal framework within all the fins do not calcify. Their counterpart, namely the actinotrichia in Osteichthyes fins will nevertheless be evoked here due to their spatial relationships with the lepidotrichia (Fig. 7).

Lepidotrichia. The lepidotrichia are located underneath the stratified epidermis and immersed in connective tissue. Lepidotrichia are organized according to a fan configuration in the paired fins (hence the word "actinopterygian") while in unpaired fins, they are parallel to each other. Each lepidotrichium (Figs. 7, 9) consists of two parallel and symmetrical bony elements called demirays (Kemp and Park, 1970) or hemisegments (Lanzing, 1976; Beccera *et al.*, 1983) easily detected in wholemounts stained with Alizarin Red S. Each lepidotrichium is made of adjacent short bony segments separated by a joint region and connected to each other by collagenous ligaments (Fig. 8). Calcification of ligaments occurs, especially in the most proximal region of the lepidotrichia and consequently, obscures the joint; finally several adjacent segments ankylose (François and Blanc, 1956; Castanet *et al.*, 1975).

The bone forming the lepidotrichia is either cellular as in the trout (Blanc, 1953) or acellular in higher Teleostei as in the Poeciliidae although its ontogenesis is similar in both cases. Lepidotrichial bone is laid at the acellular dermoepidermal interface (Géraudie and Landis, 1982; Géraudie, 1983) and secondarily it leaves its subepidermal location to move deeply within the fin mesenchyme. Lepidotrichial bone consists of woven-fibered bone. Collagen fibrils, 20–30 nm in diameter, are typically striated. Preliminary data show that type I collagen is the predominant collagen present in this bone (Cohen-Solal and Géraudie, unpub. res.).

Collagen fibrils are immersed in a fine electron-dense granular ground substance the appearance of which precedes mineralization (Fig. 29). The positive staining observed after PAS treatment suggests the presence of sugar residues within the lepidotrichial bone as well as in adjacent new bony region of the dermoepidermal interface.

Among living bony fishes, only in Polypteridae are the most proximal segments of the bony lepidotrichia incompletely covered by a layer of ganoine, a hypermineralized tissue (Géraudie, 1988). The lepidotrichia so far examined in this group are made of cellular bone that show the same structural characteristics as bone of teleostean lepidotrichia (Meunier, 1980).

Spiny rays. Spiny rays are single tapered bony rods mainly developed among "advanced" Teleostei. Unlike the flexible lepidotrichia, spiny rays (Fig. 10) are unjointed pointed rods which participate in the fins skeleton as either a unique anteriorly located ray (carp, catfish) or support the whole fins, especially in evolved Teleostei. There are two different types of spiny rays.

The first type, located anteriorly as a simple ray can be considered a transformed lepidotrichium that has lost its joints because of mineralization; besides, it has developed peripheral growth. In carp, for instance, the dorsal and anal spiny rays have maintained their two original adjacent demirays. On the contrary, in catfish they have lost their two symmetrical components and show a central medullary canal which is more or less wide, according to the species (Vaillant, 1895a,b).

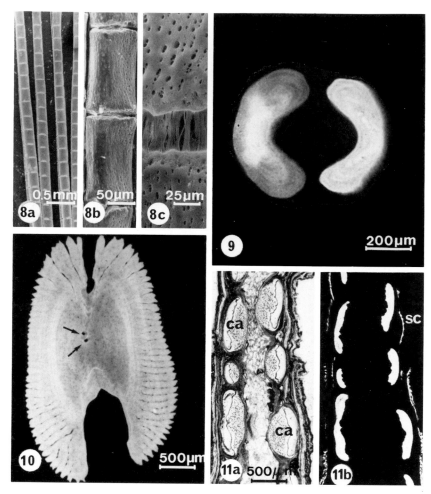

Fig. 8 *Salmo gairdneri* (Salmonidae). SEM. (a) Lateral view of four lepidotrichia. (b) High magnification of two lepidotrichial segments with three articulation areas. (c) High magnification of an articulation between two segments.

Fig. 9 *Polypterus senegalus* (Polypteridae). X-ray microradiography of a cross ground-section of a lepidotrichium. The lepidotrichial segment is made of two symmetrical parts (hemisegments). The mineralization is heterogeneous within each hemisegment.

Fig. 10 *Katsuwomus pelamis* (Thunnidae). X-ray microradiography of a cross ground-section of a spiny ray. Mineralization degree of bone is heterogeneous. Vascular canals (arrows) are present.

Fig. 11 *Neoceratodus forsteri* (Dipnoi). Ground-section of the caudal fin. (a) Normal transmitted light. Camptotrichia (ca) of different sizes are organized in two parallel rows underneath the epidermis. (b) X-ray microradiography. Only the superficial part of the camptotrichium is mineralized. The mineralized part of several scales (sc) are observed.

The second type of spiny rays supports the unpaired fins (the first dorsal fin and the anterior part of the anal one) in evolved Teleostei such as Perciformes. There, it is not possible to recognize either any symmetrical units or successive hemisegments as it is in the spiny rays of carp or catfish.

Camptotrichia.   The camptotrichia represent the original supporting elements of Dipnoi fins. They consist of single straight parallel tapered rods easily detected within the fin tissue by Alizarin Red S staining *in toto*. Their diameter is highly variable (Géraudie and Meunier, 1984) and dichotomous organization may be observed. Camptotrichia (Fig. 11) form two parallel rows which are not in register but alternate in the fin (Géraudie and Meunier, 1982).

In toto studies reveal two basic features of these bony elements; enlarged regions with dense staining suggest the presence of narrow joints and irregular staining is visible in places of bone resorption. In *Neoceratodus*, camptotrichia are cellular skeletal elements while in *Protopterus*, they are acellular. Another specificity of the camptotrichia is the heterogeneity of their mineralization (Fig. 11). The anterior part of the ray is normally calcified whereas the posterior part lacks any crystallites (Géraudie and Meunier, 1984). Comparative studies point out the possibility that camptotrichia could be derived from typical lepidotrichia (Géraudie and Meunier, 1984).

Ultrastructural studies confirmed the dual nature of the camptotrichia components as already shown by histological procedures by Goodrich (1904) and Jarvik (1959). The medial region of the subepidermal part of the camptotrichium can be described as bony in nature when opposed to the rest of the rod which is composed of unmineralized collagen fibrils packed into thick bundles oriented basically along the longitudinal axis of the camptotrichium. In the mineralized region, collagen fibrils embedded in an electron-dense granular matrix form a dense network obscured by the mineral phase.

Actinotrichia.   First reported in Teleostei by Ryder (1884), actinotrichia have been observed in Coelacanth (Géraudie and Meunier, 1980), Dipnoi fin buds (Géraudie, 1984) and Polypteridae (Géraudie, 1988). Actinotrichia are unjointed slender tapered rods that do not usually mineralize. During normal ontogenesis (Bouvet, 1974; Géraudie, 1977, 1978) they precede the formation of the lepidotrichia as during fin regenerative processes (Kemp and Park, 1970; Kirschbaum and Meunier, 1988).

The presence of the actinotrichia at the external margin of the fins is not detectable at first sight. Whole mounts of fins observed with an optical microscope through normal but reduced illumination or polarized light allow long transparent rods embedded between the distal region of the bony lepidotrichia to be detected. They have been extensively described by Goodrich (1904), Fauré-Frémiet (1936) and Garrault (1936) who suggested their homology with the ceratotrichia described earlier by Krükenberg (1885) in sharks. Actinotrichia, like ceratotrichia, are assumed to be made of elastoidin, a proteinaceous element related to collagen (Damodaran *et al.*, 1956).

The Integumental Skeleton of Amphibia and Reptilia

Scales

Two orders of living Amphibia, the Gymnophiona (Apoda) and the Anura have dermal ossifications. However, only the former are assumed to have typical "scales" (Kerr, 1955; Smith, 1960; Gabe, 1971b; Zylberberg *et al.*, 1980; Ruibal and Shoemaker, 1984). The first descriptions of the gymnophionan scales appeared in the last century (see Sarasin and Sarasin, 1887–90) and later, Taylor (1972) established an atlas of the scales based on the arrangement, size and shape of the squamulae, the only mineralized part topping the scales.

Up to now, from the structural data available on *Dermophis mexicanus*, *Hypogeophis rostratus*, *Ichthyophis kohtaoensis*, *Microcaecila unicolor*, it is obvious that all the scales share many structural features (Casey and Lawson, 1979; Perret, 1982; Zylberberg *et al.*, 1980; Fox, 1983; Wake and Nygren, 1987; Zylberberg and Wake, 1990).

Scales are small, flat disks set in large pouches forming successive rings around the body. However, each scale is located within its own pocket (Figs. 12, 13). As Gymnophiona show an evolutionary trend of reduction of the rings, concomitantly scales do also (Wake, 1975; Moodie, 1978). Ultrastructural studies (Zylberberg *et al.*, 1980) have shown that each scale is composed of two superimposed layers (Fig. 15): an unmineralized basal plate and the superficial squamulae which are the only mineralized part of the scale (Fig. 14). There are no cells within the scale, as it is also the case in most teleost elasmoid scales. The basal plate is composed of thick collagen fibrils ($\simeq$100 nm in diameter) which are organized in superimposed plies forming a plywood-like structure as in the isopedine of the elasmoid scale. In each ply, the collagen fibrils are closely packed in bundles.

At the outer surface, the squamulae are arrayed in concentric circles separated by unmineralized concentric and radial grooves. These grooves are distinct from the hypomineralized ring (Fig. 14) described by Feuer (1962). The surface of the squamulae bristles with preeminent mineralized globules which may be either isolated or aggregated in large concretions (Figs. 15, 16). The squamulae contain acid mucosubstances (Fig. 13, Table 1) (Gabe, 1971a) forming a microfibrillar meshwork often organized in a radiating pattern within the mineralized globules (Zylberberg *et al.*, 1980; Zylberberg and Wake, 1990) and also thick collagen fibrils arising from the basal plate. No distinct boundary was observed between the superficial squamulae and the underlying basal plate as in the dipoan scales.

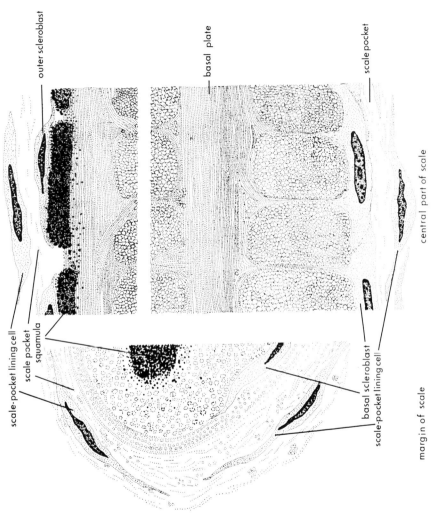

Fig. 12 Diagram of a scale section. (Adapted from Zylberberg and Wake, 1990.)

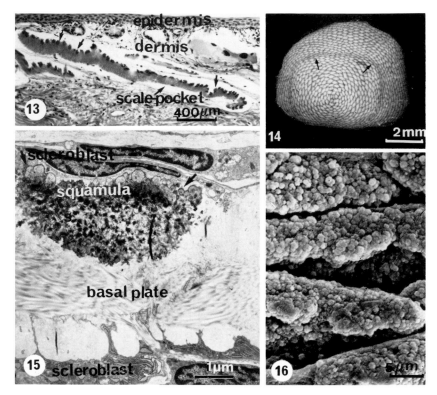

Figs. 12–16 The scales of Gymnophiona.

Fig. 13 *Dermophis mexicanus* (Caeciliidae). Section perpendicular to the skin surface. Alcian blue-PAS — hematoxylin. Each scale is located in its pocket. The squamulae (arrows) are intensely stained.

Fig. 14 *Ichthyophis kohtaoensis* (Ichthyophiidae). X-ray microradiography of a whole mounted scale. This scale shows a hypomineralized ring (arrows). The mineralized squamulae form concentric circles. They are separated by unmineralized grooves.

Fig. 15 *Microcaecilia unicolor* (Caeciliidae). TEM. Globules (arrows) located at the outer surface of the squamula.

Fig. 16 *Hypogeophis rostratus* (Caeciliidae). SEM. Detail of the outer surface of the squamulae with mineralized globules.

Osteoderms

The term osteoderm is usually used to denote the calcified dermal plates found in the integument of various unrelated families of Anura and Reptilia. One of the characteristics of osteoderms is to be located within both the deep dense dermis and the loose superficial dermis so that each osteoderm is composed of two superimposed layers, the structures of which are related to that of the surrounding dermis with which they are connected. In spite of an overall similarity in structural organization, the osteoderms vary in location, development, and histological characteristics according to anatomical and taxa specific patterns which largely remain to be explored and explained.

In Anura, the osteoderms forming the dermal armor show two forms. In some families, they are juxtaposed, small ossicles also called dermolita (Muzii, 1968) whereas in others, they form large and thick plates. These plates which are inserted in the deep dense dermis are made of a vascular or an avascular bone depending on the species (Guibé, 1970; Ruibal and Shoemaker, 1984). The calcified collagen fibrils forming the plate are organized in superimposed plies forming a plywoood-like structure. In some species such as the hylid *Phyllomedusa bicolor,* the osteoderm is ornamented with spines that protrude into the epidermis (Ruibal and Shoemaker, 1984). The presence of acid mucosubstances is revealed by histochemical tests in the dermolita (Muzii, 1968) and in the tips of some spines (Ruibal and Shoemaker, 1984) of Anura.

Among the reptiles, several lizard families have osteoderms which show variations in location, development, correlation with the epidermal keratinized scales, and general structure (reviewed in Bellairs, 1969; Moss, 1969; Guibé, 1970; Levrat-Calviac, 1986–87; Levrat-Calviac and Zylberberg, 1986). In the Gekkos, the osteoderms may be juxtaposed single ossicles (Figs. 17, 18) connected to one another and to the surrounding dermis by unmineralized collagen fibres (Figs, 19, 20, 21) resembling Sharpey's fibres (Otto, 1908; Schmidt, 1912, 1914; Levrat-Calviac, 1986–87). The distribution of these osteoderms shows no apparent relationship with the organization of the epidermal folds (Fig. 18) forming the characteristic epidermal "scales" of the reptilian skin (Otto, 1908; Levrat-Calviac, 1986–87). In the scincid *Scincus officinalis* the osteoderms fuse to form a mosaic which does not correspond with the keratinized epidermal scales (Otto, 1908). The osteoderms, which may be constituted of a large single plate in the anguiid *Anguis fragilis* (Figs. 22, 23) or composed of connected individual plates in the scincid *Chalcides viridanus* (Figs, 25, 26), are associated with the overlying epidermal folds; these osteoderms are imbricated in the same manner as the elasmoid scales of teleost fish (Figs. 23, 26) and they coincide exactly with the keratinized epidermal folds (Zylberberg and Castanet, 1985).

Reptilian osteoderms are composed of various mineralized tissues "which are not all bone" (Moss, 1969). The basal plate inserted in the dense dermis is composed of calcified collagen fibrils organized in an orthogonal plywood-like structure as in lamellar bone (Fig. 24). The superficial layer located in the loose dermis is composed of various tissues, the structure of which differs from that of bone (Moss, 1969, 1972; Levrat-Calviac and Zylberberg, 1986). For instance, in lizards such as *Tarentola mauritanica* and *T. neglecta* or in *Chalcides viridanus,* these superficial calcified layers do not contain collagen fibrils (Fig. 75) except the anchoring bundles which are made of closely packed collagen fibrils, but they are rich in acid mucosubstances (Table 1) forming a microfibrillar meshwork (Levrat-Calviac and Zylberberg, 1986).

In Anura and in Reptilia, the formation of the osteoderms occurs without differentiation of a specialized tissue structure such as the fish-scale papilla

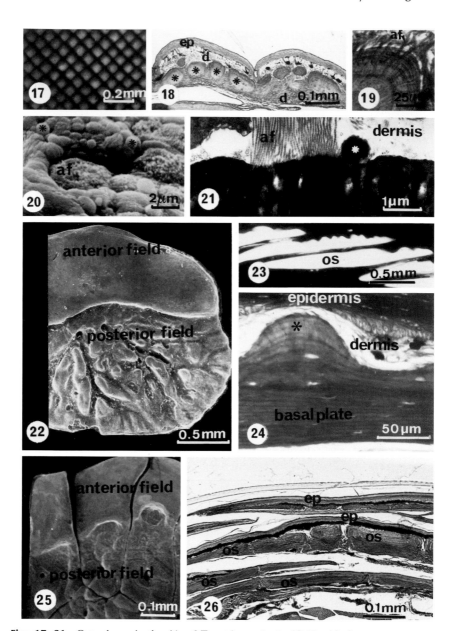

Figs. 17–21 Osteoderms in the skin of *Tarentola mauritanica* (Gekkonidae).

Fig. 17 X-ray microradiography of the skin.

Fig. 18 Several osteoderms (*) underneath a single epidermal fold (ep). One step trichrome (d = dermis).

Fig. 19 Detail of the outer surface of one osteoderm. Danielli's coupled tetrazonium reaction. Anchoring fibres (af) arise from the osteoderm.

Fig. 20 SEM. The anchoring fibres (af) are surrounded by mineralized globules (*).

Fig. 21 TEM. The anchoring fibres (af) made of collagen fibrils are surrounded by mineralized globules (*).

(Ruibal and Shoemaker, 1984; Zylberberg and Castanet, 1985). They mineralize by metaplastic ossification, i.e., more or less direct ossification of a preexisting dense connective tissue without involvement of a differentiated periostracum (Haines and Mohuiddin, 1968). Because of their structural diversity, osteoderms are thought to have appeared independently several times in unrelated taxa (Moss, 1969; Ruibal and Shoemaker, 1984).

To sum up this descriptive part, a large structural variety of mineralized tissues are found in the integumental skeleton. Several mineralization processes may coexist in a single structural element such as a scale or an osteoderm while histological processes involved in such tissue formation basically resemble those found in most other bony tissues of vertebrates. Indeed, most bone tissues contain the same basic components: osteocytes, collagen fibrils, noncollagenous proteins and other macromolecules plus apatitic crystals. Variations in the proportion of these components, e.g., in the coarseness and arrangement of the fibrils, in the size, number and location of the osteocytes, vascularity, are responsible for the differences among the various types of bony tissues (Pritchard, 1972; Ricqlès *et al.*, Volume 3 of this treatise). Nevertheless, the typological diversity of the bony tissues and some unusual mineralized tissues of the integumental skeleton show specific peculiarities unknown in the endoskeleton.

Analysis of Mineralization

Ørvig (1968) defined two different processes of mineralization depending on the relationships between the apatitic crystals and the organic matrix in the integumental skeleton: 1) inotropic mineralization occurs when the crystals are oriented along the collagen fibrils as in typical bony tissues (Glimcher, 1981); 2) spheritic mineralization is responsible for the formation of calcospherites within which the crystals show a radial arrangement. In this case, crystals are arranged without any relationships with the fibrillar collagenous framework. It may occur also in noncollagenous matrices (proteoglycans). According to Ørvig (1951, 1968), spheritic mineralization might be considered the phylogenetic precursor of the inotropic mineralization which, perhaps, represents the "ultimate stages" in a phyletic process of increasing

---

Figs. 22–24   Osteoderms in the skin of *Anguis fragilis* (Anguiidae).

Fig. 22   SEM. The superficial ornamentation of the uncovered posterier field differs from the smooth surface of the anterior field.

Fig. 23   X-ray microradiography of the imbricated osteoderms (os).

Fig. 24   Section of the posterior part of the osteoderm. The collagenous stroma is less dense in the superficial elevation (*) than in the basal plate made of lamellar bone.

Figs. 25 & 26   Osteoderms in the skin of *Chalcides viridanus* (Scincidae).

Fig. 25   SEM. Several plates constitute a single osteoderm. The superficial ornamentations of the uncovered posterior field differ from those of the covered anterior field.

Fig. 26   Section perpendicular to the skin surface. One step trichrome. Each osteoderm (os) is inserted in an epidermal fold (ep).

Table 3.
Mineralization Rate (% of the Dry Weight) of Various Bones in the Osteichthyes

Species	Bone		Scales
Cyprinus carpio	spiny ray	59.4	25.6
	rib	58.3	
Tilapia nilotica	spiny ray	68.5	35.8

Table 4.
Comparative Data for the Mineralization Degree in the Superficial Layer (S.L.) and in the Isopedine (I) of Scales

Species	Organ	Mineralization degree (g/cm^3)	Bone type	Authors
Rutilus rutilus	S.L.	1.09–1.18	+	Schönbörner, 1977
Rutilus rutilus	I	0.83–0.85	+	Schönbörner, 1977
Tilapia rendalli	S.L.	1.16–1.34	−	Schönbörner, 1977
Tilapia rendalli	I	0.88–0.91	−	Schönbörner, 1977
Eupomotis gibbosus	S.L.	1.31	−	Schönbörner, 1977
Eupomotis gibbosus	I	0.97	−	Schönbörner, 1977
Balistes conspicillum	S.L.	1.37	−	Meunier, 1983
Balistes conspicillum	I	1.12	−	Meunier, 1983

+   cellular bone
−   acellular bone

complexity of the "calcification mechanisms". The type of mineralization has been thought to depend on the abundance of calcium phosphate (Schmidt, 1971) or to be related to the spatial organization of the organic matrix (Boyde and Sela, 1978; Ben Hur and Ornoy, 1984). In the integumental skeleton, both spheritic and inotropic mineralizations can develop concomitantly.

The Mineral Phase

Few studies have dealt with the chemical characteristics of the mineral component found in the integumental skeleton. Moreover, almost all of these studies have been devoted to the scales of the Osteichthyes and particularly those of the Teleostei.

The total amount of mineral in the scales of adult Teleostei varies from 25% to 52% of dry weight depending on the species (van Oosten, 1957; Snyder, 1958; Meunier, 1983). It is noticeable that this percentage is always lower than that found in the bony tissue of the same species (Table 3). Microradiographic analysis of the distribution of the mineral within a single scale reveals that the mineralization degree of the superficial layer is almost the same as in the bony tissue of the same fish whereas it is always lower in the mineralized parts of the isopedine (Table 4).

As in the vertebrate bone, apatitic calcium phosphate is the main com-

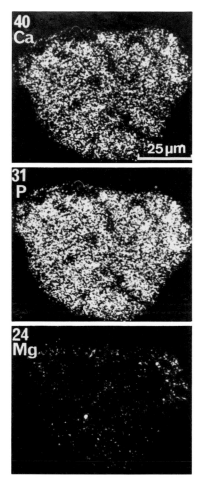

Fig. 27   Electron probe microanalysis showing the distribution of Ca, P, and Mg in a section of an osteoderm of *Tarentola mauritanica* (Gekkonidae).

ponent found in all mineralized structures constituting the integumental skeleton: ganoid scales (Meinke *et al.*, 1979), elasmoid scales (Cooke, 1967), fin-rays (Landis and Géraudie, 1990), gymnophionan scales (Zylberberg *et al.*, 1979), anuran osteoderms (Muzii, 1968) and reptilian osteoderms (Fig. 27) (Levrat-Calviac, 1986–87).

   Pioneering experiments in the last century had already shown that the osteichthyan scales contain not only calcium phosphate but also fluorine and magnesium (Jackson, 1854–56) and carbonate (Baudelot, 1873). Since these early observations, analyses using a variety of techniques showed that the mineral phase displays traces of other ions such as sodium and potassium that are known to substitute for calcium in the apatite (Posner, 1987). The amount of carbonate found in the scales by van Oosten (1957) exceeds 9.5%

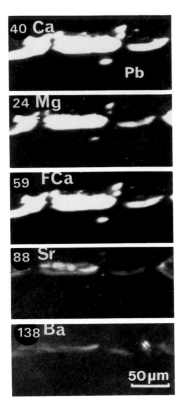

Fig. 28 Analytical ion microscopy showing the distribution of Ca, Mg, F, Sr, and Ba in a section of a scale of *Anguilla anguilla* (Anguillidae).

which is the highest content of carbonate ions found in well-crystallized apatite (Le Geros *et al.*, 1968). On the other hand, it has been demonstrated that carbonate ions are also related to non-apatitic environment (Rey *et al.*, 1989). Therefore, it can be hypothesized that a part of the important amount of carbonate indicated by van Oosten (1957) is not related to the apatitic framework.

Teleost scales contain fluorine and chlorine which can substitute for hydroxyl ions. They contain also strontium, barium, zinc, iron, lead, aluminium, bromine (Fig. 28) (van Oostren, 1957; van Coillie and Rousseau, 1974; Zylberberg *et al.*, 1984; Johnson, 1989; Sauer and Watabe, 1989) which are known to be common trace elements in biological apatites (Posner, 1987).

Metals such as cadmium, chromium, cobalt, lead, manganese, mercury, nickel, and silver known for their toxicity, are also stored in the scales of fishes collected in polluted water (van Coillie and Rousseau, 1974). These metals are thought to replace calcium in apatite. Therefore, in fish, mineral composition might be related, at least in part, to the surrounding aquatic environment, as suggested by van Coillie and Rousseau (1974). However,

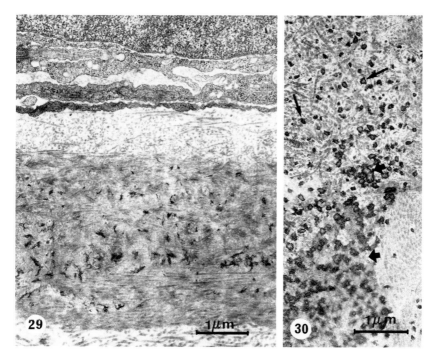

Fig. 29 *Salmo gairdneri* (Salmonidae). TEM. First stages of the mineralization of a lepidotrichium. Small crystals are located within the collagenous stroma.
Fig. 30 *Protopterus annectens* (Dipnoi). TEM. Front of mineralization in a longitudinally sectioned camptotrichia. Isolated mineral deposits (arrows) are distributed among the collagen fibrils in the apex. Then they fuse and form a continuous mineralized area (solid arrows).

recent studies dealing with the variations of the metal composition in the scale mineral related to the environment do not support this hypothesis (Johnson, 1989) even if it is known that fishes increase the calcium uptake from the ambient water to ensure the mineralization of the scales rather than from its bones in case of a dietary calcium deficiency (Berg, 1968; Ichii and Mugiya, 1983). The incorporation of environmental calcium is required for normal calcification of regenerating scales when a great number of scales are removed (Takagi *et al.*, 1989).

Mineralization Processes of Collagenous Matrices

As mentioned above, the dermal skeleton of the lower vertebrates presents a wide variety of mineralized tissues which moreover can coexist in a single element. In many cases, the mineralization processes and the relationships between the collagen fibrils (probably of type I) and the apatitic crystals are similar to those described for bony tissues. However, such relationships are not always observed even if collagen fibrils are present as in the isopedine and the external layer of the elasmoid scales. Moreover, these two layers show quite different mineralization processes (Schönbörner et al., 1979; Zylberberg and Nicolas, 1982).

Bone

Fin rays

Lepidotrichia. Mineralization of the bony tissue constituting the fin rays, lepidotrichia and spiny rays, is very similar to that of basic bone (Fig. 29). Microradiography shows that mineral is not regularly and homogeneously distributed (Fig. 9): it is generally slightly more abundant in slow growth areas (annuli) than in fast growth ones (zones) (Meunier, 1983, 1988).

The mechanism of calcification during development has been studied by techniques using unstained tissue sections obtained after samples fixed by anhydrous fluids such as ethylene-glycol which prevent fixative artifacts (Boothroyd, 1964; Landis et al., 1977; Landis and Glimcher, 1978). Electron diffraction generated in the distal growing region of the bone shows no coherent diffraction pattern, while in a more proximal one, thus in an ontogenetically older part of the same lepidotrichium, patterns characteristic of a poorly crystalline hydroxyapatite type of mineral are observed (Landis et al., 1981; Landis and Géraudie, 1990). In the same way, electron probe microanalysis detected the presence of Ca and P within the bone shaft of the lepidotrichium. Molar Ca/P ratio ranged from about 1.0 (distal) to 1.4 (proximal) along the lepidotrichial hemisegments (Landis and Géraudie, 1990). Recently, use of selected area diffraction technique associated with bright field imaging and selected-area dark field imaging (Jackson et al., 1978; Arsenault, 1988) allowed the size of the mineral particles to be determined. They range from 12–15 nm in length and eventually aggregate in larger crystals (35–40 nm) (Landis and Géraudie, 1990). Data upon the spatial distribution of the mineral within the organic matrix of the lepidotrichium suggest that the mineral is not regularly distributed along the collagen fibrils and a definitive association of the images of the crystallites with the collagen hole or its overlap regions is not clear (Landis and Géraudie, 1990).

In conclusion, it appears that the mineral deposits of calcium phosphate associated with collagen fibrils is a poorly crystalline hydroxyapatite deposited according to a proximal to distal direction along the growing hemisegment.

In Polypteridae, the mechanisms of collagen mineralization of the lepidotrichium have not yet been studied. A 1 μm-thick section studies combined with transmission electron microscopy reveal that woven bone is to be found at the surface of the segment while lamellar bone forms its core (Géraudie, 1988). Collagen-fibril diameter ranges from 50 to 70 nm and typical striation of the collagen fibrils may fade, as clearly observed in demineralized bone samples. As in teleosts, ligaments are susceptible to mineralization and ultimately two adjacent segments fused, the joint losing its function as a consequence.

Camptotrichia.   Longitudinal sections show that mineralization is a progressive event occurring in a proximal to distal direction (Fig. 30). At the apex, the mineral deposits are scattered clusters which fuse progressively and then give way to a dense mass hiding the organic phase (Géraudie and Meunier, 1984).

Bony basal plates.   Very few studies have been devoted to the fine relationships between the mineral and the collagenous matrix forming the basal plate of the ganoid scales, of the bony scutes of the Osteichthyes and of the anuran osteoderms. The thick basal plate of the ganoid scale is made of a bony tissue which shows the structural characteristics of a lamellar bone and it has a mineralization degree similar to that of the endoskeleton bony tissue. X-ray and electron microscopic studies (Ermin *et al.*, 1971; Sire, 1989; Zylberberg unpub. res.) show that the location of the apatitic crystals in the collagenous matrix resembles that of a bony tissue (Figs. 31, 32).

In anuran osteoderms, electron diffraction reveals that the apatitic crystals are oriented with their major axis parallel to the collagen fibrils (Muzii, 1968).

In reptilian osteoderms, the basal plate is made of lamellar bone which shows a mineralization degree similar to that of bone (Zylberberg and Castanet, 1985; Levrat, 1985). Ultrastructural studies reveal that the apatitic crystals are deposited along and within the collagen fibrils packed in bundles, their major axis oriented parallel to the axis of the collagen fibrils (Figs. 33, 34). Then the crystals invade the interfibrillary matrix. Mineralization starts in the upper collagen layers of the dense dermis. The osteoderms thicken while the mineralization front extends in the inner plies of the dense dermis. The mineralization progress does not appear to be related to the cells inserted within the collagenous matrix; these cells seem to become trapped in the mineralized tissue when the mineralization front progresses towards the inner part of the dermis.

In the basal plate of the scincid lizard *Chalcides viridanus*, SEM and TEM (Figs. 35, 36) have shown that numerous isolated mineralized corpuscles are localized ahead of the mineralization front (Zylberberg and Maisonneuve, unpub. res.). Because of their location, size and structure, these corpuscles resemble Mandl's corpuscles (Baudelot, 1873) which were so far considered to be a characteristic mineralization process of the isopedine of the elasmoid scales (see below: isopedine). As in the isopedine, these Mandl's corpuscle-like structures fuse with the mineralization front, increasing the thickness of the mineralized part of the basal plate.

No mineralized structures were found in the skin of juvenile *Anguis fragilis*, but numerous cells either isolated or arranged in groups, are located in areas between the dense and the loose dermis. Mineralized small-sized plates appear in the vicinity of these cells which are surrounded by small membrane-limited vesicles containing either an electron dense material or crystallites. The crystals invade the collagen fibrils and the interfibrillary ground sub-

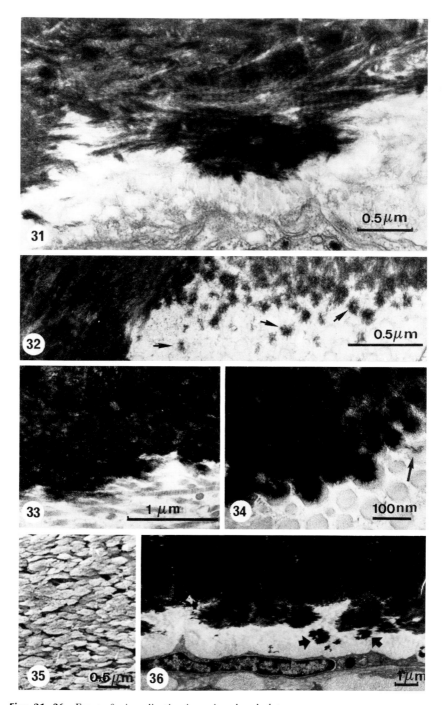

Figs. 31–36   Front of mineralization in various basal plates.
Figs. 31 & 32   *Calamoichthys calabaricus* (Polypteridae). TEM. Section of a ganoid scale.

stance so that whole bundles of collagen fibrils become entirely mineralized; these mineralized bundles fuse and form small-sized mineralized plates (Zylberberg and Castanet, 1985).

In Anura and Reptilia, the connective tissue is directly transformed into bone during the formation of the osteoderms. These results support the hypothesis that the osteoderms could be formed by metaplastic ossification defined as a "progressive mineralization of the matrix and inclusion of cells without multiplication and hypertrophy" (Haines and Mohuiddin, 1968).

Isopedine

Baudelot (1873) has reported that the basal plate of the teleostean scales is either partially mineralized or entirely unmineralized, depending on species. Many recent studies using microradiography and TEM, have confirmed these previous results, showing that in Teleostei a part of the isopedine remains unmineralized (Cooke, 1967; Brown and Wellings, 1969; Yamada and Watabe, 1979; Meunier et al., 1974; Lanzing and Wright, 1976; Onozato and Watabe, 1979; Meunier and Sire, 1981; Sire and Meunier, 1981; Meunier, 1984b). Moreover, mineral is completely lacking in the isopedine of the scales of Latimeria chalumnae (Fig. 6) (Castanet et al., 1975; Meunier, 1982) and of Neoceratodus forsteri (Meunier and François, 1980). These results explain the low amount of mineral in the scales in toto (expressed as percent of dry weight) compared to bone (Table 3).

Anhydrous techniques for electron microscopic analyses (see above, fin rays) showed that the crystals of hydroxyapatite vary from 30 to 100 nm in length and that their major axis is oriented parallel to the elongation of the collagen fibrils. The mineral deposit lies mostly in the interfibrillary matrix (Figs. 37, 39, 40) as described by Brown and Wellings (1969), Onozato and Watabe (1979), Schönbörner et al., (1979), Yamada and Watabe (1979) and Olson and Watabe (1980). The crystals do not penetrate deeply within the fibrils which appear in cross-sections as circular electron-lucent spaces, even in the oldest mineralized plies (Fig. 37) located in the vicinity of the external layer (Zylberberg and Nicolas, 1982; Landis and Zylberberg, unpub. res.). This peculiar location of the mineral might also be responsible for the lower degree of mineralization of the isopedine when compared to that of the

---

Fig. 31   The crystals are distributed along the collagen fibrils.

Fig. 32   The crystals penetrate within the fibrils (arrows).

Fig. 33   *Anguis fragilis* (Anguiidae). TEM. The crystals are oriented along the collagen fibrils in the osteoderm.

Fig. 34   *Tarentola mauritanica* (Gekkonidae). TEM. The crystals appear within the collagen fibrils (arrow) in the osteoderm.

Figs. 35 & 36   *Chalcides viridanus* (Scincidae).

Fig. 35   SEM. Numerous small-sized mineralized corpuscles are located at the deep surface of the osteoderm.

Fig. 36   TEM. Mineralized corpuscles are located ahead of the front of mineralization and resemble Mandl's corpuscles (arrows).

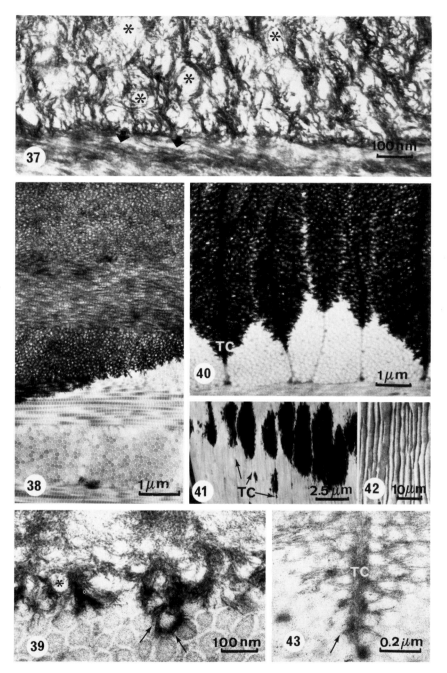

Figs. 37–43 Mineralization in the basal plate of teleost scales.

Fig. 37 *Carassius auratus* (Cyprinidae). TEM. Quick-freeze anhydrous techniques. The crystals are aligned along the collagen fibrils (arrows). The cross-sectioned collagen fibrils (*) appear as electron-lucent circular spaces surrounded by the crystals in a well-mineralized ply located in the vicinity of the external layer.

external layer of the scale or to endoskeletal bone tissue (Tables 3, 4). In the partially mineralized isopedine, the crystals are located in more or less numerous plies beneath the external layer except under the grooves (radii) (Figs. 44, 46) where isopedine remains unmineralized (Meunier *et al.*, 1974; Sire and Meunier, 1981; Meunier, 1984a).

The mineralization of isopedine starts after that of the external layer, the crystals of which are thought to initiate the formation of new crystals in the collagen fibrils of the ply of the isopedine adjacent to the external layer. Then, the extension of the mineralization is due either to the formation of secondary nucleation sites initiated by the previously formed crystals, or to the multiplication of new primary nucleation sites (Glimcher, 1989). The mineralization front progresses towards the basal part of the isopedine (Fig. 38). This mineralization process called "subsequential mineralization" (Schönbörner *et al.*, 1979), occurs without the participation of cells and matrix vesicles (Schönbörner *et al.*, 1979; Olson and Watabe, 1980; Zylberberg and Nicolas, 1982). In the isopedine of the cyprinid scales the thin TC fibers (Figs. 40, 41, 43) mineralize before the thick collagen fibrils forming the plywood-like structure (Onozato and Watabe, 1979; Schönbörner *et al.*, 1979; Zylberberg and Nicolas, 1982; Meunier, 1984b). Therefore the mineralization front resembling inverted fir trees in TEM (Fig. 40) also shows a peculiar SEM aspect (Fig. 42).

A specific characteristic of isopedine is that it mineralizes much more slowly than bone. Vital labeling studies have shown that the delay between collagen synthesis and the mineral deposition is much longer in isopedine than in the external layer of the same scale (Sire and Meunier, 1981) or in "regular" bone (Boivin and Meunier, 1978). These techniques have also revealed that the speed of mineralization varies according to the location of crystallite accretion in the isopedine; it is faster when it is close to the margins of the scale than under the focus (Table 5).

A second feature of mineralization in isopedine concerns the progression of the mineralization front at the histological level. In most Teleostei, the mineralization front is a more or less smooth surface (Figs. 44, 45). However, the mineralization front is preceded by independently mineralized Mandl's

---

Fig. 38   *Trisopterus luscus* (Gadidae). TEM. Mineralization front.

Fig. 39   *Poecilia reticulata* (Poecilidae). TEM. Quick-freeze anhydrous techniques. Detail of the mineralization front. The crystals (arrows) are located in the spaces surrounding the cross-sectioned collagen fibrils (*).

Figs. 40 & 41   *Carassius auratus* (Cyprinidae). TEM.

Fig. 40   Section perpendicular to the scale surface. Characteristic aspect of the mineralization front due to the presence of TC fibers.

Fig. 41   Aspect of the mineralization front in a section parallel to the scale surface therefore perpendicular to the TC fibers.

Fig. 42   *Cyprinus carpio* (Cyprinidae). SEM. The ridged mineralization front differs from the smooth one of scales which have no TC fibers (compare with Fig. 48).

Fig. 43   *Carassius auratus* (Cyprinidae). TEM. Quick-freeze anhydrous techniques (OsO_4 omitted). Mineralization front in an unstained section. The first deposited crystals are located along the TC collagen fibrils, then they invade the interfibrillary spaces in isopedine (arrow).

Table 5.

Rate of Progression of Mineralization in Isopedine in the Different Areas of the Scale in
Hemichromis bimaculatus

Localization	Rate of progression of mineralization (μm/days)
Anterior area	0.21 (0.10–0.33)
Focus	0.11 (0.05–0.17)
Posterior area	0.15 (0.07–0.23)

From Sire and Meunier, 1981.

corpuscles (Mandl, 1839). In a given species, even more in a single scale, the corpuscles vary in size and shape depending on their location, the smaller being close to the margin and the larger under the focus. The size of the corpuscles is also linked to the age of the fish (Baudelot, 1873; Schönbörner *et al.*, 1981; Meunier, 1983). The great variability of their shape (ovoid, cubic, polyhedral or spherical) as revealed by SEM, depends on the spatial organization of the collagenous matrix of isopedine (Schönbörner *et al.*, 1981; Meunier and Castanet, 1982; Meunier, 1984b). The morphology of Mandl's corpuscles is usually more complex in a twisted plywood than in an orthogonal one (Meunier, 1984b). Newly formed Mandl's corpuscles located in a single ply, are ovoid and parallel to each other and to the elongation of the collagen fibrils within this ply (Fig. 47). They show a ridged surface in scales with TC fibers (Fig. 50). When Mandl's corpuscles grow, they become polyhedral (Fig. 48) (Schönbörner *et al.*, 1981; Meunier, 1984b) because the mineral extends to the adjacent plies in the direction of the long axis of the collagen fibrils in each ply (Zylberberg and Nicolas, 1982). Mandl's corpuscles coalesce and fuse with the mineralization front (Figs. 48, 49), increasing the thickness of the mineralized part of isopedine (Schönbörner *et al.*, 1981; Sire and Meunier, 1981). They are particularly abundant in regenerating scales in which they are involved in fast mineralization during the first stages of regeneration (Frietsche and Bailey, 1980; Sire and Géraudie, 1984). In spite of their "globular" appearance when observed with the light microscope and SEM, Mandl's corpuscles appear in TEM to be formed by inotropic mineralization (Figs. 49, 51) (Schönbörner *et al.*, 1979, 1981; Zylberberg and Nicolas, 1982). Mandl's corpuscles form in the absence of cells and matrix vesicles and without any contact with a preexisting calcified tissue.

Mandl's corpuscles are common in the teleostean scales, but are absent in the scales of Anguillidae, Osteoglossidae and Mormyridae. In the two latter families, the mineralization front shows a characteristic aspect (Figs. 52, 53); it progresses faster at the margin of the squamulae (the mineralized

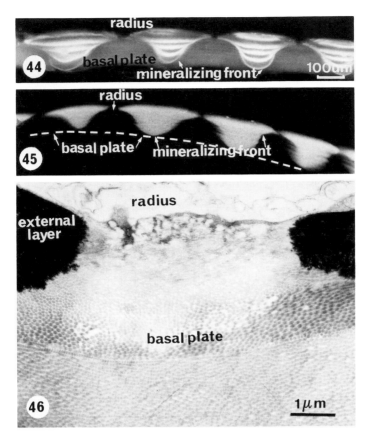

Figs. 44 & 45 *Hemichromis bimaculatus* (Cichlidae). Cross ground-section.
Fig. 44 Vital labeling. Fluorescent light. The four successive labelings show that the progression of the mineralization front is slower at the margin of the radii than under the interradii.
Fig. 45 X-ray microradiography. The basal plate remains unmineralized underneath the radii.
Fig. 46 *Trisopterus luscus* (Gadidae). TEM. No mineral is deposited in the basal plate under the radius where the external layer is lacking.

plates topping the scales) near the grooves separating two adjacent squamulae than under their center (Gayet and Meunier, 1983; Meunier, 1983, 1984a,b).

Mandl's corpuscles are also present in the elasmoid scales of the Holostean *Amia* in which they show complex shapes (Meunier, 1981). They are also found in the dipnoan *Protopterus* where they show a less complex morphology (Meunier, 1984b). The cells inserted within the isopedine of *Protopterus annectens* do not appear to participate in the formation of Mandl's corpuscles or in mineralization of isopedine which is partially mineralized. The mineral appears to be deposited first in the plies adjacent to the outer superficial layer and then spreads toward the basal part of the scale as in the acellular isopedine of the teleostean elasmoid scale (Zylberberg, 1988). Up to now,

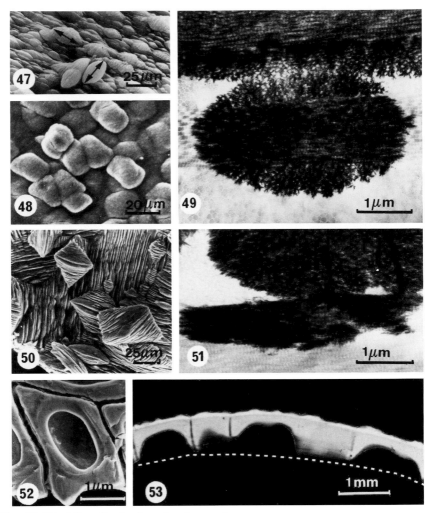

Figs. 47–53 Mineralization front in teleost scales.

Fig. 47 *Megalops atlanticus* (Elopidae). SEM. The long axes (arrows) of ovoid Mandl's corpuscles located in two adjacent plies of the orthogonal plywood-like structure forming the isopedine are at right angle.

Figs. 48 & 49 *Trisopterus luscus* (Gadidae).

Fig. 48 SEM. The mineralization front is ornamented with fused Mandl's corpuscles. Both show a smooth surface.

Fig. 49 TEM. In the Mandl's corpuscle, the crystals are oriented along the collagen fibrils in the three plies of the isopedine.

Fig. 50 *Cyprinus carpio* (Cyprinidae). SEM. Mandl's corpuscles show a squared shape and a ridged surface like the mineralization front (see also Fig. 42).

Fig. 51 *Carassius auratus* (Cyprinidae). TEM. The progression of the mineralization is related to the orientation of the collagen fibrils and varies in the two adjacent plies.

Fig. 52 *Gnathonemus petersii* (Mormyridae). SEM. Aspect of the surface of the squamula facing the isopedine with its cavited center.

Fig. 53 *Osteoglossum bicirrhosum* (Osteoglossidae). X-ray microradiography of a ground section. The mineralized margin of the squamula is thicker than its center (compare with Fig. 45). The dotted line indicates the limit of the basal plate which is not completely mineralized.

Mandl's corpuscles were considered a characteristic feature of the elasmoid scales. However, since similar corpuscles were observed in the basal plate of a lizard osteoderm *(Chalcides viridanus)* (Figs. 35, 36), their functional and/ or evolutive significance remains an open question.

External Layer of the Elasmoid Scales

This layer is well-mineralized even in the minute scales of the eel (Zylberberg *et al.*, 1984). It mineralizes first during ontogenesis (Neave, 1940; Sire, 1985) and regeneration (Frietsche and Bailey, 1980; Sire and Géraudie, 1984). Ultrastructural analysis carried out with various fixation procedures, cytochemical reactions, electron diffraction and selected-area dark field imaging, suggests that the small-sized apatitic crystals (from 30 to 100 nm in length depending on the fixation and the species) do not appear to be related to the thin collagen fibrils (Zylberberg and Nicolas, 1982; Landis and Zylberberg, unpub. res.). The crystals seem to be rather associated with the interfibrillary dense granules (Fig. 59) containing mucopolysaccharides, protein-polysaccharides and possibly acid phospholipids (Maekawa and Yamada, 1970; Olson and Watabe, 1980; Zylberberg and Nicolas, 1982). Yet, these granules where the crystals aggregate in clusters might be considered as mineralization sites as defined by Landis *et al.* (1977). In developing scales, the crystals appear in the vicinity of the marginal superficial scleroblasts (Figs. 54, 55). In several species, the crystals are observed within extracellular matrix vesicles (Fig. 56) (Maekawa and Yamada, 1970; Yamada, 1971; Kobayashi *et al.*, 1972; Schönbörner *et al.*, 1979; Zylberberg and Nicolas, 1982). The presence of matrix vesicles in the osteoid zone of developing scales is discussed by Yamada and Watabe (1979) and by Olson and Watabe (1980). In *Hemichromis bimaculatus*, matrix vesicles were identified in the regenerating scales only (Sire and Géraudie, 1984). Thus, in the scales, as in other bony tissues, matrix vesicles might be related to early fast mineralization processes (Ali, 1976; Anderson, 1976; Glimcher, 1984; Bonucci, 1987).

The crystals, which do not increase in size during mineralization, aggregate in clusters that increase in number and size by accretion of newly-formed crystals (Fig. 57). In the clusters the crystals are arranged in a radiating manner (Fig. 58). Then, the clusters fuse to form a fully mineralized layer. During the mineralization processes, the crystals do not show any relationships with the collagen fibrils. Therefore, this mineralization might not be considered as inotropic nor typically spheritic according to the definition of Ørvig (1968). But it seems to be characteristic of the external layer.

In the dipnoan *Protopterus annectens*, the structure of the external layer which forms the squamulae, differs from that of a typical elasmoid scale. It contains both mineralized collagen fibrils organized in a loose meshwork and mineralized globules which do not contain a collagenous stroma (Figs. 60, 61); so

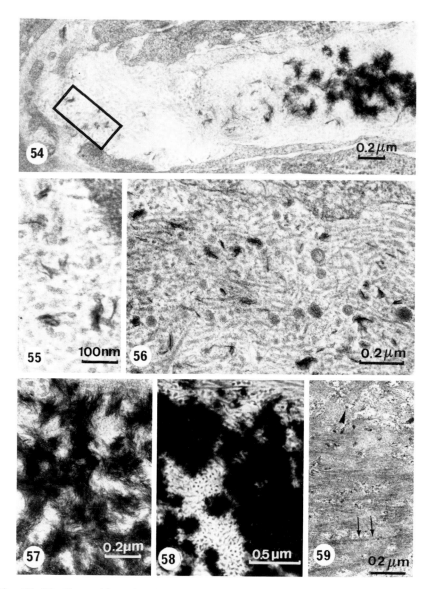

Figs. 54–59   External layer in teleost scales. TEM.

Figs. 54 & 55   *Poecilia reticulata* (Poecilidae).

Fig. 54   Quick-freeze anhydrous techniques. The first crystals are seen at the margin of the scale.

Fig. 55   Detail of the Fig. 54. Crystals do not show relationships with the collagen fibrils.

Fig. 56   *Tinca tinca* (Cyprinidae). In the margin of the scale, matrix vesicles are present in the vicinity of the scleroblasts.

Fig. 57   *Salmo gairdneri* (Salmonidae). Quick-freeze anhydrous techniques. The crystals aggregate and form clusters.

Figs. 58 & 59   *Carassius auratus* (Cyprinidae).

Fig. 58   Quick-freeze anhydrous techniques. The clusters fuse and form fully mineralized areas.

Fig. 59   Section of a demineralized scale. Ruthenium red added to the fixative. Thin collagen fibrils (arrows) are randomly oriented and electron-dense granules are present (arrowhead).

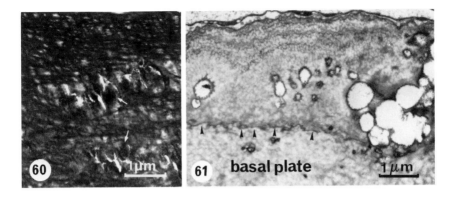

Figs. 60 & 61 External layer of the scale of *Protopterus annectens* (Dipnoi). TEM.
Fig. 60 Mineralized globules (arrows) are observed within the massive mineral deposit.
Fig. 61 Demineralized section. Ruthenium red added to the fixative. The circular electron-lucent areas are surrounded by abundant collagen fibrils. Ruthenium red positive material (arrowheads) form an obvious boundary between the external layer and the isopedine.

far a similar structure is unknown in the external layer of the typical elasmoid scales of the Teleostei (Zylberberg, 1988). Similarly the squamulae of the gymnophionan scales contain both mineralized collagen fibrils and mineralized globules (Fig. 62) within which the crystallites organized in a radiating pattern (Fig. 63) are associated with a noncollagenous organic matrix (Fig. 64) (Zylberberg *et al.*, 1980).

The uncovered posterior area of the elasmoid scales of the Teleostei and of the Dipnoi is connected to the overlying dermis by anchoring fibres which resemble Sharpey's fibres (Fig. 69). Only the part of the fibre inserted in the scale is mineralized. The crystals are oriented by the collagen fibrils within which they penetrate, obscuring the characteristic periodic structure of the collagen fibrils (Zylberberg and Meunier, 1981). Therefore, in this case, it is an inotropic mineralization.

Mineralization Processes of Noncollagenous Matrices

Ganoine

Ultrastructural data (Zylberberg *et al.*, 1985; Sire *et al.*, 1987; Meunier *et al.*, 1988) have shown that this hypermineralized layer topping the ganoid scales of primitive Actinopterygii is devoid of collagen fibrils as previously suggested by Thomson and McCune (1984). It contains microfibrils involved in the orientation of the apatitic crystals (Fig. 65). These crystals perpendicular to the scale surface are long (250 nm) and thin (8 nm) and resemble

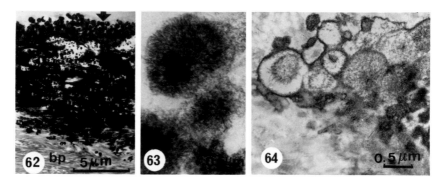

Figs. 62–64   The squamulae of the scales of Gymnophiona. TEM.

Fig. 62   *Dermophis mexicanus*. Mineralized globules (arrow) are abundant at the outer surface of a squamula (see Fig. 16 for the SEM aspect of the surface). Collagen fibrils are mineralized within the squamulae but they remain unmineralized in the basal plate (bp).

Figs. 63 & 64   *Microcaecilia unicolor*.

Fig. 63   Detail of a mineralized globule with radiating crystals.

Fig. 64   The demineralized globules show an organic matrix composed of thin noncollagenous fibrils organized in a radiating pattern.

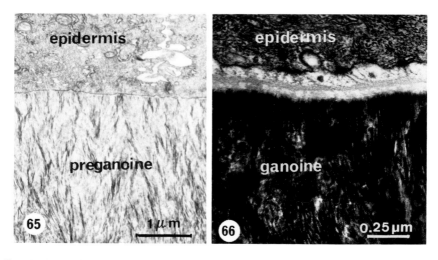

Figs. 65 & 66   Ganoine formation in the regenerating scale of *Calamoichthys calabaricus* (Polypteridae). TEM.

Fig. 65   First stages of mineralization of the ganoine layer. The preganoine long crystals are oriented along the organic fibrils which are perpendicular to the scale surface lined by the epidermal cells.

Fig. 66   Well-mineralized ganoine layer with abundant long crystals perpendicular to the scale surface.

those described in tooth enamel (Fig. 66) (Nylen *et al.*, 1963; Glimcher *et al.*, 1965; Frank and Voegel, 1977; Carlson, 1990).

In the regenerating scales of the polypterid *Calamoichthys calabaricus*, differentiated epidermal cells forming the inner epidermal layer are involved in the formation and growth of the ganoine (Sire *et al.*, 1987). Therefore, the ganoine of the integumental skeleton is considered homologous to true enamel of the tooth but with peculiar characteristics such as its stratified structure, especially in the scales (Ørvig, 1978a,b) and its permanent position below the epidermis (Géraudie, 1988).

Outer Limiting Layer of the Elasmoid Scales

This layer is not easily distinguishable from the external layer in TEM micrographs of mineralized scales because of the similar electron density and the similar size of the crystals in both layers. In the inner part of the outer limiting layer which is in contact with the external layer, the crystals do not show any preferential direction whereas at the outer surface they are perpendicular to the scale surface (Fig. 67) (Schönbörner *et al.*, 1979) as previously observed with polarizing microscopy by Schmidt (1951) and Lerner (1953). As isopedine, the outer limiting layer mineralizes after the external layer; its mineralization might be considered as subsequential (Schönbörner *et al.*, 1979). However, the mineralization processes are different from those of the isopedine because the outer limiting layer is very poor in collagen fibrils (Sire, 1985) or entirely devoid of them (Schönbörner *et al.*, 1979; Zylberberg and Meunier, 1981; Zylberberg *et al.*, 1984) but rich in acid mucosubstances (Zylberberg and Nicolas, 1982).

TEM micrographs of mineralized material showed that the outer limiting layer is stratified (Fig. 68). It is composed of superimposed bands distinguishable by their definite differences of opacity to electrons, reflecting the different organization of the subadjacent organic matrix (Schönbörner *et al.*, 1979; Zylberberg and Meunier, 1981; Sire, 1985). The presence of these superimposed bands might be related to the cyclical growth of the outer limiting layer throughout the life of the fish. Mineralized globules were observed on the outer surface of the scale mostly near the focus of the scales of Cyprinidae and of the Trout (Figs. 69, 70) and associated with the tubercles around the anchoring fibres in the scale of *Hemichromis bimaculatus* (Sire, 1985, 1988). Spheritic mineralization was found in these globules within which the microfibrillar matrix is organized in a radiating pattern (Fig. 71). In the scales of Cichlidae, mineralized globules are found in the basement membrane of the epidermal-dermal junction (Fig. 72). These spherules then migrate to the upper surface of the scales where they aggregate to the outer limiting layer increasing the thickness of this outer layer (Sire, 1988). These data reopen the question of the actual participation of the epidermis in the formation of the superficial layer of the elasmoid scales.

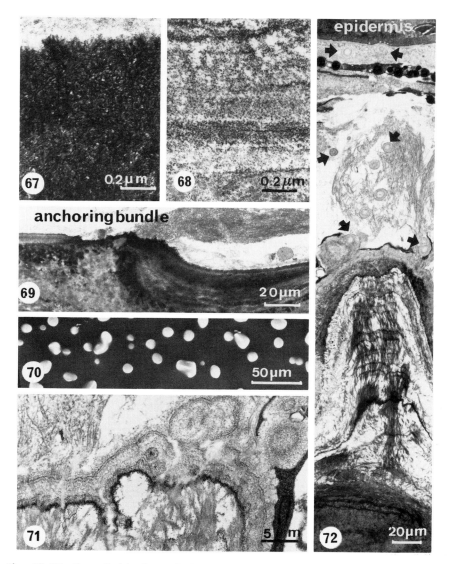

Figs. 67–72 Outer limiting layer of teleost scales.

Figs. 67 & 68 *Carassius auratus* (Cyprinidae). TEM.

Fig. 67 Small-sized crystals are perpendicular to the scale surface.

Fig. 68 Demineralized scale. Ruthenium red added to the fixative. The organic matrix is distributed in superimposed bands which are more or less dense. The presence of such super-imposed dense lines suggest that the outer limiting layer thickens by cyclic accretions. Fibrillar collagen is not found in this layer.

Fig. 69 *Cyprinus carpio* (Cyprinidae). TEM. Anchoring fibre composed of parallel-oriented collagen fibrils arise from the surface.

Fig. 70 *Salmo gairdneri* (Salmonidae). SEM. The outer surface is ornamented with mineralized globules.

Figs. 71 & 72 *Hemichromis bimaculatus* (Cichlidae). Section of a demineralized scale. Ruthenium red added to the fixative.

Outer Layer of the Osteoderms

In three species of lizards *Tarentola mauritanica, T. neglecta* and *Chalcides viridanus,* the outer part of the osteoderms contains small-sized crystals (less than 100 nm in length) which are either oriented perpendicularly to the outer surface of the osteoderm (Fig. 73) or organized in a radiating pattern forming globules of various sizes (Fig. 74). These globules can fuse to form larger aggregates.

This superficial part appears as a stratified structure since parallel electron-dense lines which correspond to more densely mineralized strata are either parallel to the osteoderm surface or form concentric lines in the mineralized globules. In demineralized thin sections, the organic matrix composed of thin microfibrils shows the same arrangements as the crystals (Fig. 75): the microfibrils are perpendicular to the surface of the osteoderm or organized in radiating patterns. Abundant electron-dense organic material reactive with ruthenium red forms dense lines as in the mineralized samples. The presence of these dense lines suggests that the outer layer thickens by cyclic accretions.

This superficial layer cannot be considered as ganoin as suggested by Moss (1969) since it is not hypermineralized and the crystals are small-sized. Moreover, this layer is made of a cellular tissue; its cells arise from the dermis whereas epidermal cells do not appear to participate to the formation of this layer.

Concluding Comments

This review highlights the diversity in shapes, organizations, structures, and mineralization processes found in the integumental skeleton of the living lower vertebrates. However, such a diversity is already found in the integumental skeleton of the earliest known vertebrates which had developed mineralized tissues showing the main characteristics still found in living forms (Hall, 1975; Kemp, 1984). Moreover, the integumental skeleton of the living vertebrates also shows specific mineralized tissues. The formation of such tissues might be related on the one hand to the general trend of reduction of the integumental skeleton during the vertebrate evolution, and on the other to functional adaptations. Indeed, the fin rays forming the supporting elements of the fins are involved in locomotion and are stiff bony sticks which obviously differ from the dermal mineralized plates ensuring the protection of the animal body.

All the mineralized plates share a basic structural organization which

Fig. 71   Globules with an organic matrix organized in a radiating pattern are located in the vicinity of an anchoring fiber.

Fig. 72   Globules (arrows) are localized in the vicinity of the basement membrane and in the dermis overlying the scale where they are associated with the anchoring fibers.

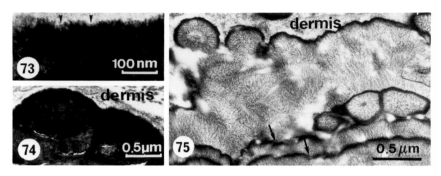

Figs. 73–75   Osteoderms of *Tarentola mauritanica* (Gekkonidae). TEM.
Fig. 73   Outer surface of the osteoderm. The crystals are oriented perpendicularly to the surface (arrowheads).
Fig. 74   Globules at the outer surface of the osteoderm (see Fig. 20 for the SEM aspect).
Fig. 75   Demineralized section. Ruthenium added to the fixative. The noncollagenous organic matrix is composed of thin fibrils either oriented perpendicularly to the surface of the osteoderm or in a radiating pattern. Superimposed dense lines (arrows) suggest that this layer thickens by cyclic accretions.

consists of two superimposed layers: the basal plate made of a more or less mineralized collagenous stroma organized in a plywood-like structure and a well-mineralized superficial layer very often composed of heterogeneous mineralized tissues, some of them are not bony tissues (Moss, 1969). It is admitted that the "primitive" basic components of the dermal plates are a bony plate topped by tooth derivatives, therefore this "conserved structural organization reflects the existence of ontogenic mechanisms responsible for both the maintenance of basic morphological arrangements and the generation of diversity within a general theme" (Burke, 1989).

At the histological and cytological levels, this review emphasizes the large spectrum of mineralized tissues found in the integumental skeleton: typical bony tissues, atypical bony tissues and mineralized tissues which are not "true" bone. This typological diversity is such that even if some unusual mineralized tissues which show specific peculiarities so far unknown in the endoskeleton and develop with regular mineralized tissues, appear to be devoid of one or more of the characteristic components of bone, they might be nevertheless recognized as bony tissues (Meunier, 1984b, 1987). Such an atypical bony tissue is represented by isopedine which is often an acellular tissue either partially mineralized or entirely unmineralized. Nevertheless according to Meunier (1984b, 1987) it might be considered as a bony tissue *sensu lato* like the permanent preosseous tissue of the camptotrichia of the fins which remains unmineralized. Both tissues represent paradoxical cases of bony tissues which lack both cells and mineral. From ultrastructural evidence, when isopedine mineralizes, the mineralization is of an inotropic type as in bone; there are close relationships between the orientation of the collagen fibrils and that of the crystallites even if the crystallites are mostly found with an extrafibrillar location. Type I collagen is probably the major component of isopedine as shown by recent biochemical analysis (unpub.

res.) but nothing is known about the degree of hydroxylation of lysine, the extent of the crosslinks and the amount of glycosylation which differentiate the type I collagen which mineralizes from the others which do not (Veis, 1985). Similarly nothing is known about the noncollagenous proteins (reviewed in Fisher and Termine, 1985) involved in the mineralizing processes.

Some unusual mineralized tissues of the integumental skeleton lacking collagen fibrils are not considered as "true" bone (Moss, 1969). Indeed, ganoine which forms an outer hypermineralized layer in the rhomboid scales is assimilated to a tooth enamel because of its epidermal origin and its structure (Sire *et al.*, 1987) but others of these mineralized tissues devoid of collagen fibrils and found at the outer surface of the teleostean scales and of the osteoderms, seems to be restricted to the integumental skeleton. These tissues, which are not hypermineralized, may not be considered as enamel like ganoine because they are not epidermal hypermineralized productions as ganoine is. Moreover, their small apatitic crystallites never reach the size of those found in the ganoine layer. These small-sized crystallites are spatially arranged as the underlying organic matrix rich in acidic proteoglycans which are known to control crystal growth (Addadi *et al.*). Thus, it might be hypothesized that both the organic matrix and the mineral are intimately associated in these peculiar mineralized tissues as in other mineralized tissues (Weiner, 1986). However, how the organic matrix controls the nucleation, growth and distribution of the crystallites, are basic questions which are still unanswered. The recent advances in the identification of the different mineralization processes occurring in the integumental skeleton support the hypothesis that several independent mechanisms may be at work in the various mineralized tissues and they suggest that the integumental skeleton could provide convenient models for a better understanding in the field of biomineralization.

Acknowledgments

The help in printing the micrographs by the Photographic Department of the "Service Accueil de Microscopie Electronique" CNRS and Université Pierre et Marie Curie, is gratefully acknowledged. Work in the authors' laboratory was supported by CNSR grants 1137 and ATP "Evolution".

References

Addadi, L., Berman, A., Moredian Oldak, J., and Weiner, S. (1989). Structural and stereochemical relations between acidic macromolecules of organic matrices and crystals. *Connect. Tissue Res.*, **21**: 127–135.

Aldinger, H. (1937). Permische ganoidfische aus Ostgrönland. *Mdd. Grönland*, **102**: 1–392.

Ali, S. Y. (1976). Analysis of matrix vesicles and their role in the calcification of epiphyseal cartilage. *Fed. Proc.*, **35**: 135–142.

Anderson, H. C. (1976). Matrix vesicle calcification. *Fed. Proc.*, **35**: 105–108.

Arsenault, A. L. (1988). Collagen relationships in calcified turkey leg tendons visualized by selected-area darkfield electron microscopy. *Calcif. Tissue Int.*, **43**: 202–212.

Baudelot, M. E. (1873). Recherches sur la structure et le développement des écailles des Poissons osseux. *Arch. Zool. Exp. Gén.*, **2**: 87–244, 429–480.

Beccera, J., Montes, G. S., Bexiga, S. R. R., and Junqueira, L. C. U. (1983). Structure of the tail fin in teleosts. *Cell Tissue Res.*, **230**: 127–137.

Bellairs, A. (1969). The skin. In: *The Life of Reptiles*, Bellairs, A., Ed., Weidenfeld and Nicholson, London, **2**: 283–331.

Bemis, W. E. (1984). Paedomorphosis and the evolution of the Dipnoi. *Paleobiology*, **10**: 293–307.

Ben Hur, H. and Ornoy, A. (1984). Ultrastructural studies of initial stages of mineralization of long bones and vertebrate fetuses. *Acta Anat.*, **119**: 33–39.

Berg, A. (1968). Studies on the metabolism of calcium and strontium in freshwater fish. I. Relative contribution of direct and intestinal absorption. *Mem. Ist. Ital. Idrobiol.*, **23**: 161–196.

Bertin, L. (1944). Modifications proposées dans la nomenclature des écailles et des nageoires. *Bull. Soc. Zool. Fr.*, **69**: 198–202.

Bertin, L. (1958). Ecailles et sclérifications dermiques. In: *Traité de Zoologie*, Grassé, P. P., Ed., Masson et Cie, Paris, **13**: 482–504.

Bhatti, H. K. (1938). The integument and dermal skeleton of Siluroidea. *Trans. Zool. Soc. Lond.*, **24**: 1–102.

Blanc, M. (1953). Contribution à l'étude de l'ostéogenèse chez les poissons téléostéens. *Mém. Mus. Natn. Hist. Nat. Paris*, **7**: 1–145.

Boivin, G. (1975). Etude chez le rat d'une calcinose cutanée induite par calciphylaxie locale. I — Aspects ultrastructuraux. *Arch. Anat. Microsc. Morphol. Exp.*, **64**: 183–205.

Boivin, G. and Meunier, F. J. (1978). Bone formation and fluorescent labelling in teleost fishes. D1-D5. In: *Symposium de recherche sur les tissus calcifiés des poissons*, CNEXO-COB, Brest.

Boivin, G., Walzer, C., and Baud, C. A. (1987). Ultrastrauctural study on the long term development of two experimental cutaneous calcinoses (topical calciphylaxix and topical calcergy) in the rat. *Cell Tissue Res.*, **247**: 525–532.

Bone, Q. (1972). Buoyancy and hydrodynamic function of the integument in the castor oil fish, *Ruvetus pretiosus* (Pisces, Gempylidae). *Copeia*, **1**: 78–87.

Bonucci, E. (1987). The structural basis of calcification. In: *Ultrastructure of the Connective Tissue Matrix*, Ruggeri, A. and Motta, P. M., Eds., Martinus Nijhoff, Boston, The Hague, 165–191.

Boothroyd, B. (1964). The problem of demineralization in thin section of fully calcified bone. *J. Cell Biol.*, **20**: 165–173.

Bouligand, Y. (1972). Twisted fibrous arrangements in biological materials and cholesteric mesophases. *Tissue Cell*, **4**: 189–198.

Bouvet, J. (1974). Différenciation et ultrastructure du squelette distal de la nageoire pectorale chez la truite indigène *(Salmo trutta fario* L.) I. Différenciation et ultrastraucture des actinotriches. *Arch. Anat. Microsc. Morph. Exp.*, **63**: 79–96.

Boyde, A. and Sela, J. (1978). Scanning electron microscope study of separated calcospherites from the matrices of different mineralizing systems. *Calcif. Tissue Res.*, **26**: 47–49.

Brien, P. (1962). Etude de la formation, de la structure des écailles des Dipneustes actuels et de leur comparaison avec les autres types d'écailles des Poissons. *Ann. Mus. Roy. Afr. Centr.*, sér. *8*, **108**: 53–129.

Brown, G. A. and Wellings, S. R. (1969). Collagen formation and calcification in teleost scales. *Z. Zellforsch.*, **93**: 571–581.

Burdak, V. D. (1979). Morphologie fonctionnelle du tégument écailleux des poissons, *La Pensée Scientifique, Kiev*, en russe). Traduction française, vol. Spécial Cybium. (1986), **10**: 1–147.

Burke, A. C. (1989). Development of the turtle carapace: Implication for the evolution of a novel Bauplan. *J. Morph.*, **199**: 363–378.

Carlson, S. J. (1990). Vertebrate dental structures. In: *Skeletal Biomineralizations: Patterns, Processes and Evolutionary Trends*, Carter, J. G., Ed., D. Van Nostrand, New York, in press.

Casey, J. and Lawson, R. (1979). Amphibians with scales: the structure of the scale in the caecilian *Hypogeophis rostratus*. *Brit. J. Herpetol.*, **5**: 831–833.

Castanet, J., Meunier, F., Bergot, C., and François, Y. (1975). Données préliminaires sur les structures histologiques du squelette de *Latimeria chalumnae*. 1 — Dents, écailles, rayons des nageoires. In: *Problèmes actuels de Paléontologie (Evolution des Vertébrés)*, Coll. Int. CNRS, 159–168.

Cooke, P. H. (1967). Fine structure of the fibrillary plate in the central head scale of the striped killifish *Fundulus majalis*. *Trans. Am. Microsc. Soc.*, **86**: 273–279.

Damodaran, M., Sivaraman, C., and Dhavalicar, R. S. (1956). Amino acid composition of elastoidin. *Biochem. J.*, **62**: 621–625.

Ermin, R., Rau, R., and Reibedanz, H. (1971). Der submikroskopische Aufbau der Ganoidschuppen von *Polypterus* in Vergleich zu den Zahngeweben der Saugetiere. *Biomineralization*, **3**: 12–21.

Fauré-Frémiet, E. (1936). La structure des fibres d'élastoîdine. *Arch. Anat. Microsc.*, **32**: 249–270.

Feuer, R. C. (1962). Structure of scales in a caecilian *(Gymnopis mexicanus)* and their use in age determination. *Copeia*, **3**: 636–637.

Fisher, L. W. and Termine, J. D. (1985). Noncollagenous proteins influencing the local mechanisms of calcification. *Clin. Orthop.*, **200**: 362–385.

Fouda, M. M. (1979a). Studies on scale structure in the common goby *Pomatoschistus microps* Kroyer. *J. Fish. Biol.*, **15**: 173–183.

Fouda, M. M. (1979b). Studies on scale regeneration in the common goby, *Pomatoschistus microps* (Pisces). *J. Zool., Lond.*, **189**: 503–522.

Fox, H. (1983). The skin of *Ichthyophis* (Amphibia: Caecilla): An ultrastructural study. *J. Zool., Lond.*, **199**: 233–248.

Francillon-Vieillot, H., Castanet, J., Géraudie, J., Meunier, F. J., Sire, J. Y., Zylberberg, L., and Ricqlès, A. de (1990). Vertebrate skeletal tissues. In: *Skeletal Biomineralizations: Patterns, Processes and Evolutionary Trends*, Carter, J. G., Ed., D. Van Nostrand, New York, 175–234.

François, Y. and Blanc, M. (1956). Sur la croissance en longueur des cayons de nageoires chez les poissons téléostéens. *Bull. Soc., Zool. Fr.*, **81**: 26–33.

Franck, R. M. and Voegel, J. C. (1977). Le cristal d'apatite biologique: son élaboration, son comportement physiologique et pathologique. *Biol. Cell.*, **28** 187–193.

Frietsche, R. A. and Bailey, C. F. (1980). The histology and calcification of regenerating scales in the blackspotted topminnow, *Fundulus olivaceus* (Storer). *J. Fish Biol.*, **16**: 693–700.

Gabc, M. (1971a). Données histologiques sur le tégument d'*Ichthyophis glutinosus* L. (Batracien, Gymnophione). *Ann. Sci. Nat., Zool.*, 12ème série, **13**: 573–608.

Gabe, M. (1971b). Apport de l'histologie à l'étude des relations phylétiques des Gymnophiones. *Bull. Biol.*, **105**: 125–157.

Garrault, H. (1936). Développement des fibres d'élastoîdine (Actinotrichia) chez les Salmonidés. *Arch. Anat. Microsc.*, **32**: 105–137.

Gayet, M. and Meunier, F. J. (1983). Ecailles actuelles et fossiles d'Ostéoglossiformes (Pisces, Teleostei). *C. R. Acad. Sci., Paris*, **297**: 867–870.

Géraudie, J. (1977). Initiation of the actinotrichial development in the early fin bud of the fish. *Salmo. J. Morph.*, **151**: 353–362.

Géraudie, J. (1978). The fin structure of the early pelvic fin bud of the trout *Salmo gairdneri* and *S. trutta fario*. *Acta Zool.*, **59**: 85–96.

Géraudie, J. (1983). Contrôles morphogénétiques du développement et de la régénération des nageoires paires des Téléostéens. Thèse de Doctorat ès Sciences, Paris. *Arch. Doc. Inst. Ethnol.*, micro-édition, *Mus. Natn. Hist. Nat.*, SN 82-600-329.

Géraudie, J. (1984). Fine structural comparative peculiarities of the developing Dipoan dermal skeleton in the fins of *Neoceratodus* larvae. *Anat. Rec.*, **209**: 115–123.

Géraudie, J. (1988). Fine structural peculiarities of the pectoral fin dermoskeleton of two Brachiopterygii, *Polypterus senegalus* and *Calamoichthys calabaricus* (Pisces, Osteichthyes). *Anat. Rec.*, **221**: 455–468.

Géraudie, J. and Landis, W. J. (1982). The fine structure of the developing pelvic fin skeleton in the trout, *Salmo gairdneri*. *Am. J. Anat.*, **163**: 141–157.

Géraudie, J. and Meunier, F. J. (1980). Elastoidin actinotrichia in coelacanth fins: a comparative study with teleosts. *Tissue Cell,* **12**: 637–645.

Géraudie, J. and Meunier, F. J. (1982). Comparative fin structure of the Osteichthyan dermotrichia. *Anat. Rec.,* **202**: 325–328.

Géraudie, J. and Meunier, F. J. (1984). Structure and comparative morphology of camptotrichia of lungfish fins. *Tissue Cell,* **16**: 217–236.

Giraud, M. M., Castanet, J., Meunier, F. J., and Bouligand, Y. (1978). The fibrous structure of coeolacanth scales: a twisted 'plywood'. *Tissue Cell,* **10**: 671–686.

Glimcher, M. J. (1981). On the form and function of bone: from molecules to organs. Wolff's Law revisited. In: *The Chemistry and Biology of Mineralized Tissues,* Veis, A., Ed., Elsevier, New York, 618–673.

Glimcher, M. J. (1984). Recent studies of the mineral phase in bone and its possible linkage to organic matrix by protein bound phosphate bond. *Phil. Trans. Roy. Soc. Lond. B.,* **304**: 479–508.

Glimcher, M. J. (1989). Mechanism of calcification: role of collagen fibrils and collagen phosphoprotein-complexes *in vivo* and *in vitro. Anat. Rec.,* **224**: 139–153.

Glimcher, M. J., Daniel, E. J., Travis, D. F., and Kamhi, S. R. (1965). Electron optical and X-ray diffraction studies of the organization of the inorganic crystals in embryonic bovine enamel. *J. Ultrastruct. Res. Suppl.* **7**: 14–77.

Goodrich, E. S. (1904). On the dermal fin-rays of fish living and extinct. *Quart. J. Microsc. Sci.,* **47**: 465–522.

Goodrich, E. S. (1907). On the scales of fish living and extinct, and their importance in classification. *Proc. Zool. Soc., Lond.,* **2**: 751–774.

Gross, W. (1935). Histologische Studien am Ausserskelett fossiler Agnathen und Fische. *Paläontographica,* **83A**: 1–60.

Gross, W. (1966). Kleine schuppenkunde. *N. Jb. Geol. Paläont.,* **125**: 29–48.

Guibé, J. (1970). La peau et les productions cutanées. In: *Traité de Zoologie,* Grassé, P.-P., Ed., Masson et Cie, Paris, **14**: 6–31.

Haines, R. W. and Mohuiddin, A. (1968). Metaplastic bone. *J. Anat.,* **103**: 527–538.

Hall, B. K. (1975). Evolutionary consequences of skeletal differentiation. *Am. Zool.,* **15**: 329–350.

Ichii, T. and Mugiya, Y. (1983). Effect of dietary deficiency in calcium on growth and calcium uptake from the aquatic environment in the goldfish *Carassius auratus. Comp. Biochem. Physiol.,* **74A**: 259–262.

Jackson, C. T. (1854–56). On the composition of the scales of the garpike. *Proc. Boston Soc. Nat. Hist.,* **5**: 92.

Jackson, S. A., Cartwright, A. G., and Lewis, D. (1978). The morphology of bone mineral crystals. *Calcif. Tissue Res.,* **25**: 217–222.

Jarvik, E. (1959). Dermal fin-rays and Holmgren's principle of delamination. *Kungl. Svenska Vetens. Akad. Handl.,* **6**: 3–51.

Johnson, M. G. (1989). Metals in fish scales collected in Lake Opeongo, Canada, from 1939 to 1979. *Trans. Am. Fish. Soc.,* **118**: 331–335.

Kemp, N. E. (1984). Organic matrices and mineral crystallites in vertebrate scales, teeth and skeletons. *Am. Zool.,* **24**: 965–976.

Kemp, N. E. and Park, J. H. (1970). Regeneration of lepidotrichia and actinotrichia in the tailfin of the teleost *Tilapia mossambica. Dev. Biol.,* **22**: 321–342.

Kerr, T. (1952). The scales of primitive living actinopterygians. *Proc. Zool. Soc. Lond.,* **122**: 55–78.

Kerr, T. (1955). The scales of modern lungfish. *Proc. Zool. Soc. Lond.,* **125**: 355–345.

Kirschbaum, F. and Meunier, F. J. (1988). South American Gymnotiform fishes as model animals for regeneration experiments. *Monogr. Dev. Biol.,* **21**: 112–123.

Klaatsch, H. (1890). Zur Morphologie der Fischenschuppen und zur Geschichte der Hartsubstanzgewebe. *Gegenbaurs Morphol. Jahrb.,* **16**: 209–258.

Kobayashi, S., Yamada, J., Maekawa, K., and Ouchi, K. (1972). Calcification and nucleation in fish-scales. *Biomineralization*, **6**: 84–90.

Krejsa, R. J. (1979). The comparative anatomy of the integumental skeleton. In: *Hyman's Comparative Vertebrate Anatomy*, Wake, M. H., Ed., The University Chicago Press, Chicago, London, 112–191.

Krükenberg, C. F. (1885). Ueber die chemische Beschaffenheit der sog. Hornfäden von *Mustelus* und über die Zusammensetzung der keratinösen Hüllen um die Eiern von *Scyllium stellare*. *Mittheil. Zool. Sta. Neapel*, **6**: 286–296.

LaMonte, F. R. (1958). Scales of the Atlantic species of *Makaira*. *Bull. Am. Mus. Nat. Hist.*, **114**: 381–395.

Landis, W. J. and Géraudie, J. (1990). Organization and development of the mineral during early ontogenesis of the bony fin rays of the trout *Oncorhynchus mykiss*. *Anat. Rec.*, **228**: 383–391.

Landis, W. J., Géraudie, J., Paine, M. C., Neuringer, J. R., and Glimcher, M. J. (1981). An electron optical and analytical study of mineral deposition in the developing fin of the trout, *Salmo gairdneri*. *Trans. Orthop. Res. Soc.*, **6**: 271.

Landis, W. J. and Glimcher, M. J. (1978). Electron diffraction and electron probe microanalysis of the mineral phase of bone tissue prepared by anhydrous techniques. *J. Ultrastruct. Res.*, **63**: 188–223.

Landis, W. J., Paine, M. C., and Glimcher, M. J. (1977). Electron microscopic observations of bone tissue prepared anhydrously in organic solvents. *J. Ultrastruct. Res.*, **59**: 1–30.

Lanzing, W. J. R. (1976). The fine structure of fins and finrays of *Tilapia mossambica* (Peters). *Cell Tissue Res.*, **173**: 349–356.

Lanzing, W. J. R. and Wright, R. G. (1976). The ultrastructure and calcification of the scales of *Tilapia mossambica* (Peters). *Cell Tissue Res.*, **167**: 37–47.

Le Geros, R. Z., Trautz, O., Le Geros, J. P., and Klein, E. (1968). Carbonate substitution in apatite structure. *Bull. Soc. Chim. Fr.*, Special number: 1693–1700.

Lerner, H. (1953). Polarisationsoptische Beitrage zur Kenntnis der Verkalkung der Knochen-fischschuppen. *Z. Zell. Anat. Mikr.*, **39**: 36–73.

Levrat, V. (1985). Structure et minéralisation des ostéodermes chez deux Gekkonidés: *Tarentola mauritanica* (Linné, 1758) et *Tarentola neglecta* (Strauch, 1887), Squamates. Thèses de 3ème cycle. Biologie animale, Paris, 52 pp.

Levrat-Calviac, V. (1986–87). Etude comparée des ostéodermes de *Tarentola mauritanica* et de *T. neglecta* (Gekkonidae, Squamata). *Arch. Anat. Microsc. Morph. Expér.*, **75**: 29–43.

Levrat-Calviac, V. and Zylberberg, L. (1986). The structure of the osteoderms in the gekko: *Tarentola mauritanica*. *Am. J. Anat.*, **176**: 437–446.

Maekawa, K. and Yamada, J. (1970). Some histochemical and fine structural aspects of growing scales of the rainbow trout. *Bull. Fac. Fish. Hokkaido Univ.*, **21**: 70–78.

Mandl, L. (1839). Recherches sur la structure intime des écailles de poissons. *Ann. Sci. Nat. Zool.*, série II, **11**: 337–371.

Matoltsy, A. G. and Bereiter-Hahn, J. (1986). 1. Introduction. 2: 1–7. In: *Biology of the Integument*, Bereiter-Hahn, J., Matoltsy, A. G., and Richards, K. S., Eds., Springer-Verlag, Berlin, Heidelberg, New York, Tokyo.

Meinke, D. K., Skinner, H. C. W., and Thomson, K. S. (1979). X-ray diffraction of the calcified tissues in *Polypterus*. *Calcif. Tissue Int.*, **28**: 37–42.

Meunier, F. J. (1980). Recherches histologiques sur le squelette dermique des Polypteridae. *Arch. Zool. Exp. Gén.*, **121**: 279–295.

Meunier, F. J. (1981). 'Twisted plywood' structure and mineralization in the scales of a primitive living fish, *Amia calva*. *Tissue Cell*, **13**: 165–171.

Meunier, F. J. (1982). Les relations isopédine-tissu osseux dans le post-temporal et les écailles de la ligne latérale de *Latimeria chalumnae* (Smith). *Zool. Scripta*, **9**: 307–317.

Meunier, F. J. (1983). Les tissus osseux des Ostéichthyens. Structure, genèse, croissance et évolution. Thèse de Doctorat ès Sciences, Paris. *Arch. Doc. Inst. Ethnol.*, micro-édition, *Mus. Natn. Hist. Nat.*, SN 82-600-328, 200.

Meunier, F. J. (1984a). Structure et minéralisation des écailles de quelques Osteoglossidae (Ostéichthyens, Téléostéens). *Ann. Sci. Nat. Zool.*, 13ème série, **13**: 111–124.

Meunier, F. J. (1984b). Spatial organization and mineralization of the basal plate of elasmoid scales in Osteichthyans. *Am. Zool.*, **24**: 953–964.

Meunier, F. J. (1987). Os cellulaire, os acellulaire et tissus dérivés chez les Ostéichthyens: les phénomènes de l'acellularisation et de la perte de minéralisation. *Ann. Biol.*, **26**: 201–233.

Meunier, F. J. (1987–88). Nouvelles données sur l'organisation spatiale des fibres de collagène de la plaque basale des écailles des Téléostéens. *Ann. Sci. Nat. Zool.*, 13ème sér., **9**: 113–121.

Meunier, F. J. (1988). Détermination de l'âge individuel chez les Ostéichthyens à l'aide de la squelettochronologie: historique et méthodologie. *Acta Œcol.*, *Œcol. Gen.*, **9**: 299–329.

Meunier, F. J. and Castanet, J. (1982). Organisation spatiale des fibres de collagène de la plaque basale des écailles des Téléostéens. *Zool. Scripta*, **11**: 141–153.

Meunier, F. J., Castanet, J., Francillon, H., and François, Y. (1974). Examen microradiographique des écailles de quelques Téléostéens. *Bull. Assoc. Anat.*, **58**: 615–624.

Meunier, F. J. and François, Y. (1980). L'organisation spatiale des fibres collagènes et la minéralisation des écailles des Dipneustes actuels. *Bull. Soc. Zool. Fr.*, **105**: 215–226.

Meunier, F. J., François, Y., and Castanet, J. (1978). Etude histologique et microradiographique des écailles de quelques Actinoptérygiens primitifs actuels. *Bull. Soc. Zool. Fr.*, **103**: 309–318.

Meunier, F. J., Gayet, M., Géraudie, J., Sire, J. Y., and Zylberberg, L. (1988). Données ultrastructurales sur la ganoïne du dermosquelette des Actinoptérygiens primitifs. In: *Teeth revisisted: Proc. VIIth Int. Symp. on Dental Morphology*, Russell, D. E., Santoro, J. P., and Sigogneau-Russell, D., Eds., *Mém. Mus. Natn. Hist. Nat., Paris*, (série C), **53**: 77–83.

Meunier, F. J. and Géraudie, J. (1980). Les structures en contre-plaqué du derme et des écailles des Vertébrés inférieurs. *Ann. Biol.*, **19**: 1–18.

Meunier, F. J. and Sire, J. Y. (1981). Sur la structure et la minéralisation des écailles du germon, *Thunnus alalunga* (Téléostéen, Perciforme, Thunnidae). *Bull. Soc. Zool. Fr.*, **106**: 327–336.

Moodie, G. E. E. (1978). Observations of the life history of the caecilian *Typhlonectes compressicaudus* (Dumeril and Bibron) in the Amazon Basin. *Can. J. Zool.*, **56**: 1005–1008.

Moss, M. L. (1964). Development of cellular dentine and lepisosteal tubules in the boowfin, *Amia calva. Acta Anat.*, **58**: 333–354.

Moss, M. L. (1968a). The origin of vertebrate calcified tissues. In: *Current Problems of Lower Vertebrate Phylogeny, Nobel Symp.*, Vol. 4, Ørvig, T., Ed., J. Wiley, New York, 359–371.

Moss, M. L. (1968b). Bone, dentin and enamel and the evolution of Vertebrates. In: *Biology of the Mouth*, Am. Assoc. Advanc. Sci. (Publisher, City) 37–65.

Moss, M. L. (1969). Comparative histology of dermal sclerifications in reptiles. *Acta Anat.*, **73**: 510–533.

Moss, M. L. (1972). The vertebrate dermis and the integumental skeleton. *Am. Zool.*, **12**: 27–34.

Muzii, E. O. (1968). Dermal calcifications of Anurans: their composition and structure. In: *Les Tissus Calcifiés*. 5ème Symposium Européen, (Publisher, City) 377–382.

Neave, F. (1936). The development of scales of *Salmo. Trans. R. Soc. Can.*, **5**: 55–72.

Neave, F. (1940). On the histology and regeneration of the teleost scale. *Quart. J. Microsc. Sci.*, **81**: 541–568.

Nickerson, W. S. (1893). Development of the scales of *Lepisosteus. Bull. Mus. Comp. Zool.*, **24**: 115–139.

Nylen, M. U. E., Eanes, E. D., and Onnell, K. A. (1963). Crystal growth in rat enamel. *J. Cell Biol.*, **18**: 109–123.

Olson, O. P. and Watabe, N. (1980). Studies on formation and resorption of fish scales. IV. Ultrastructure of developing scales in newly hatched fry of the sheepshead minnow, *Cyprinodon variegatus* (Atherinformes: Cyprinodontidae). *Cell Tissue Res.*, **211**: 303–316.

Onozato, H. and Watabe, N. (1979). Studies on fish scale formation and resorption. III. Fine structure and calcification of the fibrillary plates of the scales in *Carassius auratus* (Cypriniformes: Cyprinidae). *Cell Tissue Res.*, **201**: 409–422.

Ørvig, T. (1951). Histologic studies of Placoderms and fossil Elasmobranchs. I. The endo-skeleton, with remarks on the hard tissue of lower vertebrates in general. *Ark. Zool.*, **2**: 321–454.

Ørvig, T. (1967). Phylogeny of tooth tissues: evolution of some calcified tissues in early vertebrates. In: *Structural and Chemical Organization of Teeth*, Vol. I., Miles, A. E. W., Ed., Academic Press, New York, 45–105.

Ørvig, T. (1968). The dermal skeleton; general considerations. In: *Current Problems of Lower Vertebrate Phylogeny, Nobel Symp.*, Vol. 4., Ørvig, T., Ed., J. Wiley, New York, 373–397.

Ørvig, T. (1969). Cosmine and cosmine growth. *Lethaia*, **2**: 241–260.

Ørvig, T. (1977). A survey of odontodes ("dermal teeth") from developmental, structural, functional, and phyletic points of view. In: *Problems in Vertebrate Evolution*, Andrews, S. M., Miles, R. S., and Walker, A. D., Eds., Linnean Society Symposium 4, Academic Press, London, New York, 52–75.

Ørvig, T. (1978a). Microstructure and growth of the dermal skeleton in fossil Actinopterygian fishes: *Birgeria* and *Scanilepis*. *Zool. Scripta*, **7**: 33–56.

Ørvig, T. (1978b). Microstructure and growth of the dermal skeleton in fossil Actinopterygian fishes: *Boreosomus, Plegmolepis* and *Gyrolepis*. *Zool. Scripta*, **7**: 125–144.

Otto, H. (1908). Die Beschuppung der Brevelinguier und Ascalaboten. *Jena Zeitschr. Naturwiss.*, **44**: 193–253.

Patterson, C. (1977). Cartilage bones, dermal bones and membrane bones, or the exoskeleton versus the endoskeleton. In: *Problems in Vertebrate Evolution*, Andrews, S. M., Miles, R. S., and Walker, A. D., Eds., Linnean Society Symposium 4, Academic Press, London, New York, 77 121.

Perret, J. (1982). Les écailles de deux Gymnophiones africains (Batraciens apodes), observées au microscope électronique à balayage. *Bonn. Zool. Beitr.*, **33**: 343–347.

Posner, A. S. (1987). Bone mineral and the mineralization process. In: *Bone and Mineral Research*, Vol. 5, Peck, W. A., Ed., Elsevier, Amsterdam, New York, Oxford, 65–116.

Pritchard, J. J. (1972). General history of bone. In: *The Biochemistry and Physiology of Bone*, Bourne, G. H., Ed., Academic Press, New York, 1–20.

Rey, C., Lian, J., Grynpas, M., Shapiro, F., Zylberberg, L., and Glimcher, M. J. (1989). Non-apatitic environments in bone mineral: FT-IR detection, biological properties and changes in several disease states. *Connect. Tissue Res.*, **21**: 267–273.

Ricqlès, A. de, Meunier, F. J., Castanet, J., and Francillon-Vieillot, H. (in press). Comparative microstructure of bone. In: *Bone: Bone Matrix and Bone Specific Products*, Vol. 3, Hall, B. K., Ed., CRC Press.

Romer, A. S. (1964). Bone in early vertebrates. In: *Bone Biodynamics*, Frost, H. M., Ed., Little Brown, Boston, 13–37.

Rosen, N. (1913). Studies on the plectognaths. III. The integument. *Ark. Zool.*, **8**: 1–29.

Roth, F. (1920). Ueber den Bau und die Entwicklung des Hautpanzers von *Gastroteus aculeatus*. *Anat. Anz.*, **52**: 513–534.

Ruibal, R. and Shoemaker, V. (1984). Osteoderms in Anurans. *J. Herpetol.* **18**: 313–323.

Ryder, J. A. (1884). On the homologies and early history of the limbs of vertebrates. *Proc. Acad. Nat. Sci. Philadelphia*, **39**: 344–368.

Sarasin, P. and Sarasin P. (1887–90). Ergebnisse naturwissenschaftlicher Forschungen auf Ceylon. II. Zur Entwicklungsgeschichte und Anatomie des ceylonischen Blindwuhle *Ichthyophis glutinosus*. L. C. W. Kriedels Verlag, Wiesbaden.

Sauer, G. R. and Watabe, N. (1989). Ultrastructural and histochemical aspects of zinc accumulation by fish scales. *Tissue Cell*, **21**: 935–944.

Schaeffer, B. (1977). The dermal skeleton in fishes. In: *Problems in Vertebrate Evolution*, Andrews, S. M., Miles, R. S., and Walker, A. D., Eds., Linnean Society Symposium 4, Academic Press, London, New York, 25–52.

Schmidt, W. J. (1912). Studien am Integument der Reptilien. I. Die Haut der Geckoniden. *Zeitsch. Wiss. Zool. Leipzig.* **101**: 139–258.

Schmidt, W. J. (1914). Studien Am Integument der Reptilien. V. Anguiden. *Zool. Jahrb. Jena Anat.*, **38**: 1–120.

Schmidt, W. J. (1951). Polarisationsoptische Analyse der Schuppen des Knochenfisches *Capros aper. Zeits. Wiss. Mikrosk.*, **60**: 1–15.

Schmidt, W. J. (1971). The normal tooth tissues. I. Dentine. In: *Polarizing Microscopy of Dental Tissues*, Schmidt, W. J. and Keil, A., Eds., Pergamon Press, Oxford, 53–295.

Schönbörner, A. A., Boivin, G., and Baud, C. A. (1979). The mineralization processes in teleost fish scales. *Cell Tissue Res.*, **202**: 203–212.

Schönbörner, A. A., Meunier, F. J., and Catasnet, J. (1981). The fine structure of calcified Mandl's corpuscles in teleost fish scales. *Tissue Cell*, **13**: 589–597.

Schultze, H. P. (1966). Morphologische und histologische Untersuchungen an Schuppen mesozoischer Actinopterygier. Ubergang von Ganoid- zu Rund-Schuppen. SN. *Jahrb. Geol. Palaont.*, **126**: 232–314.

Schultze, H. P. (1977). Ausgangsform und Entwicklung der rhombischen Schuppen der Osteichthyes (Pisces). *Paläont. Z.*, **51**: 152–168.

Sewertzoff, A. N. (1932). Die Entwiclung der Knocherschuppen von *Polypterus delhesi. Jena Z. Naturwiss.*, **67**: 387–418.

Sire, J. Y. (1985). Fibres d'ancrage et couche limitante externe à la surface des écailles du Cichlidae *Hemichromis bimaculatus* (Téléostéen, Perciforme): données ultrastructurales. *Ann. Sci. Nat. Zool.*, 13ème sér., **7**: 163–180.

Sire, J. Y. (1986). Ontogenic development of surface ornamentation in the scales of *Hemichromis bimaculatus* (Cichlidae). *J. Fish Biol.*, **28**: 713–724.

Sire, J. Y. (1987). Structure, formation et régénération des écailles d'un poisson téléostéen, *Hemichromis bimaculatus* (Perciforme, Cichlidé), Thèse de Doctorat, Paris. *Arch. Doc. Inst. Ethnol.*, micro-édition, *Mus. Natn. Hist. Nat.*, SN87-600449.

Sire, J. Y. (1988). Evidence that mineralized spherules are involved in the formation of the superficial layer of the elasmoid scale in the cichlids *Hemichromis bimaculatus* and *Cichlasoma octofasciatum* (Pisces, Teleostei): an epidermal active participation? *Cell Tissue Res.*, **253**: 165–172.

Sire, J. Y. (1989). Scales in young *Polypterus senegalus* are elasmoid: new phylogenetic implications. *Am. J. Anat.*, **186**: 315–323.

Sire, J. Y. (1990). From ganoid to elasmoid scales in the actinopterygian fishes. *Neth. J. Zool.*, **40**: 75–92.

Sire, J. Y. and Géraudie, J. (1983). Fine structure of the developing scale in the Cichlid *Hemichromis bimaculatus* (Pisces, Teleostei, Perciformes). *Acta Zool.*, **64**: 1–8.

Sire, J. Y. and Géraudie, J. (1984). Fine structure of regenerating scales and their associated cells in the cichlid *Hemichromis bimaculatus* (Gill). *Cell Tissue Res.*, **237**: 537–547.

Sire, J. Y., Géraudie, J., Meunier, F. J., and Zylberberg, L. (1987). On the origin of the ganoine: histological and ultrastructural data on the experimental regeneration of the scales of *Calamoichthys calabaricus* (Osteichthyes, Brachyopterygii, Polypteridae). *Am. J. Anat.*, **180**: 391–402.

Sire, J. Y. and Meunier, F. J. (1981). Structure et minéralisation de l'écaille d' *Hemichromis bimaculatus* (Téléostéen, Perciforme, Cichlidé). *Arch. Zool. Expér. Gén.*, **122**: 133–150.

Smith, J. W. (1960). Collagen fiber patterns in mammalian bone. *J. Anat.*, **94**: 329–344.

Smith, M. M. (1977). The microstructure of the dentition and dermal ornamentation of three dipnoans from the Devonian of Western Australia: a contribution towards dipnoan interrelations and morphogenesis, growth and adaptation of the skeletal tissues. *Phil. Trans. Roy. Soc. Lond.*, B. **281**: 29–72.

Smith, M. M. and Hall, B. K. (1990). Development and evolutionary origins of vertebrate skeletogenic and odontogenic tissues. *Biol. Rev.*, **65**: 277–373.

Smith, M. M., Hobdell, M. H., and Miller, W. A. (1972). The structure of the scales of *Latimeria chalumnae. J. Zool., Lond.*, **167**: 501–509.

Snyder, D. G. (1958). Amino acid composition of the protein and inorganic constituents of the ash of pollock fish scales. *Comm. Fish Rev.*, **20**: 4–9.

Spearman, R. C. I. (1973). In: *The Integument*. Harrison, R. J., McMinn, R. M. H., and Treherne, J. E., Eds., Cambridge, University Press, Cambridge, 208.

Takagi, Y., Hirano, T., and Yamada, J. (1989). Scale regeneration of tilapia *(Oreochromis viloticus)* under various ambient and dietary calcium conditions. *Comp. Biochem. Physiol.*, **92A**: 605–608.

Taylor, E. H. (1972). Squamation in caecilians, with an atlas of scales. *Univ. Kansas Sci. Bull.*, **59**: 989–1164.

Thomson, K. S. (1975). On the biology of cosmine. *Bull. Peabody Mus. Nat. Hist.*, **40**: 1–59.

Thomson, K. S. and McCune, A. R. (1984). Development of the scales in *Lepisosteus* as a model for scale formation in fossil fishes. *Zool. J. Linn. Soc.*, **82**: 73–86.

Vaillant, L. (1895a). Sur la constitution et la structure de l'épine osseuse de la nageoire dorsale chez quelques poissons Malacoptérygiens. *C. R. Acad. Sci., Paris,* **121**: 909–911.

Vaillant, L. (1895b). Sur la structure histologique des rayons osseux chez la carpe. *C. R. Sess. 3ème Cong. Int. Zool., Leyde,* 275–278.

van Coillie, R. and Rousseau, A. (1974). Composition minérale des écailles du *Catostomus commersoni* issu de deux milieux différents: étude par microscopie électronique analytique. *J. Fish Res. Bd. Can.*, **31**: 63–66.

van Oosten, J. (1957). The skin and scales. In: *The Physiology of Fishes*, Brown, M. E., Ed., Academic Press, New York, 207–244.

Veis, A. (1985). Phosphoproteins of dentin and bone: do they have a role in matrix mineralization? In: *The Chemistry and Biology of Mineralized Tissues*, Butler, W. T., Ed., Ebsca Media, Birmingham, Alabama, 170–176.

Wake, M. H. (1975). Another scaled caecilian (Gymnophiona: Typhlonectidae). *Herpetologica*, **31**: 134–136.

Wake, M. H. and Nygren, K. M. (1987). Variation in scales in *Dermophis mexicanus* (Amphibia: Gymnophiona): Are scales of systematic utility? *Fieldiana*, **1378**: 1–8.

Wallin, O. (1956). Mucopolysaccharides and the calcification of the scale of the roach *(Leuciscus rutilus)*. *Quart. J. Microsc. Sci.*, **97**: 329–332.

Waterman, R. E. (1970). Fine structure of scale development in the teleost, *Brachydanio rerio*. *Anat. Rec.*, **168**: 361–380.

Weiner, S. (1986). Organization of extracellulary mineralized tissues: a comparative study of biological crystal growth. *CRC Critical Rev. Biochem.*, **20**: 365–408.

Weisel, G. F. (1975). The integument of the paddlefish, *Polyodon spathula*. *J. Morph.*, **145**: 143–150.

Weiss, P. and Ferris, W. (1954). Electron micrographs of larval amphibian epidermis. *Exp. Cell Res.*, **6**: 546–560.

Whitear, M. (1986). The skin of fishes including cyclostomes. Epidermis. Dermis. Vol. 2. In: *Biology of the Integument*. 2. Vertebrates. Bereiter-Hahn, J., Matoltsy, A. G., and Richards, K. S., Eds., Springer Verlag, Berlin, Heidelberg, New York, Tokyo, 8–64.

Whitear, M. and Mittal, A. K. (1986). Structure of the skin of *Agonus cataphractus* (Teleostei). *J. Zool., Lond.*, **210**: 551–574.

Williamson, W. C. (1849). On the microscopic structure of the scales and dermal teeth of some ganoid and placoid fish. *Phil. Trans. Roy. Soc. Lond.*, **139**: 435–475.

Williamson, W. C. (1851). Investigations into the structure and development of the scales and bones of fishes. *Phil. Trans. Roy. Soc. Lond.*, **141**: 643–702.

Yamada, J. (1971). A fine structural aspect of the development of scales in the chum salmon fry. *Bull. Jap. Soc. Sci. Fish.*, **37**: 18–29.

Yamada, J. and Watabe, N. (1979). Studies on fish scale formation and resorption. I. Fine structure and calcification of the scales in *Fundulus heteroclitus* (Atheriniformes: Cyprinodontidae). *J. Morph.*, **159**: 9–65.

Zylberberg, L. (1988). Ultrastructural data on the scales of the dipnoan *Protopterus annectens* (Sarcopterygii, Osteichthyes). *J. Zool., Lond.* **216**: 55–71.

Zylberberg, L., Berry, J. P., Castanet, J., Lefevre, R., and Ricqlès, A. de (1979). Apport de la microanalyse à l'étude des écailles dermiques de Batraciens Apodes. *Biol. Cell.*, **35**: 30a.

Zylberberg, L. and Castanet, J. (1985). New data on the structure and the growth of the osteoderms in the reptile *Anguis fragilis* L. (Anguidae, Squamata). *J. Morph.*, **186**: 327–342.

Zylberberg, L., Castanet, J., and Ricqlès, A. de (1980). Structure of the dermal scales in *Gymnophiona* (Amphibia). *J. Morph.*, **165**: 41–54.

Zylberberg, L., Géraudie, J., Sire, J. Y., and Meunier, F. J. (1985). Mise en évidence ultra-structurale d'une couche organique entre l'épiderme et la ganoine du dermosquelette des Polypteridae. *C. R. Acad. Sci., Paris*, III, **10**: 517–522.

Zylberberg, L. and Meunier, F. J. (1981). Evidence of denticles and attachment fibres in the superficial layer of scales in two fishes: *Carassius auratus* and *Cyprinus carpio* (Cyprinidae, Teleostei). *J. Zool., Lond.*, **195**: 459–471.

Zylberberg, L., Meunier, F. J., Escaig, F., and Halpern, S. (1984). Données nouvelles sur la structure et la minéralisation des écailles d'*Anguilla anguilla* (Osteichthyes, Anguillidae). *Can. J. Zool.*, **62**: 2482–2494.

Zylberberg, L. and Nicolas, G. (1982). Ultrastructure of scales in a teleost *(Carassius auratus* L.) after use of rapid freeze-fixation and freeze-substituion. *Cell Tissue Res.*, **223**: 349–367.

Zylberberg, L. and Wake, M. (1990). Structure of the scales of *Dermophis* and *Microcaecilia* (Amphibia: Gymnophiona), and comparison to dermal ossification of other vertebrates. *J. Morph.*, **206**: 25–43.

8

In Vitro Studies on Matrix-Mediated Mineralization

GRAEME K. HUNTER
Division of Oral Biology
Faculty of Dentistry
University of Western Ontario
London, Ontario, Canada

Introduction

Because the calcification of bone and other tissues involves deposition of a crystalline mineral phase upon a preformed organic matrix, it has long been assumed that components of the matrix play a role in determining the site and nature of mineral deposition. Ultrastructural observations appear to confirm this assumption, as sites of calcification are often associated with specific extracellular matrix structures. The classic example of this is the close spatial relationship of hydroxyapatite crystals with Type I collagen

225

fibrils (specifically, the gap zones of the fibrils) in the early stages of bone mineralization.

Over several decades, many *in vitro* model systems have been used to investigate the effect of collagen and other organic components of mineralized tissues on the formation of biologically-important mineral phases. These systems include metastable calcium phosphate solutions; gels of collagen, gelatin, agarose, silica and polyacrylamide; liposomes; and matrix macromolecules immobilized on solid phase surfaces. It is such *in vitro* studies on organic matrix effects on calcification that are the subject of this chapter. The role of matrix vesicles in biological calcification will not be discussed here, although the effects of phospholipids on hydroxyapatite formation clearly may be relevant to vesicle-mediated calcification mechanisms (see below). Also, the discussion will focus on calcium phosphates (principally hydroxyapatite), although some recent studies on other mineral phases, which illustrate general principles of organic matrix-crystal relationships, will be alluded to.

Two distinctly-different forms of calcification occur during bone development and growth: epiphyseal cartilage calcification, as part of endochondral ossification at the growth plate of long bones; and osteoid calcification, in periosteal bone formation. The organic matrices of these two tissues are quite different: osteoid consists principally of Type I collagen, with lesser amounts of non-collagenous proteins; epiphyseal cartilage matrix consists mainly of proteoglycan and Type II collagen. The calcification ultrastructures of bone and cartilage are also distinctly different, the mineral deposits being associated with collagen fibrils in osteoid but not in epiphyseal cartilage. As will be seen, the current state of knowledge suggests that matrix macromolecules perform different functions in the calcification of these two tissues.

The reader should note that a number of older studies deal with matrix effects on the formation of hydroxyapatite by transformation of amorphous calcium phosphate (ACP). These will not be discussed here, as it now has been conclusively demonstrated that ACP does not occur in bone (Grynpas *et al.*, 1984), and organic matrix molecules can have quite different effects on amorphous-crystalline transformation than on *de novo* crystal formation (Hunter *et al.*, 1987). Also, in the studies discussed below, a distinction will be drawn between factors which induce crystal formation at lower supersaturation than that at which precipitation otherwise occurs, and factors which increase the amount of crystal formation under conditions at which some precipitation would otherwise occur. For the purpose of this article, the former effect will be referred to as *nucleation*, and the latter effect as *promotion*. As will be seen, both effects may occur in biological calcification phenomena.

Effect of Collagen on *In Vitro* Calcification

Collagen Fibril Systems

Type I collagen is by far the predominant organic constituent of bone, comprising approximately 90% of the organic dry weight of cortical bone. The physical relationship between collagen fibrils and hydroxyapatite crystals in bone is still controversial, but a functional role for collagen in osteoid calcification is suggested by the preferential orientation of crystal c-axes parallel to the long axis of the collagen fibrils (Stuehler, 1937). In order to determine whether Type I collagen acts as an inducer of calcification in bone, studies first performed in the 1950's examined the effect of collagen preparations on calcification in model systems. This is well-trodden ground, and will not be covered extensively here; for a recent review of collagen effects on calcification, the reader is referred to Glimcher (1984). With regard to this literature, it is important to realize that many older studies were not performed to contemporary standards of protein chemistry, and therefore "collagen" preparations used may have contained considerable amounts of contaminants. Also, the precipitates produced were not always fully-characterized (that is, by diffraction techniques), and may not have been apatitic. A final caveat is that, for a variety of reasons, these systems are highly technique-dependent, which may "explain" some apparently contradictory findings.

Early experiments in this area typically consisted of adding reconstituted collagen fibrils or demineralized bone matrix to metastable calcium phosphate solutions. Such solutions have $Ca \times PO_4$ concentration products which, although greater than the solubility product for hydroxyapatite (and other calcium phosphates), will not produce precipitation in the absence of a nucleator. Using this approach, Glimcher *et al.* (1957) showed that skin collagen reconstituted into native (64 nm-banded) fibrils resulted in precipitation of hydroxyapatite. This effect was quite specific, as other collagen aggregates (segment long spacing and fibrous long spacing) did not nucleate hydroxyapatite formation. Other workers also reported nucleation or promotion of hydroxyapatite by native collagen fibrils (Strates *et al.*, 1957; Katz, 1969). However, in some studies a greater effect was observed with demineralized bone matrix than with reconstituted tendon collagen (Bachra and Fisher, 1968; Bachra, 1972). This apparent difference between bone and soft tissue collagens may be due, in part, to posttranslational modifications such as glycosylation, crosslinking or phosphorylation. Alternatively, there may be variable amounts of contaminants in the two preparations. Collagen purified from tendon by acid extraction and differential salt precipitation contains less noncollagenous protein and other impurities than bone matrix demineralized with EDTA, which is known to extract only a fraction of the noncollagenous protein (Goldberg *et al.*, 1988).

Collagen Gel Systems

Another system for investigating the role of collagen in calcification involves the growth of hydroxyapatite crystals in collagen gels. Because ion diffusion is restricted in semi-solid matrices, nucleation is limited; therefore, large crystals may be grown (Henisch, 1970). The effect of collagen may be determined by comparing the rate of hydroxyapatite formation in collagen gels with that in other (nonphysiological) matrices. Gelatin (heat-denatured collagen) would appear to be ideal for comparison. The rationale of this approach is that heating, which destroys the native fibrillar structure of collagen, should also cause loss of biological activity. Therefore, if collagen is in fact a nucleator of hydroxyapatite, collagen gels should induce more hydroxyapatite formation than gelatin gels. It should be noted that some workers have used the terms collagen and gelatin interchangeably. In the view of the present author, this is a significant conceptual error — gelatin preparations, which are often very impure, are composed of "random coil" collagen α-chains, and therefore are not physiological.

Comparative calcification of (tendon) Type I collagen and gelatin gels was first studied by Pokric and Pucar (1979), who found no difference in amount of precipitation in the two matrices. However, the crystal phase formed was dicalcium phosphate dihydrate (DCPD, or brushite), which subsequently matured into octacalcium phosphate (OCP).

A system for growing hydroxyapatite crystals in native Type I collagen gels was developed by the present author (Hunter et al., 1985). Collagen gels containing sodium phosphate are overlaid with a solution containing calcium chloride. Under appropriate conditions of pH and ionic strength, hydroxyapatite crystals form in the gel near the gel-solution interface. Comparative studies showed that gelatin gels support a lower amount of hydroxyapatite formation than collagen gels under otherwise-identical conditions (Hunter et al., 1986). However, gels composed of agarose (a seaweed polysaccharide) produce even higher amounts of hydroxyapatite than collagen gels. In this system, it appears that hydroxyapatite formation correlates with the rate of calcium diffusion into the gel, and not with the polymeric matrix used. Transmission electron microscopy of calcified collagen gels revealed no spatial relationship between collagen fibrils and hydroxyapatite crystals (Hunter, 1987b) (see Fig. 1). This appears to be due to the low protein concentration possible in gels — collagen gels typically contain 1–5 mg/ml protein, or approximately one one-hundredth of the collagen concentration in bone. If, as suggested by the solution phase experiments described above, pure Type I collagen is only a weak nucleator of hydroxyapatite formation, gels are not an appropriate system for studying collagen effects on calcification.

In an overview of collagen effects on calcification, Glimcher (1984) concluded that "the native aggregated state of collagen fibrils is *necessary* for their calcification but may not be *sufficient*, at least not *biologically* sufficient". That is, although fibrillar collagen can be induced to calcify *in vitro*, this process

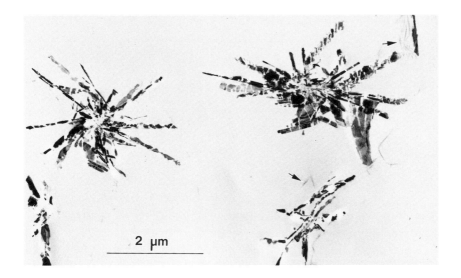

2 μm

Fig. 1 Transmission electron microscopy of hydroxyapatite crystals grown in native collagen gels. Hydroxyapatite was grown in native Type I collagen gels by diffusion of $CaCl_2$ into phosphate-containing gels. Arrows indicate collagen fibrils. Note the lack of association between crystal aggregates and fibrils in this system. (Reprinted from Hunter, 1987b.)

alone may not be rapid enough to account for the mineralization process in bone. For this reason, much recent attention has focussed on the calcification properties of the noncollagenous components of bone matrix.

Effect of Noncollagenous Proteins on *In Vitro* Calcification

Bone Proteins

In recent years, a large variety of noncollagenous proteins has been purified from bone and characterized biochemically (Termine *et al.*, 1981a; Linde *et al.*, 1983; Sato *et al.*, 1985; see also Chapter 8 of Volume 3). In general, these are acidic glycoproteins, some of which contain phosphorylated residues. Several noncollagenous bone proteins have been claimed to function in the initiation of mineralization. Before looking at specific examples, two general principles are worth stating. First, a spatial or temporal association of a matrix component with calcification foci is often used to infer a causal relationship with the mineralization process. These kinds of studies are not within the scope of the present discussion, but suffice it to say that for such an argument to be valid, the putative nucleator must be shown to be present *before* the matrix calcifies. Second, the phenomenon of calcium binding is often used to justify a role for a matrix component in calcification. However, many proteins bind calcium (albumin being a classic example), and, as pointed out by other authors (Bowness, 1968; Glimcher, 1984), binding of calcium may as easily inhibit as stimulate calcification.

The properties of three of the noncollagenous proteins of bone will be examined here, as these illustrate different aspects of the problem. Osteonectin is a 42 kD glycoprotein originally claimed to be a bone-specific protein linking collagen to mineral (Termine *et al.*, 1981b; see also Chapter 10 of Volume 3). However, as pointed out by Glimcher (1984), there is no evidence for a specific interaction of osteonectin with collagen (in fact osteonectin was originally purified on *gelatin* columns), and binding to preformed hydroxyapatite, which is a common property of proteins, is not the same thing as *nucleating* hydroxyapatite. Further, osteonectin is not bone-specific — it has been shown to be synthesized by periodontal ligament cells (Wasi *et al.*, 1984) and is now known to be identical to the endodermal cell protein SPARC, and to the BM40 protein of basement membranes (Tracy *et al.*, 1988). In addition, more recent studies have indicated that osteonectin *inhibits* hydroxyapatite formation both in solution (Menanteau *et al.*, 1982; Romberg *et al.*, 1986) and in the presence of fibrillar Type I collagen (Doi *et al.*, 1989).

Unlike osteonectin, osteocalcin (also known as bone gla protein) is specific to bone and dentin (Bronckers *et al.*, 1985), and its gamma-carboxyglutamate (gla) groups confer it with high calcium-binding affinity (Svard *et al.*, 1986; see also Chapter 7 of Volume 3). Like other calcium-binding proteins, osteocalcin is a calcification inhibitor in solution chemistry systems (Menanteau *et al.*, 1982; Romberg *et al.*, 1986). Functionally, this protein is unusually amenable to experimental investigation, as treatment of animals with the vitamin K antagonist warfarin inhibits the gamma-carboxylation reaction (and therefore presumably decreases the biological activity of osteocalcin). Warfarin-treated rats whose bone gla content was only 2% of the control level exhibited normal bone formation (Price and Williamson, 1981). Recent evidence suggests that osteocalcin production is a relatively late event in osteogenesis, and it now appears that the biological function of this protein is related to bone resorption (Lian *et al.*, 1984).

The strongest candidates for calcification-regulating factors are the phosphoproteins of bone and dentin. These are proteins or glycoproteins which are rich in aspartate, glycine and alanine, and contain phosphoserine and (in bone) phosphothreonine residues. The major phosphoprotein of dentin, termed phosphophoryn by Veis and co-workers, has been extensively characterized (Lee *et al.*, 1977). Multiple phosphorylated proteins have been isolated from bone, some of which are degradation products, and it is not yet clear how many gentically-distinct phosphoproteins exist in this tissue (Uchiyama *et al.*, 1986). Because of the harsh treatments required for their extraction, and the presence of hydroxyproline and hydroxylysine in phosphoprotein extracts, it appears that some of the phosphoproteins in bone and dentin occur covalently bound to collagen (Shuttleworth and Veis, 1972; Butler *et al.*, 1972; Uchiyama *et al.*, 1986). Phosphoproteins have extremely high densities of negative charges, and exhibit high affinity binding of calcium (Zanetti *et al.*, 1981). The addition of calcium to dentin phosphoprotein has been reported to result in conformational changes (Lee *et al.*, 1977; Marsh, 1989). In agar gels, phosphophoryn reduced the amount of hydroxyapatite precipitation, although the precipitant bands were sharpened (Fujisawa *et al.*, 1987). However, like many anionic proteins, phosphoproteins promote hydroxyapatite deposition if immobilized on solid phases. This point is explored further below.

Epiphyseal Cartilage Proteins

Several organic matrix components of epiphyseal cartilage have been suggested to function in the initiation of mineralization in that tissue. Generally, these have not been available in large enough quantities for their effects on *in vitro* calcification to be determined. However, two will be discussed briefly here. Chondrocalcin was originally described as a calcium-binding protein concentrated in the hypertrophic zone of epiphyseal cartilage (Poole *et al.*, 1984). Although it was subsequently demonstrated that this protein is in fact the C-terminal propeptide of Type II procollagen (van der Rest *et al.*, 1986), a role in cartilage calcification is suggested by the observation that addition of chondrocalcin stimulates the mineralization of epiphyseal chondrocyte cultures (Poole *et al.*, 1987).

Type X collagen is present only in the hypertrophic and calcified zones of epiphyseal cartilage, and accordingly was suggested to be a facilitator of calcification (Schmid and Linsenmayer, 1985). However, Type X collagen is concentrated in the territorial (pericellular) matrix of epiphyseal cartilage, whereas calcification typically occurs in the inter-territorial matrix. Also, Type X collagen had no effect on hydroxyapatite formation in a gelatin gel system (Boskey *et al.*, 1989).

Of the organic matrix constituents of epiphyseal cartilage thought to function in the regulation of calcification, most attention has focussed on the proteoglycans. The role of proteoglycans in calcification will be considered separately below.

Calcification in Solid-Phase and Solution-Lipid Interface Systems

Calcification on Solid-Phase Surfaces

An important breakthrough in understanding matrix-mineral interactions and reconciling contradictory observations of matrix effects on *in vitro* calcification has come from studies on crystal formation in the presence of ordered biological structures. The elegant studies of Weiner, Addadi and coworkers have been of particular conceptual importance. Although these studies involve a nonapatitic crystal phase, the phenomena elucidated are likely to be of general significance, and will therefore be described in some detail. It has been shown that an aspartate-rich protein from mollusk shell adsorbs to specific faces of growing calcium dicarboxylate crystals, inhibiting the development of these faces and hence altering the crystal morphology (Addadi and Weiner, 1985). If adsorbed onto a plastic or glass surface, the aspartate-rich protein will nucleate crystals of calcite (calcium carbonate) from a specific crystal face (001) (see Fig. 2). The (001) face of calcite is composed entirely of Ca^{2+} ions, and the underlying carbonate ions are oriented perpendicular to this plane. As the mollusk protein is in the β-sheet conformation, the carboxylate groups of the aspartate side-chains will be perpendicular to the solid-phase surface. Thus it appears that this protein can nucleate calcite crystals specifically from the (001) face because the carboxylate groups bind a layer of Ca^{2+} ions in a similar stereochemical arrangement to that in the (001) hexagonal plane of the calcite crystal. These workers have further shown that if polyaspartic acid, which also adopts the β-sheet conformation, is adsorbed onto a sulfonated polystyrene surface, the carboxylate and sulfonate groups act cooperatively in binding Ca and nucleating calcite crystals (Addadi et al., 1987). As a sulfated mollusk shell protein appears to have the same activity, these workers suggest that sulfate groups may act by inducing a locally high calcium supersaturation and carboxylates may act by nucleating the appropriate crystal face.

Calcite crystals are far more amenable to experimental study than calcium phosphates, but recent evidence suggests that phenomena similar to those described by Addadi and Weiner may be involved in bone mineralization. In particular, it has become clear that many anionic proteins which act as calcification inhibitors in solution, as described above, may act as nucleators if immobilized on solid phase surfaces. Linde and co-workers have described a system in which proteins from bone and dentin are covalently attached to Sepharose beads in a carbodiimide-catalyzed reaction, and incubated in calcium phosphate solutions of low supersaturation. Under these conditions, dentin phosphoprotein induces the formation of hydroxyapatite crystals on the bead surface (Lussi et al., 1988) (see Fig. 3). Further studies showed that beads containing dentin proteoglycan and osteocalcin also promoted calcification, but albumin-containing beads had no effect (Linde et al., 1989). Interestingly, the apparent order of hydroxyapatite-inducing potency was phosphoprotein > proteoglycan > osteocalcin, which may reflect the relative calcium-binding capacities of these proteins.

Thus, anionic proteins which are inhibitors of hydroxyapatite formation in solution, are capable of nucleating hydroxyapatite if attached to a solid surface. The nucleating activity requires very small amounts of protein: for phosphoprotein, an inductive effect is observed at a concentration of 8 μg protein/g beads, whereas inhibition requires 40-160 μg/ml (Lussi et al., 1988). Sepharose beads are not, of course, biologically-relevant, but preliminary

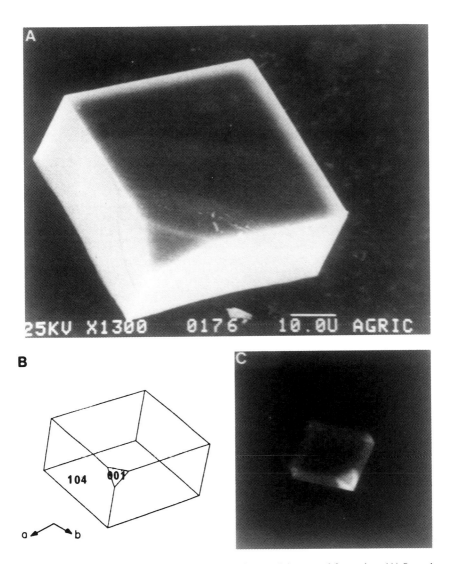

Fig. 2 Effect of mollusk shell aspartate-rich protein on calcite crystal formation. (A) Scanning electron micrograph of a calcite crystal nucleated by mollusk aspartate-rich protein adsorbed onto a glass surface. The crystal was nucleated from the small triangular (001) face. (B) Diagrammatic representation of calcite crystal in A. (C) Immunofluorescent staining of a calcite crystal, showing the presence of aspartate-rich protein on the 001 face. (Reprinted from Addadi and Weiner, 1985.)

studies suggest that phosphoprotein crosslinked to guanidine-extracted Type I collagen fibrils from rat tail tendon can also induce calcification (Linde and Lussi, 1989).

Similar results were obtained using a system in which reconstituted tendon collagen tape is treated with alkaline phosphatase and then incubated in β-

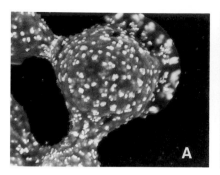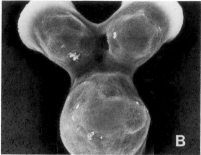

Fig. 3 Induction of hydroxyapatite by phosphoprotein covalently attached to sepharose beads. AH-Sepharose beads to which phosvitin had been covalently attached were incubated in calcium phosphate solutions of low supersaturation (Ca × PO_4 = 1.6 mM²) for 24 h. In panel A, large mineral blocks are seen on the surface of the beads. Enzymatic dephosphorylation of the phosvitin greatly reduces the amount of mineral nucleated (panel B). (Reprinted from Linde *et al.*, 1989.)

glycerol phosphate. Covalent attachment to the collagen of the egg yolk phosphoprotein, phosvitin, using the protein cross-linking agent dimethyl suberimidate, resulted in a higher level of calcification than with control tape (Banks *et al.*, 1977). Moreover, the crystals formed (a carbonated apatite) were oriented in the dimension of the collagen fibril axis.

Calcification at Aqueous Solution-Lipid Interfaces

Proteins are not unique in their ability to nucleate biological crystals on ordered surfaces — an apparently-similar phenomenon occurs with amphipathic lipids. In a recent report, Mann and co-workers have shown that monolayers of stearic acid promote calcification in adjacent supersaturated calcium carbonate solutions (Mann *et al.*, 1988). The amount of calcification is directly related to the surface pressure, suggesting that crystal formation is favoured by ordering of the lipid monolayer. Although control solutions produce calcite, the lipid monolayers induce the formation of vaterite, which is nucleated at a specific face (0001) composed entirely of Ca^{2+} ions (see Fig. 4). This is analogous to the effect of aspartate-rich protein on calcite formation described above, as the carbonate ions of the (0001) face of vaterite are oriented perpendicular to the plane of the face, whereas in the (001) face of calcite the carbonates are parallel. Mann *et al.* (1988) emphasize that this phenomenon is not due to epitaxy (crystal growth by lattice matching with a preformed structure), as the head group spacings in the stearic acid monolayer do not match those of the Ca^{2+} ions in the crystal face, but to more general stereochemical and electrostatic effects. This lack of specificity may partially explain how different chemical groups (carboxylate, sulfate and phosphate), in both proteins and polysaccharides, can induce hydroxyapatite formation in the Sepharose bead system described above.

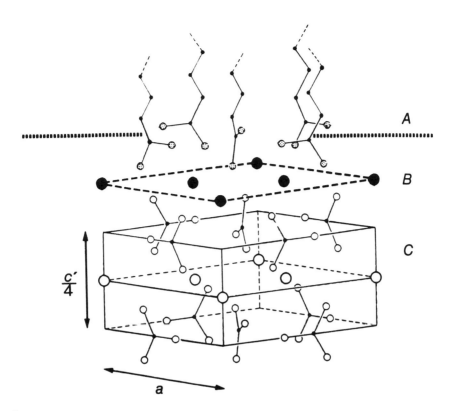

Fig. 4   Proposed mechanism of nucleation of vaterite crystals from calcium carbonate solutions adjacent to stearic acid monolayers. (A) Lipid monolayer surface showing carboxylate groups aligned perpendicular to the air/water interface. (B) Layer of Ca^{2+} ions bound to lipid carboxylate groups; this is electrostatically (although not sterically) equivalent to the 0001 face of vaterite. (C) Vaterite subcell — note that the carbonate ions are perpendicular to the 0001 face, and thus parallel to the lipid carboxylate groups. ●,○ — Ca atoms; ●,○ — O atoms; ● — C atoms. (Reprinted by permission from *Nature* vol. 334, pp. 692–695. Copyright © 1988 Macmillan Magazines Ltd.)

Formation of calcium phosphate crystals may also be induced by ordered lipid structures. There is evidence that phospholipid-containing vesicles and proteolipids from bacterial cell walls can promote hydroxyapatite formation in metastable calcium phosphate solution (Boskey and Posner, 1977; Boyan-Salyers and Boskey, 1980). Lipid vesicles preloaded with inorganic phosphate, and incubated in calcium-containing solutions in the presence of a calcium ionophore, result in calcification on the inner surface of the bilayer (Eanes and Hailer, 1985). Although the complexity of this system makes the results rather difficult to interpret, it seems reasonable to suppose that hydroxyapatite crystals are being nucleated by binding of Ca^{2+} to the phosphate head groups on the bilayer surface. If this is indeed the case, the reported ability of matrix vesicles to induce calcification *in vitro* may be due to their membrane lipids rather than to the enzymes or ions they may contain.

The above studies are consistent with a general mechanism of matrix-mediated calcification outlined by Veis (1985): "the organic matrix must be considered as a two-component system. There is a structural bulk phase which defines the architecture of the system and the ultimate orientation of crystal axes. The second phase is an interactive protein (or proteins) which has the dual role of interacting specifically with the structural component and nucleating crystallization". In bone (and dentin), the structural phase consists of Type I collagen fibrils; the interactive phase consists (probably) of phosphoprotein. However, it is the opinion of the present author that this mechanism does *not* apply to the calcification process in epiphyseal cartilage. In this tissue, there is no structural phase which can support crystal deposition, and the properties of cartilage matrix components suggest a radically-different role for the organic matrix in calcification.

Effect of Proteoglycans on *In Vitro* Calcification

Whereas most studies on osteoid calcification have concluded that collagen and/or some noncollagenous protein acts as a nucleator of hydroxyapatite formation, studies on epiphyseal cartilage calcification have mainly focused on potential *inhibitors* of hydroxyapatite formation, the proteoglycans. A considerable body of literature has been devoted to the theory that removal or modification of proteoglycans is a prerequisite for calcification of the cartilage matrix (for review, see Buckwalter, 1983). The concept that proteoglycans act as inhibitors of calcification is attributed by most modern authors to Logan (1935). Ironically, what Logan actually showed was that epiphyseal cartilage contains a far higher sulfate content than metaphyseal bone. This, of course, is irrelevant in terms of calcification mechanisms, as cartilage calcification and osteoid calcification are completely different processes. It is surprising that many contemporary authors continue to perpetuate this fallacious argument.

The modern version of Logan's hypothesis is based on observations that calcified *cartilage* has a lower proteoglycan content than noncalcified cartilage (Matukas and Krikos, 1968; Thyberg *et al.*, 1973; Lohmander and Hjerpe, 1975). Also, there is evidence to suggest that proteoglycans of the calcified zone of the epiphysis are smaller and less aggregated than those of higher zones (Axelsson *et al.*, 1983; Buckwalter *et al.*, 1987). However, other workers have found that the proteoglycan content of calcified cartilage is similar to or greater than that of uncalcified areas (Larsson *et al.*, 1973; Poole *et al.*, 1982; Shepard and Mitchell, 1985), and that no change in proteoglycan size or aggregation is associated with calcification (Vittur *et al.*, 1972; Reinholt *et al.*, 1985). Such ultrastructural and biochemical studies are out of the scope of this review, which will focus on the properties of cartilage proteoglycans in *in vitro* calcification model systems. In this context, Howell and Pita (1976) found that aspirates of epiphyseal cartilage interstitial fluid inhibited calcification in a "synthetic lymph" solution. The greatest inhibitory activity copurified with a rapidly-sedimenting aggregated proteoglycan fraction (Cuervo *et al.,* 1973). However, the low proteoglycan and calcium concentrations in the micropuncture fluid suggest that this technique produces an aspirate which is not entirely characteristic of the cartilage matrix.

More recent studies, mainly performed by Boskey, Rosenberg and co-workers, have used highly-purified and well-characterized preparations of proteoglycans from bovine nasal septum and other cartilages. The effects of these preparations on hydroxyapatite formation have been determined using metastable calcium phosphate solutions of approximately serum concentrations, and of physiological ionic strength, pH and temperature. Using this approach, it was shown that bovine nasal septum proteoglycans delay the *de novo* formation of hydroxyapatite in calcium phosphate solution, but do not affect the final amount of precipitation (Blumenthal *et al.,* 1979). A partially-aggregated proteoglycan preparation was a more effective inhibitor than a monomer preparation. Cartilage proteoglycan also inhibited the growth of hydroxyapatite seed crystals, as did a commercial chondroitin sulfate (CS) preparation, but to a lesser extent (Chen *et al.,* 1984). (However, it should be noted that commercial glycosaminoglycan preparations may differ in size and/or sulfation, depending on the source and purification methodology used, from those of intact proteoglycans.) The inhibitory activity of CS was reduced by chemical desulfation (Chen and Boskey, 1985). In agreement with the finding of Cuervo *et al.* (1973), it was shown that epiphyseal proteoglycans were more effective inhibitors of calcification than proteoglycans from non-calcifying cartilages (Chen and Boskey, 1986). From these experiments it was concluded that degradation or disaggregation of proteoglycans could facilitate the calcification of epiphyseal cartilage.

Two limitations in this hypothesis bear mentioning. First, the difference in hydroxyapatite inhibition displayed by aggregates and monomers is slight. This led Blumenthal *et al.* (1979) to conclude that further breakdown of proteoglycan would be necessary to produce calcification. However, the difference between the inhibitory activities of proteoglycan monomers and CS appears to be even less dramatic (Chen *et al.,* 1984; Chen and Boskey, 1985). It is difficult to see how such a small difference in inhibitory potential could explain the sudden and massive calcification which occurs in hypertrophic cartilage. A further limitation of the traditional view of proteoglycans as inhibitors of cartilage calcification is that, of course, removal of an inhibitor is not sufficient to initiate calcification. After all, most tissues contain much less proteoglycan than even calcified cartilage, and do not normally undergo calcification.

The high concentrations of proteoglycan required to inhibit hydroxyapatite formation *in vitro* (typically 5 or 10 mg/ml, corresponding to approximately 10 or 20 mM disaccharide) suggest that the inhibitory activity is relatively nonspecific. In comparison, a crystal poison such as the bisphosphonate EHDP inhibits hydroxyapatite formation at concentrations as low as 1 μM (Lussi *et al.*, 1988). Therefore, the possibility that inhibition of hydroxyapatite formation and/or growth by proteoglycan was due to calcium binding by the proteoglycan sulfate and carboxylate groups has been considered. Cuervo *et al.* (1973) determined that the concentration of proteoglycan required for inhibition of hydroxyapatite bound approximately one-third of the calcium in the synthetic lymph solution, but calculated that this amount of calcium binding would not affect hydroxyapatite formation. Chen and Boskey (1985) claimed that calcium binding by CS was negligible under conditions which inhibited seeded growth of hydroxyapatite, and showed that the growth of seed crystals was inhibited by pretreatment with proteoglycan.

In attempting to determine the importance (if any) of calcium binding in the hydroxyapatite-inhibiting activity of proteoglycans, a disadvantage of solution chemistry systems is that they are not amenable to simultaneous measurement of calcium binding and hydroxyapatite formation. This problem is circumvented by the collagen gel model system described above. In this system, addition of CS was found to delay the onset and decrease the amount of hydroxyapatite precipitation (Hunter *et al.*, 1985). However, by measuring the uptake of calcium in phosphate-free gels, it was shown that the degree of hydroxyapatite inhibition correlated with the amount of sequestration of calcium by the CS-containing gels — for example, gels containing 30 mg/ml CS reached equilibrium with twice the calcium concentration of the overlay solution. Therefore, the inhibition of hydroxyapatite formation by CS, if not by proteoglycan, is associated with a reduction in the available calcium concentration. This Ca-GAG interaction was further investigated using other techniques, and was shown to be of low affinity but high capacity, and apparently electrostatic in nature (Hunter, 1987a; Hunter *et al.*, 1988).

It is still not clear, therefore, to what extent proteoglycans inhibit calcification by binding calcium, and to what extent by other mechanisms. In a sense, though, the point is moot, because proteoglycans in epiphyseal cartilage certainly *do* bind calcium, and this effect has to be taken into account in determining the role of proteoglycans in calcification. The calcium concentration in noncalcified epiphyseal cartilage matrix is several times higher than the (total) calcium concentration in serum (for a discussion of the composition of epiphyseal cartilage matrix, see Hunter and Bader, 1989). Studies on the equilibration of ions between cartilage and surrounding fluids indicate that the selectivity coefficient for Ca^{2+} is much higher than for Na^+, because of calcium binding to the fixed negative charges of proteoglycans (Maroudas, 1980). This is in agreement with polyelectrolyte theory, which predicts that polyions of sufficient linear charge density will "discriminate" between monovalent and divalent counterions (Manning, 1969). Conversely, the concentration of phosphate and other anions will be *lower* in cartilage than in adjacent fluids (Maroudas, 1980).

Experiments on proteoglycan effects on hydroxyapatite formation in solution are therefore typically performed under ionic conditions more resembling serum than cartilage matrix. A more serious problem is that *in vitro* studies are typically performed under equilibrium conditions, whereas *in vivo* conditions are nonequilibrium. That is, proteoglycans, by binding calcium, will lower the free calcium concentration of *in vitro* solutions, but will not lower the free calcium concentration *in vivo*, because Ca^{2+} ions can diffuse into cartilage from adjacent tissue fluids. This crucial distinction is seldom recognized, but was clearly stated two decades ago by Bowness: "The presence of (proteoglycan) in solution . . . will result in a decreased amount . . . of precipitated calcium phosphate. However, in a nonequilibrium system, such as that in living organisms, where there is a continual supply of calcium and phosphate, . . . the formation of calcium phosphate will be faster in the presence of (proteoglycan)" (Bowness, 1968).

Investigation of the effect of proteoglycans on calcium phosphate precipitation under nonequilibrium conditions has produced contradictory results. By pumping calcium- and phosphate-containing solutions past opposite sides of polyacrylamide films, de Jong *et al.* (1980) showed that 1% (w/v) CS *decreased* the minimum $Ca \times PO_4$ product for precipitation of an unidentified calcium phosphate phase. However, proteoglycan monomer and aggregate preparations inhibited hydroxyapatite formation in a similar system recently described by Boskey (1989). Further studies will be required to determine whether proteoglycans act as promoters or inhibitors of calcification under nonequilibrium (physiological) conditions.

The ability of proteoglycans to inhibit hydroxyapatite formation is probably due to steric or electrostatic interference with the growth of crystal nuclei. The ability to promote hydroxyapatite formation is presumably due to the sequestration of high concentrations of calcium into the vicinity of the proteoglycan molecule. Because of the high capacity, low affinity mode of binding, calcium bound to proteoglycan constitutes a large reservoir of Ca^{2+} ions which can easily be made available for precipitation.

A means by which proteoglycan-bound calcium could be displaced has recently become clear. As originally pointed out by Dunstone (1962), the fixed negative charges of proteoglycans confer cartilage with ion-exchange properties. Accordingly, Ca^{2+} ions bound to proteoglycan may be displaced by cations which compete for the anionic binding "sites", or by anions capable of complexing calcium. In the latter category is phosphate, which was shown to inhibit the Ca-proteoglycan interaction (Hunter, 1987b). Further, the ability of GAGs to inhibit hydroxyapatite formation is dependent upon the phosphate/GAG ratio; at a sufficiently-high phosphate concentra-

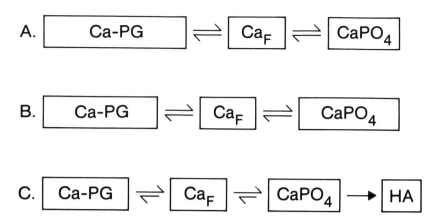

Fig. 5 Proposed interactions of calcium, proteoglycan, and phosphate involved in the calcification of epiphyseal cartilage. (A) In pre-calcified cartilage, most calcium is bound to proteoglycan (Ca-PG), some is free (Ca_F), and some is complexed with phosphate ($CaPO_4$). (B) An increase in extracellular phosphate concentration increases the proportion of $CaPO_4$ complexes by shifting the Ca-PG = Ca_F equilibrium to the right. (C) At sufficiently-high Ca-PO$_4$ concentration, hydroxyapatite precipitates, introducing an essentially-irreversible step into the equilibria. As calcification proceeds, the Ca-PG complex dissociates by mass-action effects.

tion, hydroxyapatite formation in collagen gels is identical in the absence and presence of CS (Hunter, 1987b).

The properties of the Ca-proteoglycan-phosphate interaction are consistent with the view that proteoglycans in epiphyseal cartilage, far from acting as calcification inhibitors, may function as a cation-exchanging calcium reservoir (Hunter, 1987b). In order to initiate calcification of cartilage, phosphate must be supplied, and calcium bound to proteoglycan must be released. These two processes may occur simultaneously, as increasing the extracellular phosphate concentration may displace sufficient calcium from proteoglycan to raise the Ca $\times$ PO$_4$ product above the hydroxyapatite precipitation threshold. These interactions are shown diagramatically in Fig. 5.

In order to determine whether this mechanism is quantitatively feasible, mathematical modeling of the interactions between proteoglycan, Ca^{2+}, Na^+ and phosphate was performed. This led to the prediction that spontaneous precipitation of hydroxyapatite would be initiated by an approximate doubling of the extracellular phosphate concentration (Hunter and Bader, 1989). Therefore, release of a fraction of the total intracellular phosphate stores of hypertrophic chondrocytes may initiate calcification of epiphyseal cartilage. In apparent agreement with this mechanism, a turnover of intracellular organic phosphate compounds into inorganic phosphate occurs prior to calcification of the epiphyseal cartilage matrix (Kakuta *et al.*, 1985).

It may be concluded that proteoglycans have two potential effects on the calcification of cartilage. First, by acting as a calcium "sink", proteoglycans greatly increase the (total) Ca $\times$ PO$_4$ product in cartilage matrix. Second, proteoglycans may, depending on their state of aggregation, inhibit the growth of hydroxyapatite crystals. Most studies done in this area to date have not been able to distinguish between these two effects.

Implications for the Mineralization of Bone and Epiphyseal Cartilage, and Future Perspectives

In vitro studies of organic matrix effects on biological crystal formation have proved a powerful complement to ultrastructural approaches in the ongoing attempt to determine the mechanisms of calcification in bone and epiphyseal cartilage. However, much confusion has been generated by the fact that anionic matrix molecules often act as calcification inhibitors in these systems by complexing calcium ions and (in some cases) inhibiting crystal growth by adsorption onto specific crystal faces. An important conceptual breakthrough has been the recent realization that macromolecules having a high density of negatively-charged groups may act as crystal nucleators if immobilized onto solid-phase surfaces. Similarly, amphipathic lipid monolayers or bilayers may promote calcification in an adjacent solution phase. This phenomenon is not epitaxy, and in fact appears to be quite nonspecific in terms of the nature and spacing of the anionic groups. At least in the case of the better-characterized calcium carbonate systems, matrix-mediated crystal growth appears to represent an electrostatic and stereospecific interaction between a negatively-charged surface and a specific face of the nascent crystal: electrostatic, because a layer of Ca^{2+} ions bound to the anionic surface appears to be the first step in forming the crystal; sterospecific, because the specific crystal faces nucleated have the carbonate ions perpendicular to the face, and therefore parallel to the anionic groups of the ordered surface.

What are the implications of these studies for bone mineralization? It now appears clear that Type I collagen alone is biologically insufficient to induce mineralization. However, collagen is *necessary* for mineralization, and this is apparently because the large, highly-periodic Type I fibrils constitute an ordered solid-phase surface onto which anionic molecules can be adsorbed. Many anionic proteins occur in bone, some of which are synthesized specifically by bone cells, others concentrating in the tissue because of an affinity for hydroxyapatite. At this time, the strongest candidate for a role in nucleating hydroxyapatite would appear to be one or more of the phosphoproteins: these are highly-charged, specific for bone (and dentin), bind to collagen fibrils, and have nucleating ability in appropriate *in vitro* assay systems. As poly-carboxylate compounds can nucleate calcium carbonate crystals in a stereospecific fashion, the intriguing possibility exists that phosphoprotein-collagen complexes may nucleate calcium phosphate crystals in an analogous way. If this is the case, it may explain why the hydroxyapatite crystal c-axes are oriented parallel to the collagen fibril axis in bone. The challenge for researchers interested in mammalian calcification is to devise approaches similar to the elegant studies of Addadi and Weiner, and of Mann and co-workers, to study a crystal phase (hydroxyapatite) characterized by a complex unit cell and (in biological systems) small crystal size. It should be emphasized that simplistic approaches often used in the past, such as adding a purified soluble protein to a metastable calcium phosphate solution, are no longer justified. The relationship between hydroxyapatite and the organic matrix of bone will only be elucidated by studies capable of resolving the stereochemical relationship of organic surfaces and specific crystal faces.

Another important unsolved problem in bone mineralization relates to the spatial distribution of hydroxyapatite deposition. Specifically, it is unclear by what means calcification is induced at the mineralization front, but prevented in the osteoid seam. In dentin, phosphoprotein appears to be deposited directly at the predentin-dentin boundary via the odontoblast process (Weinstock and Leblond, 1973; Dimuzio and Veis, 1978). However, no comparable mechanism is known in bone. Further work is necessary to determine how the osteoid matrix is rendered calcifiable at the mineralization front.

Epiphyseal cartilage contains a major anionic macromolecule, the aggregating proteoglycan. As sulfate and carboxylate groups can act cooperatively in nucleating calcite crystals, it has been suggested that proteoglycan may act as a hydroxyapatite nucleator in epiphyseal cartilage calcification (Addadi *et al.*, 1987). Indeed, dentin proteoglycans can induce calcification when covalently attached to Sepharose beads (Linde *et al.*, 1989). However, in the view of the present author, this effect is unlikely to be significant in calcifying cartilage. First, there is no evidence to suggest that cartilage proteoglycans, or any structure with which they are associated, have a sufficient degree of structural order to nucleate crystal formation. Second, there is no evidence to suggest a preferential orientation of hydroxyapatite crystals in epiphyseal cartilage. Third, proteoglycan is present in cartilage in concentrations far higher than would be required for a nucleation function.

What, then, is the role of proteoglycan in epiphyseal cartilage calcification? As argued above, the traditional view of proteoglycans as inhibitors of cartilage calcification suffers from serious limitations: the calcium-binding properties of proteoglycans are not taken into account, and the removal of an inhibitor is not sufficient to induce calcification. In fact, proteoglycans may *facilitate* the calcification process in cartilage by concentrating calcium in a form which can readily be liberated for hydroxyapatite formation. According to the definition given above, proteoglycans may be promoters, but not nucleators, of calcification in epiphyseal cartilage.

To differentiate between conflicting ideas of the role of proteoglycans in epiphyseal cartilage calcification, it will be necessary to use systems, such as constant composition and flow systems, in which availability of ions (particularly calcium) is essentially infinite. Also, because of the reported differences in calcification inhibitor activity between proteoglycan aggregates, monomers and free GAG chains, it is desirable that these experiments involve proteoglycans in their physiological (that is, aggregated) state. If these two stipulations are observed, it should be possible to determine the true function of proteoglycans in the calcification of epiphyseal cartilage.

Concluding Remarks

Despite decades of active investigation on the *in vitro* properties of organic matrix macromolecules, the role of the matrix in initiating the calcification of bone and epiphyseal cartilage remains elusive. However, it appears that significant theoretical advances have recently been made. Specifically, it has become clear that many model systems used in the past deviate significantly from physiological conditions, and therefore have produced misleading results. Most previous studies on bone calcification failed to recognize either the importance of solid phase surfaces in providing a template for ordered hydroxyapatite deposition or the danger of studying matrix components in isolation. Most previous studies on epiphyseal cartilage calcification ignored the large calcium-binding capacity of proteoglycans and hence the potential of these molecules to act as calcification promoters under physiological conditions.

Even with these new insights, it is not yet possible to determine the precise role of the organic matrix in the mineralization processes of bone and epiphyseal cartilage. However, it can be stated that the mechanisms of calcification in these two tissues appear to be quite different. In bone, an interaction between anionic proteins and Type I collagen fibrils may provide a stereochemical orientation of negatively-charged groups which acts as a hydroxyapatite nucleator. In epiphyseal cartilage, no such nucleating agent has been identified, and recent studies suggest that the role of the organic matrix in calcification is to sequester large amounts of calcium into the cartilage matrix. Therefore, cartilage calcification may result from a "booster" mechanism (local increase in calcium phosphate supersaturation) rather than a nucleation event. Biological calcification phenomena have proved remarkably resistant to experimental elucidation: it is to be hoped that the studies described above will provide a conceptual framework within which the role of matrix-mineral interactions in bone and cartilage calcification can finally be elucidated.

Acknowledgments

The author wishes to thank Dr. A. L. Boskey and Dr. A. Linde for kindly providing access to unpublished material. The original studies described here were supported by the Medical Research Council of Canada.

References

Addadi, L. and Weiner, S. (1985). Interactions between acidic proteins and crystals: stereo-chemical requirements in biomineralization. *Proc. Natl. Acad. Sci. U.S.A.*, **82**: 4110–4114.

Addadi, L., Moradian, J., Shay, E., Maroudas, N. G., and Weiner, S. (1987). A chemical model for the cooperation of sulfates and carboxylates in calcite crystal nucleation: relevance to biomineralization. *Proc. Natl. Acad. Sci. U.S.A.*, **94**: 2732–2736.

Axelsson, I., Berman, I., and Pita, J. C. (1983). Proteoglycans from rabbit articular and growth plate cartilage. Ultracentrifugation, gel chromatography and electron microscopy. *J. Biol. Chem.*, **258**: 8915–8921.

Bachra, B. N. (1972). Calcification *in vitro* of demineralized bone matrix: electron microscopic and chemical aspects. *Calcif. Tissue Res.*, **8**: 287–303.

Bachra, B. N. and Fisher, H. R. A. (1968). Mineral deposition in collagen *in vitro*. *Calcif. Tissue Res.*, **2**: 343–352.

Banks, E., Nakajima, S., Shapiro, L. C., Tilevitz, O., Alonzo, J. R., and Chianelli, R. R. (1977). Fibrous apatite grown on modified collagen. *Science*, **198**: 1164–1166.

Blumenthal, N. C., Posner, A. S., Silverman, L. D., and Rosenberg, L. C. (1979). Effect of proteoglycan on *in vitro* hydroxyapatite formation. *Calcif. Tissue Res.*, **27**: 75–82.

Boskey, A. L. (1989). Hydroxyapatite formation in a dymanic gel system: effects of type I collagen, lipids and proteoglycans. *J. Phys. Chem.*, **93**: 1628–1633.

Boskey, A. L. and Posner, A. S. (1977). The role of synthetic and bone extracted Ca-phospho-lipid-PO₄ complexes in hydroxyapatite formation. *Calcif. Tissue Res.*, **23**: 251–258.

Boskey, A. L., Maresca, M., and Appel, J. (1989). The effect of noncollagenous matrix proteins on hydroxyapatite formation and proliferation in a collagen gel system. In: *Proceedings of the Third International Conference on Mineralized Tissues*, Glimcher, M. J., Ed.

Bowness, J. M. (1968). Precent concepts of the role of ground substance in calcification. *Clin. Orthop.*, **59**: 233–247.

Boyan-Salyers, B. D. and Boskey, A. L. (1980). Relationship between proteolipids and calcium-phospholipid-phosphate complexes in *Barterionema matruchotii* calcification. *Calcif. Tissue Int.*, **30**: 167–174.

Bronckers, A. L. J. J., Gay, S., DiMuzio, M., and Butler, W. T. (1985). Immunolocalization of gamma-carboxyglutamic acid containing proteins in developing rat bones. *Collagen Rel. Res.*, **5**: 273–281.

Buckwalter, J. A. (1983). Proteoglycan structure in calcifying cartilage. *Clin. Orthop.*, **172**: 207–232.

Buckwalter, J. A., Rosenberg, L. C., and Ungar, R. (1987). Changes in proteoglycan aggregates during cartilage mineralization. *Calcif. Tissue Int.*, **41**: 228–236.

Butler, W. T., Finch, J. E., and Desteno, C. V. (1972). Chemical character of proteins in rat incisors. *Biochim. Biophys. Acta*, **257**: 167–171.

Chen, C.-C. and Boskey, A. L. (1985). Mechanisms of proteoglycan inhibition of hydroxyapatite growth. *Calcif. Tissue Int.*, **37**: 395–400.

Chen, C.-C. and Boskey, A. L. (1986). The effects of proteoglycans from different cartilage types on *in vitro* hydroxyapatite proliferation. *Calcif. Tissue Int.*, **39**: 324–327.

Chen, C.-C., Boskey, A. L., and Rosenberg, L. C. (1984). The inhibitory effect of cartilage proteoglycans ono hydroxyapatite growth. *Calcif. Tissue Int.*, **36**: 285–290.

Cuervo, L. A., Pita, J. C., and Howell, D. S. (1973). Inhibition of calcium phosphate mineral growth by proteoglycan aggregate fractions in a synthetic lymph. *Calcif. Tissue Res.*, **13**: 1–10.

De Jong, A. S. H., Hak, T. J., and Van Duijn, P. (1980). The dynamics of calcium phosphate precipitation studied with a new polyacrylamide steady state matrix model: influence of pyrophosphate, collagen and chondroitin sulfate. *Connect. Tissue Res.*, **7**: 73–79.

DiMuzio, M. T. and Veis, A. (1978). The biosynthesis of phosphophoryns and dentin collagen in the continuously erupting rat incisor. *J. Biol. Chem.*, **253**: 6845–6852.

Doi, Y., Okuda, R., Takezawa, Y., Shibata, S., Moriwaki, Y., Wakamatsu, N., Shimizu, N., Moriyama, K., and Shimokawa, H. (1989). Osteonectin inhibiting *de novo* formation of apatite in the presence of collagen. *Calcif. Tissue Int.*, **44**: 200–208.

Dunstone, J. R. (1962). Ion-exchange reactions between acid mucopolysaccharides and various cations. *Biochem. J.*, **85**: 336–351.

Eanes, E. D. and Hailer, A. W. (1985). Liposome-mediated calcium phosphate formation in metastable solutions. *Calcif. Tissue Int.*, **37**: 390–394.

Fujisawa, R., Kuboki, Y., and Sasaki, S. (1987). Effects of dentin phosphophoryn on precipitation of calcium phosphate in gel *in vitro*. *Calcif. Tissue Int.*, **41**: 44–47.

Glimcher, M. J. (1984). Recent studies of the mineral phase in bone and its possible linkage to the organic matrix by protein-bound phosphate bonds. *Phil. Trans. R. Soc. Lond. B*, **304**: 479–508.

Glimcher, M. J., Hodge, A. J., and Schmitt, F. O. (1957). Macromolecular aggregation states in relation to mineralization: the collage-hydroxyapatite system as studied *in vitro*. *Proc. Natl. Acad. Sci. U.S.A.*, **43**: 860–867.

Goldberg, H. A., Maeno, M., Domenicucci, C., Zhang, Q., and Sodek, J. (1988). Identification of small collagaenous proteins with properties of $\alpha_1(I)$ pN-propeptide in fetal porcine calvarial bone. *Collagen Rel. Res.*, **8**: 187–197.

Grynpas, M. D., Bonar, L. C., and Glimcher, M. J. (1984). X-ray diffraction radial distribution function studies on bone mineral and synthetic calcium phosphate. *J. Mater. Sci.*, **19**: 723–736.

Henisch, H. K. (1970). Crystal growth in gels, Pennsylvania State University Press.

Howell, D. S. and Pita, J. C. (1976). Calification of growth plate cartilage with special reference to studies on micropuncture fluids. *Clin. Orthop.*, **118**: 208–229.

Hunter, G. K. (1987a). Chondroitin sulfate-derivatized agarose beads: a new system for studying cation binding to glycosaminoglycans. *Anal. Biochem.*, **165**: 435–441.

Hunter, G. K. (1987b). An ion-exchange mechanism of cartilage calcification. *Connect. Tissue Res.*, **16**: 111–120.

Hunter, G. K. and Bader, S. M. (1989). A mathematical modelling study of epiphyseal cartilage calcification. *J. Theor. Biol.*, **138**: 195–211.

Hunter, G. K., Allen, B. L., Cheng, P.-T., and Grynpas, M. D. (1985). Inhibition of hydroxyapatite formation in collagen gels by chondroitin sulfate. *Biochem. J.*, **228**: 463–469.

Hunter, G. K., Nyburg, S. C., and Pritzker, K. P. H. (1986). Hydroxyapatite formation in collagen, gelatin and agarose gels. *Collagen Rel. Res.*, **6**: 229–238.

Hunter, G. K., Grynpas, M. D., Cheng, P.-T., and Pritzker, K. P. H. (1987). Effect of glycosaminoglycans on calcium pyrophosphate crystal formation in collagen gels. *Calcif. Tissue Int.*, **41**: 164–170.

Hunter, G. K., Wong, K. S., and Kim, J. J. (1988). Binding of calcium to glycosaminoglycans: an equilibrium dialysis study. *Arch. Biochem. Biophys.*, **260**: 161–167.

Kakuta, S., Golub, E. E., and Shapiro, I. M. (1985). Morphochemical analysis of phosphorus pools in calcifying cartilage. *Calcif. Tissue Int.*, **37**: 293–299.

Katz, E. P. (1969). The kinetics of mineralization *in vitro*. I. The nucleation properties of 640 A collagen at 25°. *Biochim. Biophys. Acta*, **194**: 121–129.

Larsson, S.-E., Ray, R. D., and Kuettner, K. E. (1973). Microchemical studies on acid glycosaminoglycans of the epiphyseal zones during endochondral calcification. *Calcif. Tissue Res.*, **13**: 271–285.

Lee, S. L., Veis, A., and Glonek, T. (1977). Dentin phosphoprotein: an extracellular calcium-binding protein. *Biochemistry*, **16**: 2971–2979.

Lian, J. B., Tassinari, M., and Glowacki, J. (1984). Resorption of implanted bone from normal and warfarin-treated rats. *J. Clin. Invest.*, **73**: 1223–1226.

Linde, A. and Lussi, A. (1989). Mineral induction by polyanionic dentin and bone proteins at physiological ionic conditions. In: *Proceedings of the Third International Conference on Mineralized Tissues*, Glimcher, M. J., Ed.

Linde, A., Jontell, M., Lundgren, T. Nilson, B., and Svanberg, U. (1983). Noncollagenous proteins of rat compact bone. *J. Biol. Chem.*, **258**: 1698–1705.

Linde, A., Lussi, A., and Crenshaw, M. A. (1989). Mineral induction by immobilized polyanionic proteins. *Calcif. Tissue Int.*, **44**: 286–295.

Logan, M. A. (1935). Composition of cartilage, bone, dentin and enamel. *J. Biol. Chem.*, **110**: 375–389.

Lohmander, S. and Hjerpe, A. (1975). Proteoglycans of mineralizing rib and epiphyseal cartilage. *Biochim. Biophys. Acta*, **404**: 93–109.

Lussi, A., Crenshaw, M. A., and Linde, A. (1988). Induction and inhibition of hydroxyapatite formation by rat dentine phosphoprotein *in vitro*. *Arch. Oral Biol.*, **33**: 685–691.

Mann, S., Heywood, B. R., Rajam, S., and Birchall, J. D. (1988). Controlled crystallization of $CaCO_3$ under stearic acid monolayers. *Nature*, **334**: 692–695.

Manning, G. S. (1969). Limiting laws and counterion condensation in polyelectrolyte solutions I. Colligative properties. *J. Chem. Phys.*, **51**: 924–933.

Maroudas, A. (1980). Physical chemistry of articular cartilage and the intervertebral disc. In: *The Joints and Synovial Fluid*, Volume II, Sokoloff, L., Ed., Academic Press, New York, 239–291.

Marsh, M. E. (1989). Self-association of calcium and magnesium complexes of dental phosphophoryn. *Biochemistry*, **28**: 339–345.

Matukas, V. J. and Krikos, G. A. (1968). Evidence for changes in protein polysaccharide associated with the onset of calcification in cartilage. *J. Cell Biol.*, **39**: 43–48.

Menanteau, J., Neuman, W. F., and Neuman, M. W. (1982). A study of bone proteins which can prevent hydroxyapatite formation. *Metab. Bone Dis. Rel. Res.*, **4**: 157–162.

Pokric, B. and Pucar, Z. (1979). Precipitation of calcium phosphates under conditions of double diffusion in collagen and gels of gelatin and agar. *Calcif. Tissue Int.*, **27**: 171–176.

Poole, A. R., Pidoux, I., and Rosenberg, L. (1982). Role of proteoglycans in endochondral ossification: immunofluorescent localization of link protein and proteoglycan monomer in bovine epiphyseal growth plate. *J. Cell Biol.*, **92**: 249–260.

Poole, A. R., Pidoux, I., Reiner, A., Choi, H., and Rosenberg, L. C. (1984). Association of an extracellular protein (chondrocalcin) with the calcification of cartilage in endochondral bone formation. *J. Cell Biol.*, **98**: 54–65.

Poole, A. R., Lee, E. R., Hinek, A., and Rosenberg, L. C. (1987). Studies on the calcification of cartilage matrix in endochondral ossification. In: *The Biology of Tooth Movement*, Norton, L. and Burstone, C., Eds., CRC Press.

Price, P. A. and Williamson, M. K. (1981). Effect of warfarin on bone. Studies on the vitamin K-dependent protein of rat bone. *J. Biol. Chem.*, **256**: 12754–12759.

Reinholt, F. P., Engfeldt, B., Heinegard, D., and Hjerpe, A. (1985). Proteoglycans and glycosaminoglycans of normal and strontium rachitic epiphyseal cartilage. *Collagen Rel. Res.*, **5**: 41–53.

Romberg, R. W., Werness, P. G., Riggs, B. L., and Mann, K. G. (1986). Inhibition of hydroxyapatite crystal growth by bone-specific and other calcium-binding proteins. *Biochemistry*, **25**: 1176–1180.

Sato, S., Rahemtulla, F., Prince, C. W., Tomana, M., and Butler, W. T. (1985). Acidic glycoproteins from bovine compact bone. *Connect. Tissue Res.*, **14**: 51–64.

Schmid, T. M. and Linsenmayer, T. F. (1985). Immunohistochemical localization of short chain cartilage collagen (type X) in avian tissues. *J. Cell Biol.*, **100**: 598–605.

Shepard, N. and Mitchell, N. (1985). Ultrastructural modifications of proteoglycans coincident with mineralization in local regions of rat growth plate. *J. Bone Joint Surg.*, **67A**: 455–464.

Shuttleworth, A. and Veis, A. (1972). The isolation of anionic phosphoproteins from bovine cortical bone via the periodate solubilization of bone collagen. *Biochim. Biophys. Acta*, **257**: 414–420.

Strates, B. S., Newman, W. F., and Levinskas, G. J. (1957). The solubility of bone mineral II. Precipitation of near-neutral solutions of calcium and phosphate. *J. Phys. Chem.*, **61**: 279–282.

Steuhler, R. (1937). Ueber den Feinbau des Knochens. Fortschr. a. d. Geb. der Roentgenstrahlen, **57**: 231–264.

Svard, M., Drakenbearg, T., Andersson, T., and Fernlund, P. (1986). Calcium binding to bone gamma-carboxyglutamic acid protein from calf studied by ^{43}Ca NMR. *Eur. J. Biochem.*, **158**: 373–378.

Termine, J. D., Belcourt, A. B., Conn, K. M., and Kleinman, H. K. (1981a). Mineral and collagen-binding proteins of fetal calf bone. *J. Biol. Chem.*, **256**: 10403–10408.

Termine, J. D., Kleinman, H. K., Whitson, S. W., Conn, K. M., McGarvey, M. L., and Martin, G. R. (1981b). Osteonectin, a bone-specific protein linking mineral to collagen. *Cell*, **26**: 99–105.

Thyberg, J., Lohmander, S., and Friberg, U. (1973). Electron microscopic demonstration of proteoglycans in guinea pig epiphyseal cartilage. *J. Ultra. Res.*, **45**: 407–427.

Tracy, R. P., Shull, S., Riggs, B. L., and Mann, K. G. (1988). The osteonectin family of proteins. *Int. J. Biochem.*, **20**: 653–660.

Uchiyama, A., Suzuki, M., Lefteriou, B., and Glimcher, M. (1986). Isolation and chemical characterization of the phosphoproteins of chicken bone matrix: heterogeneity in molecular weight and composition. *Biochemistry*, **25**: 7572–7583.

van der Rest, M., Rosenberg, L. C., Olsen, B. R., and Poole, A. R. (1986). Chondrocalcin is identical with the C-propeptide of type II procollagen. *Biochem. J.*, **237**: 923–925.

Veis, A. (1985). Phosphoproteins of dentin and bone — do they have a role in matrix mineralization? In: *The Chemistry and Biology of Mineralized Tissues*, Butler, W. T., Ed., Ebsco Press, 170–176.

Vittur, F., Pugliarello, M. C., and de Bernard, B. (1972). Some properties of proteoglycans of pre-osseous cartilage. *Biochim. Biophys. Acta*, **257**: 389–397.

Wasi, S., Otsuka, K., Yao, K.-L., Tung, P. S., Aubin, J. E., Sodek, J., and Termine, J. D. (1984). An osteonectin-like protein in porcine periodontal ligament and its synthesis by periodontal ligament fibroblasts. *Can. J. Biochem. Cell Biol.*, **62**: 470–478.

Weinstock M. and Leblond, C. P. (1973). Radioautographic visualization of the deposition of a phosphoprotein at the mineralization front in the dentin of the rat incisor. *J. Cell Biol.*, **56**: 838–845.

Zanetti, M., de Bernard, B., Jontell, M., and Linde, A. (1981). Ca^{2+}-binding studies of the phosphoprotein from rat-incisor dentine. *Eur. J. Biochem.*, **113**: 541–545.

Index

A

H